D1046816

IMPROVING HEALTH IN THE COMMUNITY

A Role for Performance Monitoring

Committee on Using Performance Monitoring
to Improve Community Health

Jane S. Durch, Linda A. Bailey, and Michael A. Stoto, *Editors*

Division of Health Promotion and Disease Prevention

INSTITUTE OF MEDICINE

NATIONAL ACADEMY PRESS
Washington, D.C. 1997

NATIONAL ACADEMY PRESS • 2101 Constitution Avenue, N.W. • Washington, D.C. 20418

NOTICE: The project that is the subject of this report was approved by the Governing Board of the National Research Council, whose members are drawn from the councils of the National Academy of Sciences, the National Academy of Engineering, and the Institute of Medicine. The members of the committee responsible for the report were chosen for their special competences and with regard for appropriate balance.

This report has been reviewed by a group other than the authors according to procedures approved by a Report Review Committee consisting of members of the National Academy of Sciences, the National Academy of Engineering, and the Institute of Medicine.

The Institute of Medicine was chartered in 1970 by the National Academy of Sciences to enlist distinguished members of the appropriate professions in the examination of policy matters pertaining to the health of the public. In this, the Institute acts under the Academy's 1863 congressional charter responsibility to be an adviser to the federal government and its own initiative in identifying issues of medical care, research, and education. Dr. Kenneth I. Shine is president of the Institute of Medicine.

Funding for this project was provided by the Office of the Assistant Secretary for Health, U.S. Department of Health and Human Services (contract no. 282-94-0032); The Robert Wood Johnson Foundation (grant no. 024336); and the Kellogg Endowment Fund of the National Academy of Sciences and the Institute of Medicine. The views presented in this report are those of the Committee on Using Performance Monitoring to Improve Community Health and are not necessarily those of the funding organizations.

Library of Congress Cataloging-in-Publication Data

Institute of Medicine (U.S.). Committee on Using Performance
Monitoring to Improve Community Health.
Improving health in the community : a role for performance
monitoring / Committee on Using Performance Monitoring to Improve
Community Health ; Jane S. Durch, Linda A. Bailey, and Michael A.
Stoto, editors.
p. cm
Includes bibliographical references and index.
ISBN 0-309-05534-2
1. Community health services—United States—Evaluation.
2. Health status indicators—United States. 3. Health promotion—
United States. I. Durch, Jane. II. Bailey, Linda A. III. Stoto,
Michael A. IV. Title.
[DNLM: 1. Community Health Services—standards—United States.
2. Quality Assurance, Health Care—organization & administration—
United States. 3. Community Health Planning—methods—United
States. 4. Health Status Indicators—United States. WA 546 AA1
I59i 1997]
RA445.I575 1997
362.1′2—dc21
DNLM/DLC
for Library of Congress 97-6336
CIP

Additional copies of this report are available for sale from the National Academy Press, Box 285, 2101 Constitution Avenue, N.W., Washington, D.C. 20055. Call (800) 624-6242 or (202) 334-3313 (in the Washington metropolitan area), or visit the NAP online bookstore at **http://www.nap.edu**

Printed in the United States of America

The serpent has been a symbol of long life, healing, and knowledge among almost all cultures and religions since the beginning of recorded history. The image adopted as a logotype by the Institute of Medicine is based on a relief carving from ancient Greece, now held by the Staatlichemuseen in Berlin.

COMMITTEE ON USING PERFORMANCE MONITORING TO IMPROVE COMMUNITY HEALTH

BOBBIE A. BERKOWITZ[*] (*Co-Chair*), Deputy Secretary, Washington State Department of Health, Olympia, Washington

THOMAS S. INUI[†] (*Co-Chair*), Professor and Chair, Department of Ambulatory Care and Prevention, Harvard Medical School and Harvard Pilgrim Health Care, Boston, Massachusetts

ALAN W. CROSS (*Vice Chair*), Professor of Social Medicine and Pediatrics and Director, Center for Health Promotion and Disease Prevention, University of North Carolina, Chapel Hill, North Carolina

LARRY W. CHAMBERS, Epidemiology Consultant, Hamilton-Wentworth Regional Public Health Department, and Professor, Department of Clinical Epidemiology and Biostatistics, McMaster University, Hamilton, Ontario, Canada

THOMAS W. CHAPMAN,[‡] Chief Executive Officer, George Washington University Hospital, and Senior Vice President for Network Development, George Washington University Medical Center, Washington, D.C.

ELLIOTT S. FISHER, Co-Director, Veterans Affairs Outcomes Group, Veterans Affairs Medical Center, White River Junction, Vermont, and Associate Professor of Medicine and Community and Family Medicine, Dartmouth Medical School, Hanover, New Hampshire

JAMES L. GALE, Professor, Department of Epidemiology, School of Public Health and Community Medicine, and Director, Northwest Center for Public Health Practice, University of Washington, Seattle; Health Officer, Kittitas County, Washington

KRISTINE GEBBIE[†] (*Liaison, Board on Health Promotion and Disease Prevention*), Assistant Professor of Nursing, Columbia University School of Nursing, New York, New York

FERNANDO A. GUERRA, Director of Health, San Antonio Metropolitan Health District, San Antonio, Texas

---

[*] As of July 1, 1996, Deputy Director, Turning Point Program, University of Washington School of Public Health and Community Medicine, Seattle.

[†] Member, Institute of Medicine.

[‡] Served through December 1995.

GARLAND H. LAND, Director, Center for Health Information Management and Epidemiology, Missouri Department of Health, Jefferson City, Missouri

SHEILA LEATHERMAN, Executive Vice President, United HealthCare Corporation, Minneapolis, Minnesota

JOHN R. LUMPKIN, Director, Illinois Department of Public Health, Springfield, Illinois

WILLIAM J. MAYER, President and General Manager, Functional Foods Division, Kellogg Company, Battle Creek, Michigan

ANA MARIA OSORIO, Chief, Occupational Health Branch, California Department of Health Services, Berkeley, California

SHOSHANNA SOFAER, Associate Professor and Associate Chair for Research, Department of Health Care Sciences, George Washington University Medical Center, Washington, D.C.

DEBORAH KLEIN WALKER, Assistant Commissioner, Bureau of Family and Community Health, Massachusetts Department of Public Health, Boston, Massachusetts

JOHN E. WARE, Jr.,[‡] Senior Scientist, The Health Institute, New England Medical Center, Boston, Massachusetts

RICHARD A. WRIGHT, Director, Community Health Services, Denver Department of Health and Hospitals, Denver, Colorado

Study Staff

Linda A. Bailey, Senior Program Officer (*Co-Study Director*)

Jane S. Durch, Program Officer (*Co-Study Director*)

Stephanie Y. Smith, Project Assistant

Michael A. Stoto, Director, Division of Health Promotion and Disease Prevention

Marissa W. Fuller, Research Associate

Sarah H. Reich, Project Assistant

Susan Thaul, Senior Program Officer

[‡] Served through December 1995.

Preface

An interest in understanding how health care and public health activities might be coordinated and directed toward improving the health of entire communities was the basis for this study by the Institute of Medicine (IOM) Committee on Using Performance Monitoring to Improve Community Health, which we jointly chaired.

The IOM was asked by the U.S. Department of Health and Human Services and The Robert Wood Johnson Foundation to undertake a two-year study to examine the use of performance monitoring and develop sets of indicators that communities could use to promote the achievement of public health goals. The study was originally approved in mid-1994 when passage of federal health care reform legislation was anticipated. Part of the task outlined at that time was to identify public health indicators that could be measured through the national information network that was envisioned in the proposed Health Security Act.

By the committee's first meeting, comprehensive federal legislation was no longer expected and attention had shifted to opportunities for collaborative public–private activities at state and local levels. This change in the national policy environment resulted in further discussion with the study's sponsors to reframe the committee's task. After the committee's second meeting, a "vision statement" and work plan reflecting this modified context were developed in consultation with the sponsors. The vision statement appears in Appendix C of this report along with the summary of the committee's first workshop.

The revised task called for the committee to examine how a performance monitoring system could be used to improve the public's health by identifying the range of actors that can affect community health, monitoring the extent to which their actions make a constructive contribution to the health of the community, and promoting policy development and collaboration between public and private sector entities. The committee was also asked to develop prototypical sets of indicators for specific public health concerns that communities could use to monitor the performance of public health agencies, personal health care organizations, and other entities with a stake in community health.

The committee appointed to conduct the study brought together expertise in state and local health departments, epidemiology, public health indicators, health data, environmental health, adult and pediatric clinical medicine, managed care, community health and consumer interests, quality assessment, health services research, and employer concerns. The group met six times between February 1995 and April 1996. Workshops held in conjunction with our meetings in May and December 1995 gave us the opportunity to hear about a variety of community experiences and to learn more about work on performance monitoring being done by academic researchers and public and private organizations. Summaries of these workshops appear as Appendixes C and D of this report and also are posted on the World Wide Web (*http://www.nap.edu/readingroom/*).

The committee reviewed critical issues in using performance monitoring and the role it can play in community-based health improvement efforts. Our work pointed to the need for a broad view of the determinants of health and of the stakeholders that share responsibility for maintaining and enhancing health in a community. In this report, we propose an iterative and evolving community process for health improvement efforts in which performance monitoring is a critical tool for establishing meaningful stakeholder accountability. We also propose a set of indicators as the basis of a community profile that can provide background information needed to understand a community's health issues and can help communities identify specific issues that they might want to address. In addition, the committee developed prototypes of sets of performance indicators for some of those specific health issues (see Appendix A). The committee's work in developing these indicator sets illustrates how communities might apply the approach described in our report.

In the course of the committee's work a shared awareness evolved of the ways in which the public health and health care systems contribute to a community's well-being. Beyond the usual tasks of IOM committees—always complicated by subject complexity, relevance of multiple legitimate perspectives, and the need to forge multidisciplinary consensus—the committee's work required bridging what Kerr White has called the "schism" between the public health and personal care systems.[1] Furthermore, we also needed to bring together three conceptual domains that have arisen separately—determinants of health, continuous improvement, and social activism. Finally, if these circumstances were not sufficiently daunting, a conceptual process that we entered into required major envisioning of systems not yet established, partnerships not yet forged, and the way in which individuals in organizations from different social sectors might choose to work together both for the common good and out of enlightened self-interest.

Our committee's principal "product" was a community health improvement process (CHIP), a method by which, on a community-wide basis, the health of the population might be improved. However complex this process of assessment, analysis, strategy formation, evaluation, and reassessment might be, we heard in our workshops individual presentations on programs and activities that seemed to us to represent the major features of our conceptual scheme at work in communities today. These current activities were never as holistically conceived, adequately resourced, thoroughly documented, and effective as our idealized vision of a possible future. They nevertheless represented steps toward a system of community-level effort that we believe will be necessary if the health of our community populations is ever to be truly maximized within available resources. Seeing and hearing about actual community cases in the present day encouraged us to think that the larger, more systemic achievement of a community health improvement process might yet be within our grasp.

For too long, the personal health care and public health systems have shouldered their respective roles and responsibilities for curing and preventing separately from each other, and often

[1]K.L. White. 1991. *Healing the Schism: Epidemiology, Medicine, and the Public's Health.* New York: Springer-Verlag.

from the rest of the community as well. However, working alone and independently, our formal health systems cannot substantially improve population health at the level of fundamental determinants. The burden on these systems and the lost opportunities in our society from this fragmentation, segmentation, and isolation are evident in the resources consumed in repeatedly responding to the health consequences of persistent problems that can be traced to a variety of factors.

Instead, we need to invest in a process that mobilizes expertise and strategic action from a variety of community, state, and organizational entities if we are to substantially improve community and population health. The committee's experience over the course of this study suggests that developing a strategy for performance monitoring for health improvement at a community level constitutes a lens through which all potential contributors to community health become visible, their legitimate domain for action can be examined, and a virtually unlimited array of specifiable indicators of performance can be considered. In a complex, cross-sectorial collaborative strategy, indicators for successful contributions to the overall strategy can help assure all parties that the effort each is making is having its intended effects. The challenge to communities will be to choose such measures wisely, using a method of choice-making that the committee hopes we have made explicit in this report.

No complete working model of the committee's vision will emerge quickly or easily. In particular, the emergence of partnerships to improve the health of communities, when that process entails the assumption of real accountability for measured performance, is likely to proceed slowly at first. However, the committee looks forward to seeing its proposed CHIP translated into practical applications, tested in a variety of community contexts, and improved. This will require a blend of imagination and creativity that will challenge, and we hope energize, all involved.

In closing, we note that this committee's work complements that of several other current or recently completed studies at the IOM and the National Research Council. A particularly closely related study, being conducted by the National Research Council's Panel on Performance Measures and Data for Public Health Performance Partnership Grants, is examining technical issues involved in establishing state-level performance measures for federal grants in eight substantive areas. The panel's first report, *Assessment of Performance Measures in Public Health*, which was released for comment in draft form in September 1996, is scheduled for completion in early 1997. A second report will address data and data system development needs.

Three related IOM reports were released in November 1996. *Healthy Communities: New Partnerships for the Future of Public Health*, from the Committee on Public Health, examines the evolving role of public health agencies, particularly in relation to community-focused activities and the growing prominence of managed care. *The Hidden Epidemic: Confronting Sexually Transmitted Diseases*, from the Committee on Prevention and Control of Sexually Transmitted Diseases, focuses on a specific health issue for which community-level efforts are recommended along with broader state and national strategies. *Managing Managed Care: Quality Improvement in Behavioral Health*, the report of the Committee on Quality Assurance and Accreditation Guidelines for Managed Behavioral Health Care, presents a framework for accreditation standards and quality improvements for managed behavioral health care and for developing, using, and evaluating performance indicators. We also note that our study is one of several that are part of the IOM Special Initiative on Health Care Quality, a three-year effort with goals that include evaluating and promoting appropriate use of tools for quality assessment and improvement.

We want to express our appreciation to the many people—listed by name in the Acknowledgments—who aided the committee in its work. As co-chairs of this difficult but rewarding study, we also want to commend the members of the committee for their thoughtful and insightful approach to the task put before them. Finally, on behalf of the entire committee, we want to thank the members of the IOM staff whose efforts successfully translated the committee's work into this report. Susan Thaul and Sarah Reich guided us through the initial meetings and workshop. Linda Bailey, Jane Durch, and Stephanie Smith, who joined the study staff in the midst of this process, saw us through additional meetings and another workshop as well as writing the report. Michael Stoto has been a valued contributor throughout the project.

Bobbie A. Berkowitz
Thomas S. Inui
Co-Chairs

Acknowledgments

The Committee on Using Performance Monitoring to Improve Community Health and the study staff are grateful for the generous assistance received from many individuals and organizations over the course of the study.

We particularly want to thank the speakers (listed here) and other participants (listed in Appendixes C and D) at the committee's two workshops. The speakers at the May 1995 workshop were Bill Beery, Group Health Cooperative of Puget Sound; Linda Demlo, Agency for Health Care Policy and Research; Richard Garfield, Columbia University School of Nursing; Randolph Gordon, Virginia Department of Health (Centers for Disease Control and Prevention at the time of the workshop); Claude Hall, Jr., American Public Health Association; James Krieger, Seattle–King County Department of Health; Roz Lasker, New York Academy of Medicine (Office of the Assistant Secretary for Health, Department of Health and Human Services, at the time of the workshop); Carl Osaki, Seattle–King County Department of Health; Nancy Rawding, National Association of County and City Health Officials; Cary Sennett, National Committee for Quality Assurance; Bernard Turnock, University of Illinois at Chicago; Margaret VanAmringe, Joint Commission on Accreditation of Healthcare Organizations; Elizabeth Ward, Washington State Department of Health; and Ronald Wilson, National Center for Health Statistics.

The speakers at the December 1995 workshop were J. Maichle Bacon, McHenry County (Illinois) Department of Health; Laurie L. Carmody, Group Health Association of America; Ann Casebeer, University of Calgary; Jonathan E. Fielding, University of California at Los Angeles School of Public Health; Dennis J. Kelso, Escondido (California) Health Care and Community Services Project; Bonnie Rencher, Calhoun County (Michigan) Health Improvement Program; Tony Traino, consultant, (Visiting Nurse Association of Greater Salem [Massachusetts] at the time of the workshop); and Edward H. Wagner, Group Health Cooperative of Puget Sound. The summary of this workshop was drafted by Ellen Weissman, Johns Hopkins School of Hygiene and Public Health.

The committee also wants to thank the individuals who reviewed and commented on initial drafts of the performance indicator sets that appear in Appendix A. These reviewers are Peter Briss, Centers for Disease Control and Prevention; Tim Byers, University of Colorado Health Sciences Center; Joseph Cassells; Gary Chase, Georgetown University Medical Center; Graham Colditz, Harvard Medical School; Margo Edmunds, Institute of Medicine; Steven Epstein, Georgetown University Medical Center; Amy Fine, Association of Maternal and Child Health Programs; Bernard Guyer, Johns Hopkins School of Hygiene and Public Health; Marie McCormick, Harvard School of Public Health; Paul Melinkovich, Denver Department of Community Health Services; Ricardo Muñoz, University of California at San Francisco; John Pinney, Pinney Associates; Lance Rodewald, Centers for Disease Control and Prevention; Harold Sox, Dartmouth-Hitchcock Medical Center; Robert Wallace, University of Iowa; and Kenneth Warner, University of Michigan School of Public Health. Reviewers from state health departments included Alan Weil, Colorado Department of Health Care Policy and Financing; Clinton C. Mudgett and Stephen E. Saunders, Illinois Department of Health; Bruce Cohen, Daniel Friedman, and Mary Ostrem, Massachusetts Department of Public Health; Sherri Homan, Bert Malone, and Marianne Ronan, Missouri Department of Health; Mimi Fields and Dan Rubin, Washington State Department of Health; and Richard Aronson and Katherine Kvale, Wisconsin Office of Maternal and Child Health.

Others whose assistance we would like to acknowledge are Richard Bogue, Hospital Research and Educational Trust, American Hospital Association; Erin Kenney, consultant (San Diego, California); Anne Klink, California Smoke-Free Cities; David Lansky, Foundation for Accountability; James McGee, Pennsylvania Health Care Cost Containment Council; Nancy Rigotti, Massachusetts General Hospital; Julie Trocchio, Catholic Health Association; Joan Twiss, California Healthy Cities Project; and Abraham Wandersman, University of South Carolina. The committee also expresses its appreciation to the National Research Council Panel on Performance Measures and Data for Public Health Performance Partnership Grants and to Jeffrey Koshel, the panel's study director, for sharing materials and for allowing members of the committee staff to listen to some of their discussions.

The study was undertaken with funding from The Robert Wood Johnson Foundation and the U.S. Department of Health and Human Services. We appreciate the support of these organizations and the assistance provided by project officers Nancy Kaufman at The Robert Wood Johnson Foundation, Susanne Stoiber and James Scanlon in the Office of the Assistant Secretary for Planning and Evaluation at the U.S. Department of Health and Human Services, and Roz Lasker who served as project officer in the Office of the Assistant Secretary for Health until her move to the New York Academy of Medicine. In addition, we are grateful for additional funding received from the Kellogg Endowment Fund of the National Academy of Sciences and the Institute of Medicine.

Several members of the Institute of Medicine and National Academy of Sciences staff in addition to those listed with the committee made important contributions to the successful completion of this project: Mona Brinegar, Claudia Carl, Michael Edington, Sharon Galloway, Linda Kilroy, Dorothy Majewski, Amy O'Hara, Dan Quinn, Donna Thompson, and the staff of the National Academy Press. In addition, Florence Poillon provided copy editing for the report. We thank them for their assistance.

Contents

Executive Summary

In communities, health is a product of many factors, and many segments of the community can contribute to and share responsibility for its protection and improvement. Changes in public policy, in public- and private-sector roles in health and health care, and in public expectations are presenting both opportunities and challenges for communities addressing health issues. Performance monitoring offers a tool to assess activities in the many sectors that can influence health and to promote both collaboration and accountability in working toward better health for the whole community, especially within the framework of a community-based health improvement process. This report from the Institute of Medicine (IOM) Committee on Using Performance Monitoring to Improve Community Health draws on lessons from a variety of current activities to outline the elements of a community health improvement process, discuss the role that performance monitoring can play in this process, and propose tools to help communities develop performance indicators.

BACKGROUND

The report reflects three important developments: (1) a broadening of our understanding of the nature of health and its determinants, (2) a greater appreciation of the importance of a community perspective, and (3) a growing interest in the use of performance measurement to improve the quality of health and other services in public and private settings.

A Broader Understanding of Health

There is a wider recognition in many settings that health is a dynamic state that embraces well-being as well as the absence of illness. The committee defined health as "a state of well-being and the capability to function in the face of changing circumstances." Health is, therefore, a positive concept emphasizing social and personal resources as well as physical capabilities. This definition also underscores the important contributions to health that are made outside the formal medical care and public health systems.

For both individuals and populations, health depends not only on medical care but also on other factors including individual behavior and genetic makeup and social and economic conditions for individuals and communities. The *health field model*, as described by Evans and Stoddart (1994) and discussed further in Chapter 2, presents these multiple determinants of health in a dynamic relationship (see Figure 1). The model's feedback loops link social environment, physical environment, genetic endowment, an individual's behavioral and biologic responses, disease, health care, health and function, well-being, and prosperity. This multidimensional perspective reinforces the value of public health's traditional emphasis on a population-based approach to community health issues.

A Community Perspective

The array of influences on health identified by the field model also suggests that there are many public and private entities that have a stake in or can affect the community's health. These stakeholders can include health care providers (e.g., clinicians, health plans, hospitals), public health agencies, and community organizations explicitly concerned with health. They can also include various other government agencies, community organizations, private industry, and other entities that may not see themselves as having any explicit health-related role such as schools, employers, social service and housing agencies, transportation and justice agencies, and faith communities. Many of these entities have a local base and focus. Others that may play an essential role in shaping health at the local level such as state health de-

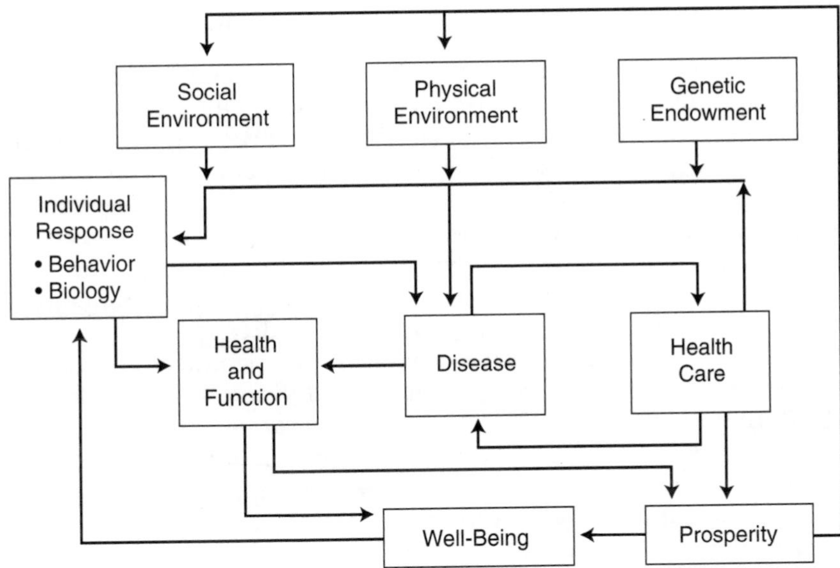

FIGURE 1 A model of the determinants of health. Source: Reprinted from R.G. Evans and G.L. Stoddart, 1990, Producing Health, Consuming Health Care, *Social Science and Medicine* 31:1347–1363, with permission from Elsevier Science Ltd, Kidlington, UK.

partments, federal agencies, managed care organizations, and national corporations have a broader scope than a single community.

As communities try to address their health issues in a comprehensive manner, all of the stakeholders will need to sort out their roles and responsibilities, which will vary from community to community. These interdependent sectors must address issues of shared responsibility for various aspects of community health and individual accountability for their actions. They also must participate in a process of community-wide social change that is necessary for health improvement efforts and related performance monitoring to succeed (Green and Kreuter, 1990). Most communities will have only limited experience with collaborative or coordinated efforts among these diverse groups. Effective collaboration will require a common language, an understanding of the multidimensional nature of the determinants of health, and a way to accommodate diversity in values and goals.

Growing Interest in Performance Monitoring

Performance monitoring has gained increasing attention as a tool for evaluating the delivery of personal health care services and for examining population-based activities addressing the health of the public (see Chapter 4 and Appendixes C and D). Although many performance monitoring activities are focused on specific health care organizations, only at the population level is it possible to examine the effectiveness of health promotion and disease prevention activities and to determine whether the needs of all segments of the community are being addressed.

As used by the committee, the term "performance monitoring" applies to a continuing community-based process of selecting indicators that can be used to measure the process and outcomes of an intervention strategy for health improvement, collecting and analyzing data on those indicators, and making the results available to the community to inform assessments of the effectiveness of an intervention and the contributions of accountable entities. Performance monitoring should promote health in a context of shared responsibility and individual accountability for achieving desired outcomes.

The monitoring process will depend on a limited number of indicators that can track critical processes and outcomes. A variety of tools are available for public health assessment. Some set, or provide a mechanism for setting, measurable health objectives and thus have some characteristics of performance measures (e.g., see APHA et al., 1991; NACHO, 1991; USDHHS, 1991). They are not, however, explicitly linked to the performance of specific entities in the community. To address this concern, the committee looked to evolving concepts of performance monitoring from the health services sector (e.g., NCQA, 1993); continuous quality improvement, particularly its application at the community level (e.g., Nolan and Knapp, 1996; Zablocki, 1996); and government reform (e.g., Osborne and Gaebler, 1992).

A FRAMEWORK FOR COMMUNITY HEALTH IMPROVEMENT

As the analysis and examples in this report demonstrate, a wide array of factors influence a community's health, and many entities in the community share the responsibility of maintaining and improving its health. Responsibility shared among many entities, however, can easily become responsibility ignored or abandoned. It is at the level of actions that can be taken to protect and improve health that it becomes possible to hold specific entities accountable. The committee proposes that accountability for those actions be established within a collaborative process, not assigned. Performance monitoring is the tool that communities can then use to hold community entities accountable for actions for which they have accepted responsibility.

Based on its review of the determinants of health, the community-level forces that can influence them, and community experience with performance monitoring, the committee finds that a *community health improvement process* (CHIP) that includes performance monitoring, as outlined in this report, can be an effective tool for developing a shared vision and supporting a planned and integrated approach to improve community health. It offers a way for a community to address a collective responsibility and marshal resources of specific, accountable entities to improve the health of its members. The committee concluded, however, that individual communities will have to determine the specific allocation of responsibility and accountability. No universal approach can be prescribed. The committee's recommendations for operationalizing a CHIP are based on a variety of theoretical and practical models for community health improvement, continuous quality improvement, quality assurance, and performance monitoring in health care, public health, and other settings. However, the specifics of the committee's proposal have never been tested, in toto, in community settings. Therefore, attention is also given in this report to ways in which the proposed process can be evaluated.

The committee suggests that a CHIP should include two principal interacting cycles based on analysis, action, and measurement (see Figure 2). This process is described in more detail in Chapter 4. The *problem identification and prioritization cycle* focuses on identification and prioritization of health problems in the community, and the *analysis and implementation cycle* on a series of processes intended to devise, implement, and evaluate the impact of health improvement strategies to address the problems. The overall process differs from standard models primarily because of its emphasis on measurement to link performance and accountability on a community-wide basis.

This process can be applied to a variety of community circumstances, and communities can begin working at various points in either cycle, with varying resources in place. It is an iterative and evolving process rather than linear or short term. One-time activities or short-term coalitions will not be adequate. There must

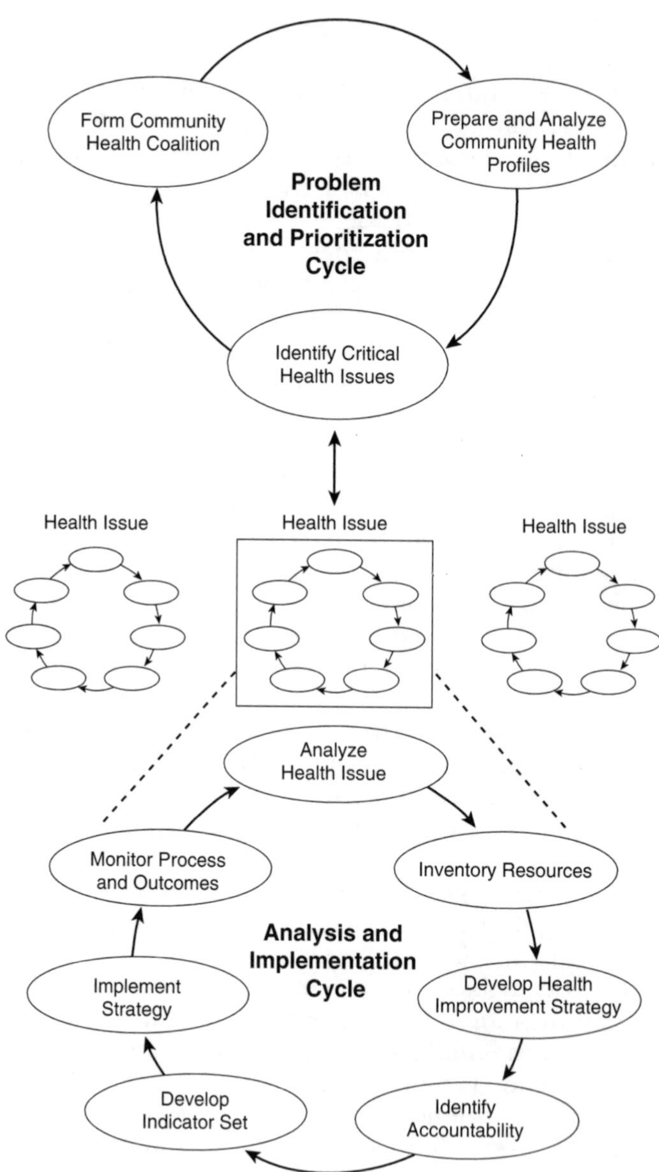

FIGURE 2 The community health improvement process (CHIP).

be support for effective and efficient operation of the accountable entities in the community that are expected to respond to specific health issues. A CHIP must also accommodate the dynamic nature of communities and the interdependence of community activities. It should facilitate the flow of information among accountable entities and other community groups and help them structure complementary efforts. The information provided by health indicators for the community and by performance indicators for specific health issues must feed back into the system on a continuing basis to guide subsequent analysis and planning. That information loop is also a critical element in establishing a link between performance and accountability.

Problem Identification and Prioritization Cycle

As proposed by the committee, the problem identification and prioritization cycle has three main phases: forming a community health coalition, collecting and analyzing data for a community health profile, and identifying critical health issues. Community efforts can begin with *any* phase of the cycle. For example, the availability of data about the community might lead to action on a specific health issue and the subsequent emergence of a more broadly based coalition. Alternatively, a general interest in health might stimulate formation of a coalition, data collection activities, and development of options for strategic actions.

The health assessment activities that are part of the problem identification and prioritization cycle should include production of a *community health profile* that can provide basic information to a community about its demographic and socioeconomic characteristics and its health status and health risks. This profile would provide background information that can help a community interpret other health data and identify issues that need more focused attention. The committee's proposed indicators for a community health profile are listed in Table 1.

Analysis and Implementation Cycle

Once an issue has been targeted by a community, the health improvement process proposed by the committee moves on to a series of steps for analysis, strategy development, implementation, and monitoring the outcome of efforts by accountable entities (see Figure 2). These steps are displayed and described as sequential, but in practice they interact and are likely to be re-

TABLE 1 Proposed Indicators for a Community Health Profile

Sociodemographic Characteristics

1. Distribution of the population by age and race/ethnicity
2. Number and proportion of persons in groups such as migrants, homeless, or the non–English speaking, for whom access to community services and resources may be a concern
3. Number and proportion of persons aged 25 and older with less than a high school education
4. Ratio of the number of students graduating from high school to the number of students who entered 9th grade three years previously
5. Median household income
6. Proportion of children less than 15 years of age living in families at or below the poverty level
7. Unemployment rate
8. Number and proportion of single-parent families
9. Number and proportion of persons without health insurance

Health Status

10. Infant mortality rate by race/ethnicity
11. Numbers of deaths or age-adjusted death rates for motor vehicle crashes, work-related injuries, suicide, homicide, lung cancer, breast cancer, cardiovascular diseases, and all causes, by age, race, and gender as appropriate
12. Reported incidence of AIDS, measles, tuberculosis, and primary and secondary syphilis, by age, race, and gender as appropriate
13. Births to adolescents (ages 10–17) as a proportion of total live births
14. Number and rate of confirmed abuse and neglect cases among children

peated a varying number of times while a community is engaged in a particular initiative. A community may have a portfolio of health improvement activities, each progressing through this cycle at its own pace.

Analyze the Health Issue

A community, through its health coalition or a designated agent such as the health department, must analyze the health issue to understand the contributing factors and how they operate in the community. A framework such as the field model should be used to ensure consideration not only of behavioral risks and health care issues but also of factors in the social and physical environments.

TABLE 1 *Continued*

Health Risk Factors

15. Proportion of 2-year-old children who have received all age-appropriate vaccines, as recommended by the Advisory Committee on Immunization Practices
16. Proportion of adults aged 65 and older who have ever been immunized for pneumococcal pneumonia; proportion who have been immunized in the past 12 months for influenza
17. Proportion of the population who smoke, by age, race, and gender as appropriate
18. Proportion of the population aged 18 and older who are obese
19. Number and type of U.S. Environmental Protection Agency air quality standards not met
20. Proportion of assessed rivers, lakes, and estuaries that support beneficial uses (e.g., fishing and swimming approved)

Health Care Resource Consumption

21. Per capita health care spending for Medicare beneficiaries (the Medicare adjusted average per capita cost [AAPCC])

Functional Status

22. Proportion of adults reporting that their general health is good to excellent
23. During the past 30 days, average number of days for which adults report that their physical or mental health was not good

Quality of Life

24. Proportion of adults satisfied with the health care system in the community
25. Proportion of persons satisfied with the quality of life in the community

Inventory Health Resources

A community must assess the resources available for health improvement efforts. Relevant resources include those that can be applied to required tasks (e.g., organizations, influence, expertise, funding); protective factors within the community that can mitigate the impact of adverse conditions; and support available from public- and private-sector sources outside the community (e.g., funding, technical assistance).

Develop a Health Improvement Strategy

Health improvement strategies should seek to apply available resources as effectively as possible, given a community's specific features. Priority should be given to actions for which evidence of effectiveness is available and for which costs are considered appropriate in relation to expected health benefits. For many health issues, however, evidence for effective interventions will be limited. A community should not ignore those issues but will have to consider carefully what actions will make the best use of its resources. Communities should also consider the implications of not acting on a health issue.

Establish Accountability for Activities

Establishing accountability through a collaborative approach is a key to using performance monitoring in the health improvement process proposed by the committee. Specific entities must be willing to be accountable to the community for undertaking activities that are expected to contribute to achieving desired health outcomes. The committee sees a collective responsibility among all segments of a community to contribute to health improvements, but each entity must accept individual responsibility for performing those tasks that are consistent with its capabilities.

Develop a Set of Performance Indicators

Performance indicators are needed to help community stakeholders monitor whether the health improvement strategy is being implemented as intended and whether it is having the intended impact. These quantitative measures must apply to specific entities in the community that have accepted responsibility for some aspect of the health improvement effort. Because health issues have many dimensions and can be addressed by various sectors in the community, *sets* of indicators will be needed to assess performance.

Implement the Improvement Strategy

Implementation of health improvement strategies and interventions requires action by many segments of a community. The particular mix of activities and participants will depend on the health issue being addressed and on a community's organization and resources. In most instances, these activities will require the involvement of both public- and private-sector entities and often of entities that may not traditionally be seen as part of the health system.

Monitor Process and Outcomes

Once a health improvement program is under way, performance monitoring becomes an essential guide. Information provided by the selected performance indicators should be reviewed regularly and used to inform further action. In assessing progress, a community coalition or other designated agent should consider whether accountable entities are taking appropriate actions and whether appropriate strategies and interventions have been adopted. The quantitative data provided by performance indicators should be interpreted in combination with qualitative information from the community. As current goals are achieved and new ones adopted, the analysis and implementation cycle of a CHIP should support initiation of new activities and selection of new indicators. Over time, a community, through its health coalition and the broader aspects of a CHIP, should reexamine its priorities and health improvement portfolio, adding new issues as progress is made on others.

OPERATIONALIZING THE CHIP CONCEPT

In developing a health improvement program, every community must consider its particular circumstances (e.g., health concerns, resources, social and political perspectives). The committee cannot prescribe what actions individual communities should take to address their health concerns or who should be responsible for what, but it does believe that communities need to address these issues and that an organized approach to health improvement that makes use of performance monitoring tools will help them achieve their goals.

Given the different perspectives and activities of personal health service, public health, and other organizations that can contribute to the health of communities and given differing views of the meaning of "health" in the community context, the committee recommends that

- **communities should base a health improvement process on a broad definition of health and a comprehensive conceptual model of how health is produced within the community.**

In the committee's view, the field model, as elaborated by Evans and Stoddart (1994), is a good starting point. Drawing on evidence from social and behavioral as well as health sciences, this comprehensive model of the determinants of health can promote creative thinking about interventions to improve a community's health. The field model perspective makes it clear that most public and private organizational entities in a community, as well as individuals, share an interest in their community's health and are collectively responsible for it. Among these stakeholders in the community's health, those that can influence health outcomes can be thought of as "accountable entities." The field model's multifactorial nature clarifies the need for careful analysis to specify (1) what *individual entities* can contribute and thus be accountable for contributing and (2) where *collaborative action* and shared responsibility are essential.

To operationalize the concept of shared responsibility and individual accountability for community health, stakeholders need to know, jointly and as clearly as possible, how the actions of each potentially accountable entity can contribute to the community's health. Thus, the committee recommends that

- **a CHIP should develop its own set of specific, quantitative performance measures, linking accountable entities to the performance of specific activities expected to lead to the production of desired health outcomes in the community.**

Selecting these indicators will require careful consideration of how to gain insight into progress achieved in the health improvement process. A set of indicators should balance population-based measures of risk factors and health outcomes and health systems-based measures of services performed. To encourage full participation in the health improvement process, the selected performance measures should also be balanced across the interests and contributions of the various accountable entities in the community, including those whose primary mission is not health specific. Selection of performance indicators is discussed in Chapter 5, and prototype indicator sets for several health issues are presented in Appendix A. One example, for vaccine-preventable diseases, is shown in Table 2.

Because stakeholder-level performance measures will generally be unique to a particular community and to the circumstances of stakeholders in that community, the committee focused on developing community-level performance indicators. Such performance measures would permit communities and their health coalitions to ask, "How are we, as a community, performing in assuring the health of our citizenry?" The prototype indicators

TABLE 2 Sample Prototype Indicator Set: Vaccine-Preventable Diseases

1. Immunization rate for children at 24 months of age
2. Immunization rate at 24 months of age for children currently enrolled in managed care organizations
3. Immunization rate at 24 months of age for children currently enrolled in Medicaid
4. Existence in the community of a computerized immunization registry that provides automated appointment reminders; if a registry exists, the percentage of children in the community included
5. Among children with commercial health insurance coverage, percentage with full coverage for childhood immunizations
6. Percentage of Medicare enrollees who received an influenza immunization during the previous calendar year; percentage who have ever received a pneumococcal pneumonia immunization
7. Pneumonia and influenza death rates for persons age 65 and older
8. Existence in the community of an active childhood immunization coalition, involving health service providers, the local health department, parents, and interested community organizations

include measures for specific sectors in the community (e.g., managed care organizations, schools, employers, public health agencies), but a community may want measures for individual entities within those sectors.

Communities will need criteria to guide the selection of indicators. Criteria proposed by the committee include consistency with a conceptual framework (such as the field model) for understanding factors that contribute to the production of health, salience to community stakeholders, and support for the social change processes needed to achieve health improvements. Other proposed criteria are validity and reliability, availability of evidence linking performance and health improvement, sensitivity to changes in community health status, and availability of timely data at a reasonable cost. An operational definition should be developed for each measure to determine what data are needed and how (or if) they can be obtained. A review of existing indicator sets may suggest measures that could be adapted for community use and may be a source of tested operational definitions.

Many of the important underlying influences on health that the field model helps identify are often not amenable to change in the short run. For example, interventions aimed at critical developmental periods, such as educational programs in early childhood, may have long-term health benefits but produce little measurable effect in the near term. A desire to make observable progress could lead a CHIP to focus on other more immediately measurable problems or problems that may be high on the political agenda but of uncertain importance to the community's overall health (e.g., a new renal dialysis unit). A CHIP must also guard against becoming paralyzed by focusing on the undoable. To maintain momentum for community health coalitions, it may be reasonable to select some problems that are amenable to change and success in the short term. Thus, the committee recommends that

- **a CHIP should seek a balance between strategic opportunities for long-term health improvement and goals that are achievable in the short term.**

This balance might be achieved by including interim goals, such as risk reduction strategies, for major health problems. If a community were interested in reducing cancer mortality, for instance, reductions in smoking initiation among teenagers and the implementation of workplace smoking restrictions might be appropriate intermediate goals.

The proposed health improvement process and performance monitoring activities will require that communities have a sustainable system that provides for participation by major stakeholders and accountable entities. Thus, the committee recommends that

- **community coalitions guiding CHIPs should strive for strategic inclusiveness, incorporating individuals, groups, and organizations that have an interest in health outcomes, can take actions necessary to improve community health, or can contribute data and analytic capabilities needed for performance monitoring.**

Participants should assume responsibility for contributing to the health of the community, not just furthering the goals of the organizations they represent.

As described in Chapters 3 and 4, a CHIP focuses on horizontal peer relationships in a community rather than vertical hierarchical relationships. Experience suggests that performance monitoring used as a basis for inspection and discipline of those not producing as expected is less effective in achieving improvements than is monitoring used as a tool for learning and process change (Berwick, 1989; Osborne and Gaebler, 1992). Rather, a CHIP should use performance monitoring to encourage productive action and collaboration from many sectors. Because the proposed community health improvement process is new, groups that carry it out should be "learning organizations" in the sense that the people, agencies, and community involved are organized to learn from their own experience and improve their operations.

All community initiatives require leadership, which may come from the public or the private sector. To institutionalize the health improvement process as a multiparty effort, the committee recommends that

- **a CHIP should be centered in a community health coalition or similar entity.**

Some communities will have appropriate coalitions in place, but others will have to expand existing groups or establish a workable forum for collective action for the first time. Strategies for improving the effectiveness of community coalitions for health improvement are discussed in Chapter 3.

ENABLING POLICY AND RESOURCES

Federal, state, and local public health agencies and boards of health are all stakeholders in a community's health and capable of taking action to improve it. Indeed, *The Future of Public Health* (IOM, 1988) implies that public health agencies have a responsibility to assure that something like a CHIP is in place. Thus, the committee recommends that

- **state and local public health agencies should assure that an effective community health improvement process is in place in all communities. These agencies should at a minimum participate in CHIP activities and, in some communities, should provide its leadership and/or organizational home.**

For the CHIP to be effective, communities need data for community health profiles and performance measures. Since all parties share in the goal of improving community health, it is reasonable to combine public and private resources to support the data collection and analysis needed for communities to obtain health profile information, to conduct health status assessments and communicate results, and to sustain performance monitoring programs. Such resources could include funding, personnel, data, data processing, and analysis.

Both public and private sectors can contribute critical data for performance monitoring. Public health agencies, as part of the public health assessment function called for in *The Future of Public Health*, should promote, facilitate, and—where necessary and appropriate—perform community health assessments and monitor changes in key performance measures. Much of the necessary data and expertise exist at the state health department. Thus, the committee recommends that

- **in support of community-level health improvement processes, state health agencies, in cooperation and collaboration with local health departments, should assure the availability of community-level data needed for health profiles.**

Currently, most of these data are aggregated by standard geopolitical units such as counties and municipalities. The committee encourages making community health data available in a form that allows communities to prepare health profiles and performance measures according to their own definitions of "community" (e.g., geographic, socioeconomic, cultural). Geocoding of health-related data gathered for other purposes would be an important step toward improving the data for performance monitoring. For data available only at the community level, state health departments should provide models and technical assistance that communities can use in their own data collection activities.

Because data on and from all accountable entities are essential for effective performance monitoring, states and the federal government (in their policy development and regulatory roles) can assist communities by facilitating access to relevant data held by the private sector. In particular, the committee recommends that

- **states and the federal government, through health departments or other appropriate channels, should require that health plans, indemnity insurers, and other private entities report standard data on the characteristics and health status of their enrolled populations, on services provided, and on outcomes of those services, as necessary for performance monitoring in the community health improvement process.**

Providing these data should be seen as part of the responsibility that these private-sector organizations have to the community

(IOM, 1996; Showstack et al., 1996). Adequate safeguards for privacy and confidentiality must be provided for all CHIP data (IOM, 1994).

The relationship between the CHIP and public or private health service and other community organizations should be reciprocal. In addition to data that these organizations can provide to a CHIP, the organizations can use the other community data that are gathered, and this in turn should reinforce CHIP goals. For instance, state agencies designing publicly funded health services programs such as Medicaid managed care can specify the performance measures to be used in evaluating the contractors and the data that contractors must report. Alternatively, private health service organizations could use CHIP data to assess their contributions to the community's health under "community benefit" guidelines and regulations or in their own service planning and resource allocation decisions.

DEVELOPING THE COMMUNITY HEALTH IMPROVEMENT PROCESS

The community health improvement process and its use of performance monitoring, as laid out in this report, are a work in progress. As noted, the committee's recommendations reflect consideration of a variety of theoretical and practical models from health care, public health, and other settings. The committee also reviewed existing efforts at the national, state, and community levels and found much of value. Not found, however, was a conceptual framework for using performance monitoring concepts to improve community health as a whole (as opposed to monitoring the performance of specific entities such as managed care organizations or public health agencies). The development of a conceptual framework, and the illustration of its application through prototype indicator sets, is the major contribution of this report, but the framework remains largely untested. The overall community health improvement process, its performance monitoring component, and the indicator sets should be tested and improved over time. Thus, the committee recommends that

- **the CHIP concept developed in this report should be implemented in a variety of communities across the country, and these efforts should be carefully documented and independently assessed.**

The assessment process should strive to include sites that vary both in the nature of the community and in the structures and processes used for performance monitoring. The assessment should also include estimates of the full range of public and private costs of carrying out the CHIP and should explore ways to achieve efficiencies in these efforts. These "natural experiments" should be studied to learn how local circumstances affect the way the CHIP is adapted by different communities; to identify the "necessary and desirable conditions" for implementation of the CHIP; and to assess whether or not the CHIP indeed results in a refocusing of attention on root causes of health problems and, ultimately, in important improvements in community health.

The current evaluations of a variety of community health interventions (e.g., Wagner et al., 1991; Elder et al., 1993; Wickizer et al., 1993; COMMIT, 1995a,b; Fortmann et al., 1995; Murray, 1995) can be expected to inform the development of specific interventions to address health problems, the community intervention process itself, and analytic techniques to apply to community studies. The recently established Task Force on Community Preventive Services, organized by the Centers for Disease Control and Prevention, will compile evidence on a variety of community-level activities. The CHIP in its entirety can also be thought of as a "comprehensive community initiative," and ideas regarding the evaluation of such initiatives can be applied (see Connell et al., 1995).

For the community health improvement process to be effective, appropriate performance measurement tools must be developed further. Thus, the committee recommends that

- **the Public Health Service, in conjunction with state and local health agencies, national professional organizations, and foundations, should develop standard measures for community health profiles and topic-specific model indicator sets that perform well in individual communities and are suitable for cross-community comparison.**

These standard measures would be a resource available to communities, not a set of prescribed measures. The prototype indicator sets described in Appendix A of this report should be viewed as a starting point. Particular attention should be given to issues for which valid measures are not currently available, but the refinement of existing measures should also be addressed. The development of measures of "quality of life" and consumer satisfaction for use in community surveys is particularly important. Research to develop and improve techniques of measurement and analysis (e.g., small area analysis) that can be applied to community-level performance monitoring should be supported as well.

More generally, technical expertise based on experience with the community health improvement process must be developed and shared. Thus, the committee recommends that

- **the Public Health Service, in conjunction with state and local health agencies, national professional organizations, and foundations, should develop workbooks, seminars, and other forms of technical assistance to catalog and convey to communities information on best CHIP practices, specific model performance measures for a variety of health issues and ways to interpret changes in these measures, and available data resources.**

Universities can, in a variety of activities and through a variety of disciplines, play an important role in helping communities implement a CHIP and in developing and sharing technical expertise. They should also contribute to the effective dissemination of the CHIP concept through their role in the development of a workforce whose attitudes, values, and skills support its implementation. Thus, the committee recommends that

- **educational programs for professionals in public health, medicine, nursing, health administration, public management, and related fields should include CHIP concepts and practices in their curriculum for preservice and midcareer students.**

These programs should introduce the concept of CHIP as a way of thinking about the application of a group of academic disciplines (epidemiology, biostatistics, environmental health, health behavior, and so on) to the practice of community health improvement. Among the other fields in which CHIP might be addressed are maternal and child health, behavioral sciences, and mental health and substance abuse counseling and program administration.

REFERENCES

APHA (American Public Health Association), Association of Schools of Public Health, Association of State and Territorial Health Officials, National Association of County Health Officials, United States Conference of Local Health Officers, Department of Health and Human Services, Public Health Service, Centers for Disease Control. 1991. *Healthy Communities 2000: Model Standards.* 3rd ed. Washington, D.C.: APHA.

Berwick, D.M. 1989. Continuous Improvement as an Ideal in Health Care. *New England Journal of Medicine* 320:53–56.

COMMIT (Community Intervention Trial for Smoking Cessation). 1995a. I. Cohort Results from a Four-Year Community Intervention. *American Journal of Public Health* 85:183–192.

COMMIT. 1995b. II. Changes in Adult Cigarette Smoking Prevalence. *American Journal of Public Health* 85:193–200.

Connell, J.P., Kubisch, A.C., Schorr, L.B., and Weiss, C.H., eds. 1995. *New Approaches to Evaluating Community Initiatives: Concepts, Methods, and Contexts.* Washington, D.C.: Aspen Institute.

Elder, J.P., Schmid, T.L., Dower, P., and Hedlund, S. 1993. Community Heart Health Programs: Components, Rationale, and Strategies for Effective Interventions. *Journal of Public Health Policy* 14:463–479.

Evans, R.G., and Stoddart, G.L. 1994. Producing Health, Consuming Health Care. In *Why Are Some People Healthy and Others Not? The Determinants of Health of Populations.* R.G. Evans, M.L. Barer, and T.R. Marmor, eds. New York: Aldine De Gruyter.

Fortmann, S.P., Flora, J.A., Winkleby, M.A., Schooler, C., Taylor, C.B., and Farquhar, J.W. 1995. Community Intervention Trials: Reflections on the Stanford Five-City Project Experience. *American Journal of Epidemiology* 142:576–586.

Green, L. W., and Kreuter, M. W. 1990. Health Promotion as a Public Health Strategy for the 1990s. *Annual Review of Public Health* 11:319–334.

IOM (Institute of Medicine). 1988. *The Future of Public Health.* Washington, D.C.: National Academy Press.

IOM. 1994. *Health Data in the Information Age: Use, Disclosure, and Privacy.* M.S. Donaldson and K.N. Lohr, eds. Washington, D.C.: National Academy Press.

IOM. 1996. *Healthy Communities: New Partnerships for the Future of Public Health.* M.A. Stoto, C. Abel, and A. Dievler, eds. Washington, D.C.: National Academy Press.

Murray, D. 1995. Design and Analysis of Community Trials: Lessons from the Minnesota Heart Health Program. *American Journal of Epidemiology* 142:569–575.

NACHO (National Association of County Health Officials). 1991. *APEXPH: Assessment Protocol for Excellence in Public Health.* Washington, D.C.: NACHO.

NCQA (National Committee for Quality Assurance). 1993. *Health Plan Employer Data and Information Set and User's Manual, Version 2.0 (HEDIS 2.0).* Washington, D.C.: NCQA.

Nolan, T.W., and Knapp, M. 1996. Community-wide Health Improvement: Lessons from the IHI-GOAL/QPC Learning Cooperative. *The Quality Letter for Healthcare Leaders* 8(1):13–20.

Osborne, D., and Gaebler, T. 1992. *Reinventing Government: How the Entrepreneurial Spirit Is Transforming the Public Sector.* Reading, Mass.: Addison-Wesley.

Showstack, J., Lurie, N., Leatherman, S., Fisher, E., and Inui, T. 1996. Health of the Public: The Private Sector Challenge. *Journal of the American Medical Association* 276:1071–1074.

USDHHS (U.S. Department of Health and Human Services). 1991. *Healthy People 2000: National Health Promotion and Disease Prevention Objectives.* DHHS Pub. No. (PHS) 91-50212. Washington, D.C.: Office of the Assistant Secretary for Health.

Wagner, E.H., Koepsell, T.D., Anderman, C., et al. 1991. The Evaluation of the Henry J. Kaiser Family Foundation's Community Health Promotion Program: Design. *Journal of Clinical Epidemiology* 44:685–699.

Wickizer, T.M., Von Korff, M., Cheadle, A., et al. 1993. Activating Communities for Health Promotion: A Process Evaluation Method. *American Journal of Public Health* 83:561–567.

Zablocki, E. 1996. Improving Community Health Status: Strategies for Success. *The Quality Letter for Healthcare Leaders* 8(1):2–12.

1

Introduction

In communities, health is a product of many factors, and many segments of the community have the potential to contribute to and share responsibility for its protection and improvement. Changes in public policy, in public- and private-sector roles in health and health care, and in public expectations are presenting opportunities and challenges for communities addressing both the overall health status of the population and more specific health issues. Performance monitoring can be used as a tool to assess activities in many sectors and to promote collaboration and accountability in working toward better health for the whole community, especially within the framework of a community-based health improvement process.

This report from the Institute of Medicine (IOM) Committee on Using Performance Monitoring to Improve Community Health outlines the elements of an ongoing and evolving health improvement process, discusses the role that performance monitoring can play, and offers tools to help communities develop and use performance indicators. In its proposals and recommendations, the committee is responding to the need it sees to introduce a conceptual framework for using performance monitoring concepts to improve community health as a whole—as opposed to monitoring performance within specific community entities. This report also addresses the need to look beyond community health assessment to ways to establish accountability for health improvement.

Drawing on lessons from a variety of current activities, the committee brings to community health improvement an approach that focuses on integrating the roles of clinical personal health services, public health, and a broad array of other elements in the community, and on developing monitoring systems that can function in this integrated context. The committee is not attempting to prescribe what communities should do to address their health concerns or who should be responsible for what, but it is encouraging communities to adopt a systematic approach to health improvement that makes use of performance monitoring tools to help them achieve their goals.

A BROADER UNDERSTANDING OF HEALTH

Contributing to the interest in health improvement and performance monitoring is a wider recognition that health embraces well-being as well as the absence of illness. For both individuals and populations, health depends not only on health care but also on other factors including individual behavior, genetic makeup, exposure to health threats, and social and economic conditions. The *health field model*, as described by Evans and Stoddart (1994) and discussed further in Chapter 2, presents these multiple determinants of health in a dynamic relationship. The model's feedback loops link social environment, physical environment, genetic endowment, an individual's behavioral and biologic responses, disease, health care, health and function, well-being, and prosperity. The committee found this model to be an effective basis for its work.

Health in the community can be seen as the product of the changing mix and interactions of these factors over time. The multidimensional perspective reinforces the value of public health's traditional emphasis on a population-based approach to community health issues. It also provides a basis for looking to many segments of the community to address factors affecting health and well-being, making it appropriate to bring a wide array of parties to the table as interested stakeholders and accountable partners.

A COMMUNITY PERSPECTIVE

The committee adopted as a starting point for its discussions of "community" a definition offered by Labonte (1988): individuals with shared affinity, and perhaps a shared geography, who organize around an issue, with collective discussion, decision making, and action. Geography emerged as a critical point of reference in the committee's discussions. Although geographic (or civic) boundaries cannot adequately capture all of the potentially meaningful communities to which individuals might belong, they are a practical basis for analysis within the limitations of current data systems. Depending on the health issue, the relevant geographic unit (e.g., county, city, census tract) may vary.

A wide range of individuals, organizations, and agencies, many of whose roles are not within the traditional domain of health care or public health, have an effect on and a stake in a community's health (Patrick and Wickizer, 1995). These entities can include individual health care providers, public health agencies, health care organizations, purchasers of health services, and community organizations explicitly concerned with health. They can also include other government agencies (e.g., housing, human services, public safety), schools, business and industry, faith communities, and other community groups that may not usually be seen as having any explicit health-related role. Entities such as state health departments, federal agencies, managed care organizations, and national corporations have a broader scope than a single community but often have an important role at the local level.

As communities respond to the multiple factors involved in various health issues, all parties will have to sort out their roles and responsibilities. The specific pattern will vary over time and from community to community, depending on the mix and interaction of factors contributing to health. To optimize the unique contributions of these interdependent sectors, it will be important to address issues of accountability and shared responsibility for various aspects of community health. In most communities, there will be only limited experience with widespread collaborative or coordinated efforts among these diverse groups. A common language and an understanding of the multidimensional nature of the determinants of health will help community stakeholders work together effectively. Finding a way to accommodate diversity in values and goals will be another important task. Participation in the process of community-wide social change will also be needed for performance monitoring to succeed in improving health (Green and Kreuter, 1990).

The committee recognizes that there are limitations in a community-based approach to health improvement. Some of the factors affecting health in a community will originate elsewhere and may not be modifiable by efforts within the community. "Outside" influences are also a factor because of the geographic mobility of the population of most communities. Current health status in any given community reflects the combined and cumulative effects of factors operating over time in many other communities. These confounding influences must be taken into account in developing and implementing health improvement efforts based on accountable performance.

GROWING INTEREST IN PERFORMANCE MONITORING

Performance monitoring has gained increasing attention as a tool for managing processes and improving their outcomes. It is an important component of the activities characterized as "reinventing government" (Osborne and Gaebler, 1992; Gore, 1993; Hatry et al., 1994), and increasingly, it is being used to evaluate the delivery of personal health care services and to examine population-based activities addressing the health of the public.

As used by the committee, the term "performance monitoring" applies to a continuing and evolving process—anchored in a context of shared responsibility and accountability for health improvement—for (1) selecting and using a limited number of indicators that can track critical processes and outcomes over time and among accountable stakeholders; (2) collecting and analyzing data on those indicators; and (3) making the results available to inform assessments of the effectiveness of an intervention and the contributions of accountable entities.

Although many performance monitoring activities are focused on specific organizations such as health plans or hospitals, there is a growing appreciation of the importance of a dynamic, population-based perspective. Only at the population level is it possible to look at the impact of a broad range of health determinants, among which a specific element such as health care services may play only a limited role. Furthermore, a population-based perspective is necessary to see whether health improvement efforts are meeting the needs of all segments of the community.

Performance Monitoring in Health Care

Developments in private-sector health care, particularly in the area of managed care, are contributing to the interest in and tools available for performance monitoring. Managed care and integrated health systems are expanding rapidly in most parts of the country, and in some markets there is strong competition. They are serving not only the privately insured but also Medicaid programs and a growing share of the Medicare population. Throughout the country, employers and other major purchasers of health services are demanding, and receiving, information on costs and performance that will help them select among plans. Less widely, consumers are seeking information that can help them make informed choices about their health care and health care providers. Individual health plans, consumer groups, and national organizations have developed a variety of reporting systems, often with summary "report cards."

Various initiatives are under way to develop and promote standardized performance indicators. One of these is the Health Plan Employer Data and Information Set, HEDIS, produced by the National Committee for Quality Assurance (NCQA, 1993, 1996). HEDIS is a defined set of performance measures used by employers and managed care organizations to compare health plans on the basis of quality, access and patient satisfaction, delivery of preventive services, membership and utilization, financing, and descriptive management information. In the newer versions, special consideration has been given to identifying measures appropriate for monitoring services for Medicaid beneficiaries. In another national-level activity, the Joint Commission on Accreditation of Healthcare Organizations (JCAHO, 1996) has promulgated standards, the focus of which in recent years has been in keeping with a broader philosophy of performance monitoring and outcomes. More recently, the Foundation for Accountability (FAcct, 1995) is reviewing and recommending other sets of indicators that employers and consumers can use to assess health plan performance. A more specialized set of performance measures has been developed by the American Managed Behavioral Healthcare Association (AMBHA, 1995), specifically for the mental health and chemical dependency services offered by its members.

In many ways these activities build on work being done in the health care sector on quality assessment and quality improvement and on outcomes research. For example, the definition of quality of care formulated by the IOM (1990) directs attention to the importance of good performance in achieving good health outcomes.[1] Quality improvement techniques, which have been

---

[1]Quality of care is defined as "the degree to which health services for individuals and populations increase the likelihood of desired health outcomes and are consistent with current professional knowledge" (IOM, 1990, p. 21).

adapted from their industrial origins for use in individual health care settings, rely on repeated measurements of performance and outcomes to identify problems and assess the effectiveness of corrective actions (e.g., see Berwick et al., 1990). Community-wide performance monitoring would extend these principles and techniques beyond individual health care settings. Several cities have been part of a demonstration project to test just such an approach (Nolan and Knapp, 1996).

Performance Monitoring in the Public Sector

In the public sector, two primary themes have emerged: assessing the performance of local health departments and assessing the population's health status. The "core functions" of public health identified in *The Future of Public Health* (IOM, 1988)—assessment of health needs and resources, policy development, and assurance that needed activities are performed—have become the basis for judging the performance of local health departments. Tools such as PATCH (Planned Approach to Community Health) (Kreuter, 1992; CDC, 1995), *APEXPH: Assessment Protocol for Excellence in Public Health* (NACHO, 1991), *Healthy Communities 2000: Model Standards* (APHA et al., 1991), and the Healthy Cities/Healthy Communities model (National Civic League, 1993; Flynn, 1996) are available to help health departments assess their ability to perform those functions. These materials also provide guidance on efforts to assess and respond to community health needs.

Formal measures of effective performance by health departments are being developed and tested (Miller et al., 1994a,b; Studnicki et al., 1994; Turnock et al., 1994a,b, 1995). The initial focus on health departments is now widening to include other elements of the community (Richards et al., 1995). Still needed are research and evaluation to determine the impact that performance of activities related to the core functions of public health, by health departments or other entities, has on health in the community.

Other activities have focused on health status measurement. *Healthy People 2000: The National Health Promotion and Disease Prevention Objectives* (USDHHS, 1991) outlines 22 categories of measurable health objectives in health status, risk reduction, and services and protection, including both process and outcome measures. Many state and local health departments have adapted the national objectives to their own circumstances. *Healthy Commu-*

nities 2000: Model Standards (APHA et al., 1991) is designed specifically to assist this process. In addition, agencies and organizations with an interest in a specific health issue or a specific population group have made use of particular subsets of the *Healthy People 2000* objectives (e.g., American College Health Association, 1990; MCHB, 1991).

Some federal block grant programs (e.g., in prevention and public health services, maternal and child health, and substance abuse) have reporting requirements for states that include health status and outcomes measures, often drawn from or similar to those in *Healthy People 2000*. Proposals by the U.S. Department of Health and Human Services for Public Health Performance Partnership Grants would require new reporting measures that are intended to focus on the link between grant-supported activities and health outcomes (USDHHS, no date). In general, however, health status assessments have provided baseline information about community health needs but have not explicitly addressed the performance of specific entities in the community, which raises different measurement and community action issues.

Accountability for Efficient and Effective Action

Performance monitoring is also a response to concerns about ensuring the efficient and effective use of resources, particularly financial resources. Overall, higher levels of health care spending in the United States than in most other countries have not produced higher levels of health, measured in terms such as life expectancy or infant mortality. Both public- and private-sector decision makers see a need to use limited funds in ways that optimize health outcomes. This concern is consistent with a heightened interest in accountability for the use of those funds and the outcomes produced.

There is a need to account for performance and outcomes within individual organizations (e.g., a health department or a health plan), but from the committee's perspective, there must also be a way to monitor performance and outcomes for communities as a whole. Looking at the results of many separate efforts will not provide a comprehensive community picture, and those separate efforts cannot, by themselves, ensure that health improvement achieves its goals.

A FRAMEWORK FOR COMMUNITY HEALTH IMPROVEMENT

The committee has based its work on a vision for community health improvement that relies on shared responsibility across a broad range of community stakeholders, combined with individual accountability to ensure that responsibilities are not ignored or abandoned. This has led to a proposal for a *community health improvement process* (CHIP), described in more detail in Chapter 4, through which a community can assess health needs in the population and also develop interventions and monitor performance and outcomes.

A Process to Support Health Improvement

A CHIP would operate through two primary interacting cycles, both of which rely on analysis, action, and measurement (see Figure 1-1). A broad *problem identification and prioritization cycle* focuses on building a community stakeholder coalition, monitoring community-level health indicators, and identifying specific health issues as community priorities. The second cycle—*an analysis and implementation cycle*—is a series of processes to devise, implement, and evaluate the impact of health improvement strategies for priority health issues. More than one analysis and implementation cycle may be operating at the same time if a community is responding to multiple health issues. The overall process differs from other health assessment and health-related performance monitoring models primarily because of its emphasis on measurement to link performance and accountability.

As envisioned by the committee, a CHIP can be implemented in a variety of community circumstances, and communities can begin working at various points in either cycle and with varying resources in place. The process must be seen as iterative and evolving rather than linear or short term. One-time activities, briefly assembled coalitions, and isolated solutions will not be adequate. The process must also be able to accommodate the dynamic nature of communities and the interdependence of community activities. Both community-level monitoring data and more detailed information related to specific health issues must feed back into the system on a continuing basis to guide subsequent analysis and planning. This information loop is also the means by which a CHIP links performance to accountable entities among the community stakeholders.

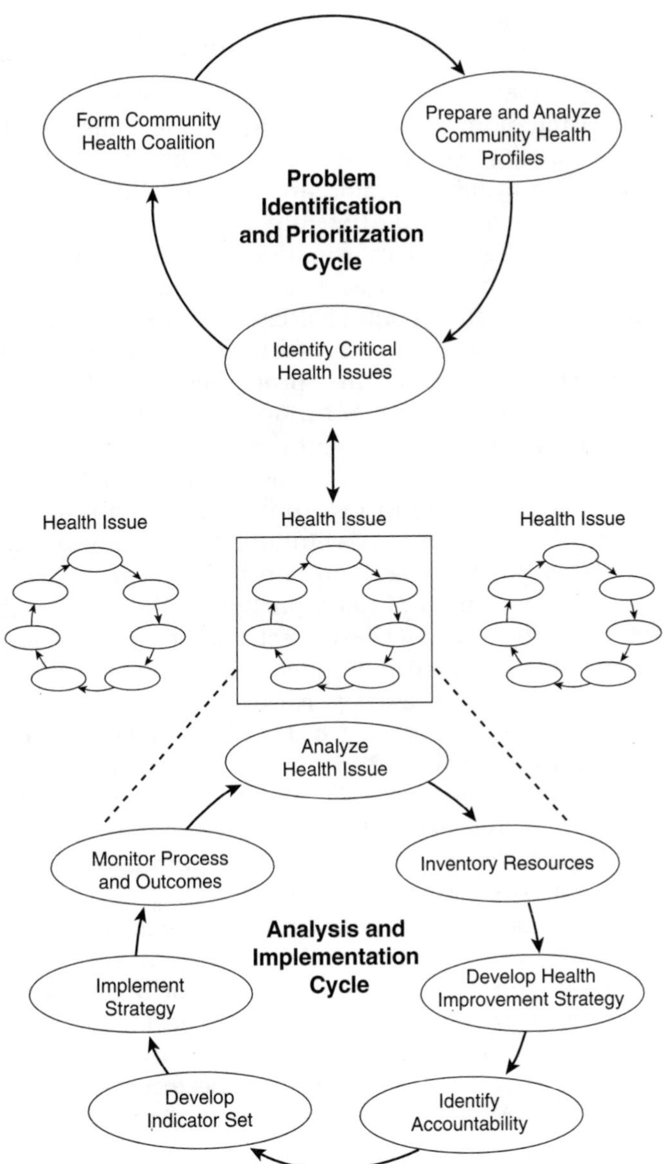

FIGURE 1-1 The community health improvement process (CHIP).

Selecting and Using Indicators

The CHIP cycles make use of two kinds of indicators. The problem identification and prioritization cycle calls for development of a *community health profile* that can provide basic information about a community's demographic and socioeconomic characteristics and its health status and health risks. This profile would provide background information that can help a community interpret other health data. Comparing these data over time or with data from other communities may help identify health issues that should receive more focused attention. The committee's proposal for a community profile appears in Chapter 5.

The analysis and implementation cycle operationalizes accountability for health improvement through sets of concrete, specific, and quantitative performance indicators linked to "accountable entities" in the community that can contribute to health improvement. A key element is linking "performance" to health outcomes. This requires both an understanding of the factors that function as determinants of a particular outcome and of scientific evidence to support the expectation that specific actions will have the desired health impact. Scientifically sound (i.e., reliable and valid) measures of performance and outcomes must also be possible. In the context of the committee's broad definition of health, appropriate indicators can be diverse.

Selecting indicators requires careful consideration of how to gain insight into progress achieved in the health improvement process. A set of indicators should balance population-based measures of risk factors and health outcomes and health systems-based measures of services performed and should also include measures for the various accountable entities in the community, including those whose primary mission is not health specific. A balance is needed among indicators that reflect short-term gains and those that measure more fundamental changes in community health. In selecting health issues and performance indicators, communities must make strategic choices that are consistent with their specific aims and circumstances. In Chapter 5, the committee reviews criteria to guide the selection of indicators, and Appendix A illustrates the application of the committee's proposals with prototype sets of community-level performance indicators for several specific health issues.

Data and Measurement Concerns

The committee found that existing indicators and data collection tools (e.g., HEDIS or state and national health surveys) are often not available for use at the community level and that available information systems are not adequate for identifying or analyzing problems, making choices for action among alternative problems and interventions, or tracking the effectiveness of interventions. Even when tools for health indicator development and implementation exist, communities may not have the necessary resources and circumstances for creating an operational health improvement process.

As envisioned by the committee, a community-based performance monitoring program will require an enhanced information infrastructure that can support monitoring diverse phenomena in the many sectors that contribute to the health of populations, including clinical care, environmental services, individual and public education, community social services, and public policy that promotes behavioral change. In some settings, it may be possible to build on information systems developed to support functions such as the delivery of health or human services or to establish links among existing data systems.

Also needed will be the capability to provide information on the health status of a community, including threats to its future health; to inform decisions about how to improve the health of the public; and to document change in community health and in performance of health-related functions. The value of the information technologies will depend on the ability of some segment of the community to analyze and understand the data produced and make them accessible to diverse community audiences.

ISSUES FOR CONSIDERATION

It is in this context that the IOM Committee on Using Performance Monitoring to Improve Community Health was charged with examining the use of performance monitoring to protect and improve the health of communities and with developing prototypical sets of performance indicators for specific health concerns. As discussions progressed during the course of the study, performance monitoring emerged as a critical tool in a broader health improvement process. Thus, the committee aims to explicate its vision for a community health improvement process that applies the techniques of performance monitoring and to demonstrate the value of the process to a diverse set of community stakeholders with an interest in and influence on health. Emphasized in this is the importance of improving our understanding of the factors that contribute to health in communities, particularly within the field model framework (Evans and Stoddart, 1994). Current limitations in that understanding often make it difficult to establish whether changes in performance will lead to improvements in health in the community, as measured through assessments of individuals.

The implications of the current social, scientific, and policy climate for community health improvement efforts and the further development of health-related performance monitoring are also a consideration. For example, some question whether meaningful responsibility and accountability for community health can be established across a range of largely autonomous entities, none of which controls all of the elements that may be critical to success (Nerenz, 1996). A different concern is that the diversity of performance monitoring developments will not achieve sufficient coordination to provide the kind of comprehensive approach that the committee believes is needed. Because performance monitoring will generally require some degree of change in the way institutions or communities make decisions and take actions, the committee also explored the processes that lead to such changes.

The committee addressed some of the challenges that must be met if performance monitoring is to progress. Despite the recognition of its value, the implementation of performance monitoring may be hindered by lack of community capacity to mount such an effort or to overcome the measurement demands it can create (see Chapter 4). There may also be concerns that rigorous monitoring could reveal poor or ineffective performance or that newer, more diverse approaches to health improvement will alter traditional patterns of responsibility and control for some sectors of the community.

The committee faced the challenge of identifying and presenting essential elements of a health improvement process and performance monitoring activities while avoiding a prescription for specific actions. It has, however, developed tools that communities can apply or adapt to their needs. In particular, the committee focused on the process of indicator selection and the development of prototypical indicator sets to use in an ongoing effort to evaluate performance and health outcomes related to specific health issues. It also presents a proposal for a set of indicators that could form the core of a community profile.

Every community will have to look at health questions from its own perspective and scrutinize its priorities and opportunities to respond. Those priorities and opportunities will vary depending on a community's particular health and social environment. Practical matters of budget and timing will also influence the way in which communities choose health priorities and performance indicators. The committee presents specific recommendations intended to address essential elements of what needs to be done to support effective performance monitoring and its integration into a community health improvement process. It has, however, avoided recommendations on how communities should go about these tasks.

The committee seeks to reach a wide audience with this report: public health agencies at the local, state, and federal levels; health care providers and organizations in the public and private sectors; employers; important public-sector purchasers of health care services for their employees and for programs such as Medicare and Medicaid; agencies and organizations with responsibilities in areas such as child health, elder health, mental health, and substance abuse; agencies with diverse community responsibilities including social services, education, and criminal justice; and a wide variety of community organizations. Others for whom the committee expects the report to have value are accrediting organizations, educators, and those who set research agendas, including foundations and other funding organizations.

UNDERLYING ASSUMPTIONS

The committee's examination of the issues related to community health improvement and performance monitoring reflects underlying assumptions on several issues.

- *Effective use of limited resources:* Limited resources, long a factor in much of the public sector and increasingly a concern in the private sector, make it necessary to improve the efficiency and effectiveness with which those resources are used. That is, resources must be used for appropriate purposes and in ways that efficiently promote desired results. The health improvement process outlined by the committee will provide a broad perspective from which to guide and assess resource use in a community. This process and its performance monitoring elements can contribute to efficiency and effectiveness by providing information on what is being done in the community, what sectors of the community are taking action, and what the impact is on community health status.

• *A conceptual model of the determinants of health:* The committee believes that the health improvement process and its performance monitoring component will be more effective if they are based on a conceptual model that can frame the interacting factors contributing to a community's health and can direct attention to the broad array of actions that could be expected to improve health.

• *Shared responsibility among diverse stakeholders:* Fundamental to the committee's work is the recognition that a wide range of individuals and organizations will have to recognize and accept that they have a shared and interdependent role in community health. Action in many sectors of society, not merely improvements within public health or health care delivery systems, will be necessary, and no one group will be able to successfully address community-wide health issues alone. Broad inclusiveness across stakeholders should be a starting point in a community's approach to the health improvement process, but it may have to be balanced by expectations for more selective involvement with specific health issues.

Although acceptance of shared responsibility is an essential element of the committee's framework, many communities may find it challenging to establish a sufficiently collaborative environment. There must also be a willingness to act. Motivation for action may come from sources such as good will, self-interest, regulation, or a combination of these.

• *Trust and equity:* By documenting actions and outcomes, performance monitoring can support increased public trust that "the system" is working. It can also, as part of a broader health improvement process, guide community actions toward minimizing major discrepancies in health status among subpopulations to promote greater equity in health throughout the community.

THE COMMITTEE'S REPORT

This report presents the committee's assessment of conceptual and operational considerations in community-based health improvement efforts and the contribution that performance monitoring can make. Chapter 2 examines the determinants of health from the broad perspective offered by the field model. This broad perspective is an essential element of the committee's approach to health improvement and performance monitoring. Chapter 3 examines issues in managing social change, the role of coalitions, and challenges in achieving consensus on accountability and responsibility.

In Chapter 4, the committee outlines its framework for a community health improvement process to help communities monitor overall health status, establish priorities, and assess progress in issue-specific efforts; the chapter also examines capacities needed to support this process. Chapter 5 presents the committee's proposal for a community health profile and discusses issues in selecting performance indicators to be used in addressing specific health issues. Presented in Appendix A are prototype sets of issue-specific indicators developed by the committee to illustrate how communities might apply the concepts outlined in this report.

Chapter 6 concludes the report with the committee's recommendations for steps to be taken by various parties to move toward the health improvement and performance monitoring processes envisioned by the committee.

REFERENCES

AMBHA (American Managed Behavioral Healthcare Association). 1995. *Performance Measures for Managed Behavioral Healthcare Programs.* Washington, D.C.: AMBHA Quality Improvement and Clinical Services Committee.

American College Health Association. 1990. *Healthy Campus 2000: Making It Happen.* Baltimore: American College Health Association.

APHA (American Public Health Association), Association of Schools of Public Health, Association of State and Territorial Health Officials, National Association of County Health Officials, United States Conference of Local Health Officers, Department of Health and Human Services, Public Health Service, Centers for Disease Control. 1991. *Healthy Communities 2000: Model Standards.* 3rd ed. Washington, D.C.: APHA.

Berwick, D.M., Godfrey, A.B., and Roessner, J. 1990. *Curing Health Care: New Strategies for Quality Improvement.* San Francisco: Jossey-Bass.

CDC. 1995. *Planned Approach to Community Health: Guide for the Local Coordinator.* Atlanta, Ga.: CDC, National Center for Chronic Disease Prevention and Health Promotion.

Evans, R.G., and Stoddart, G.L. 1994. Producing Health, Consuming Health Care. In *Why Are Some People Healthy and Others Not? The Determinants of Health of Populations.* R.G. Evans, M.L. Barer, and T.R. Marmor, eds. New York: Aldine De Gruyter.

Flynn, B.C. 1996. Healthy Cities: Toward Worldwide Health Promotion. *Annual Review of Public Health* 17:299–309.

FAcct (Foundation for Accountability). 1995. Guidebook for Performance Measurement: Prototype. Portland, Ore.: FAcct. September 22.

Gore, A. 1993. *From Red Tape to Results: Creating a Government That Works Better and Costs Less.* Report of the National Performance Review. Washington, D.C.: U.S. Government Printing Office.

Green, L.W., and Kreuter, M.W. 1990. Health Promotion as a Public Health Strategy for the 1990s. *Annual Review of Public Health* 11:319–334.

Hatry, H., Wholey, J.S., Anderson, W.F., et al. 1994. *Toward Useful Performance Measurement: Lessons Learned from Initial Pilot Performance Plans Prepared Under the Government Performance and Results Act.* Washington, D.C.: National Academy of Public Administration.

IOM (Institute of Medicine). 1988. *The Future of Public Health.* Washington, D.C.: National Academy Press.

IOM. 1990. *Medicare: A Strategy for Quality Assurance.* Vol. I. K.N. Lohr, ed. Washington, D.C.: National Academy Press.

JCAHO (Joint Commission on Accreditation of Healthcare Organizations). 1996. *Joint Commission Standards* [WWW document]. URL http://www.jcaho.org/stds.html

Kreuter, M.W. 1992. PATCH: Its Origin, Basic Concepts, and Links to Contemporary Public Health Policy. *Journal of Health Education* 23:135–139.

Labonte, R. 1988. Health Promotion: From Concepts to Strategies. *Health Care Management Forum* 1(3):24–30.

MCHB (Maternal and Child Health Bureau). 1991. *Healthy Children 2000: National Health Promotion and Disease Prevention Objectives Related to Mothers, Infants, Children, Adolescents, and Youth.* Pub. No. HRSA-M-CH 91-2. Rockville, Md.: U.S. Department of Health and Human Services, Health Resources and Services Administration.

Miller, C.A., Moore, K.S., Richards, T.B., and McKaig, C. 1994a. A Screening Survey to Assess Local Public Health Performance. *Public Health Reports* 109:659–664.

Miller, C.A., Moore, K.S., Richards, T.B., and Monk, J.D. 1994b. A Proposed Method for Assessing the Performance of Local Public Health Functions and Practices. *American Journal of Public Health* 84:1743–1749.

NACHO (National Association of County Health Officials). 1991. *APEXPH: Assessment Protocol for Excellence in Public Health.* Washington, D.C.: NACHO.

National Civic League. 1993. *The Healthy Communities Handbook.* Denver: National Civic League.

NCQA (National Committee for Quality Assurance). 1993. *Health Plan Employer Data and Information Set and User's Manual, Version 2.0 (HEDIS 2.0).* Washington, D.C.: NCQA.

NCQA. 1996. HEDIS 3.0 Draft for Public Comment. Washington, D.C.: NCQA. July 15.

Nerenz, D.R. 1996. Who Has Responsibility for a Population's Health? *Milbank Quarterly* 74:43–49.

Nolan, T.W., and Knapp, M. 1996. Community-wide Health Improvement: Lessons from the IHI-GOAL/QPC Learning Cooperative. *The Quality Letter for Healthcare Leaders* 8(1):13–20.

Osborne, D., and Gaebler, T. 1992. *Reinventing Government: How the Entrepreneurial Spirit Is Transforming the Public Sector.* Reading, Mass.: Addison-Wesley.

Patrick, D.L., and Wickizer, T.M. 1995. Community and Health. In *Society and Health.* B.C. Amick, S. Levine, A.R. Tarlov, and D.C. Walsh, eds. New York: Oxford University Press.

Richards, T.B., Rogers, J.J., Christenson, G.M., Miller, C.A., Taylor, M.S., and Cooper, A.D. 1995. Evaluating Local Public Health Performance at a Community Level on a Statewide Basis. *Journal of Public Health Management and Practice* 1(4):70–83.

Studnicki, J., Steverson, B., Blais, H.N., Goley, E., Richards, T.B., and Thornton, J.N. 1994. Analyzing Organizational Practices in Local Health Departments. *Public Health Reports* 109:485–490.

Turnock, B.J., Handler, A., Dyal, W.W., et al. 1994a. Implementing and Assessing Organizational Practices in Local Health Departments. *Public Health Reports* 109:478–484.

Turnock, B.J., Handler, A., Hall, W., Potsic, S., Nalluri, R., and Vaughn, E.H. 1994b. Local Health Department Effectiveness in Addressing the Core Functions of Public Health. *Public Health Reports* 109:653–658.

Turnock, B.J., Handler, A., Hall, W., Lenihan, D.P., and Vaughn, E. 1995. Capacity Building Influences on Illinois Local Health Departments. *Journal of Public Health Management and Practice* 1(3):50–58.

USDHHS (U.S. Department of Health and Human Services). 1991. *Healthy People 2000: National Health Promotion and Disease Prevention Objectives.* DHHS Pub. No. (PHS) 91-50212. Washington, D.C.: Office of the Assistant Secretary for Health.

USDHHS. No date. Performance Measurement in Selected Public Health Programs: 1995–1996 Regional Meetings. Washington, D.C.: Office of the Assistant Secretary for Health.

2

Understanding Health and Its Determinants

What is health? Multiple definitions of health exist, ranging from a precise biomedical or physical definition such as the absence of negative biologic circumstances (altered DNA, abnormal physiologic states, abnormal anatomy, disease, disability, or death) to the broad definition of the World Health Organization: "Health is a state of complete physical, mental and social well-being and not merely the absence of disease or infirmity" (WHO, 1994). The former definition offers the advantages of easy measurement and relatively clarity of the causal connections between the medical and public health care systems and the measured outcomes. The latter definition views health more broadly but risks assigning to the "health" system full responsibility for the economic and social welfare of members of society. Neither definition explicitly takes account of how individuals experience disease. Individuals can feel ill in the absence of disease and vary dramatically in their responses to a disease. Indeed, what matters to individuals is not simply the absence of disease, disability, or death, but also their responses to symptoms or diagnoses; their capacity to participate in work, family, and community; and their sense of well-being in many spheres (e.g., physical, psychosocial, spiritual).

A BROADER DEFINITION OF HEALTH

The successful implementation of initiatives to improve community health requires an understanding of the complex and diverse processes that produce health in communities. For both individuals and populations, health can be seen to depend not only on medical care, but also on other factors including individual behavior and genetic makeup, and social and economic conditions. The committee has adopted a broad definition of health, echoing a WHO (1986) health promotion perspective, that acknowledges multiple possible goals for the health system and underscores the important contributions to health that occur outside the formal medical care and public health systems. The committee definition allows improvement efforts to target not only the reduction of disease, disability, or death, but also an improvement in individuals' response to and perceptions of their illnesses; their functional capacity both now and in the future; and their overall sense of physical, emotional, and social well-being. The value of a broad measure thus rests in part upon the value attached to it by the population. Working within a definition of health that explicitly relies, in some measure, on community values is particularly important in a context of decision making for the allocation of limited resources.

Committee definition of health:

Health is a state of well-being and the capability to function in the face of changing circumstances.

Health is, therefore, a positive concept emphasizing social and personal resources as well as physical capabilities. Improving health is a shared responsibility of health care providers, public health officials, and a variety of other actors in the community who can contribute to the well-being of individuals and populations.

As Syme (1996) notes, viewing health as a biomedical construct has limited our ability to integrate processes that produce health and to address the underlying causes of disease. Death, disability, and disease incidence—ascertained by using traditional biologic or epidemiologic measures—are all important and valid indicators of the health of a population. A broader definition, however, allows efforts to measure community health to go beyond traditional public health measures, incorporating measures of functional status and general health perceptions. Communities embarking on health improvement initiatives should consider carefully their definition of health and ground their work in an evidence-based conceptual model of the determinants of health. Three arguments supporting such action are discussed below.

1. *The origins of good health are multiple and cross-sectorial.* Origins of good health include factors such as genetic makeup, environmental conditions, nutrition and exercise, access to health care, social support systems, and many others. Some of the factors, such as genetic makeup, are nearly impossible to alter whereas others are amenable to change. In addition, some of the factors influence a variety of health outcomes (e.g., on a population basis, dietary habits and education are known to influence multiple health outcomes). Careful consideration of what is known about the determinants of health highlights the tension between factors that are easily measurable now (e.g., hospitalization rates) and factors that may be equally or more important in the long run (e.g., teenagers' perception of their future) but are much more difficult to measure and monitor. Grounding community health improvement in a broad model of the determinants of health can remind communities to consider multiple and cross-sectorial influences when selecting health issues to target and when designing possible interventions.

2. *A focus on the origins of health emphasizes the need for cross-sectorial assumptions of responsibilities.* For various stakeholders to be accountable, the roles of those stakeholders in producing illness or health must be defined. A broad conceptual model of the determinants of health includes the full spectrum of possible influences on health. Such a model provides a valuable framework for communities to use as they consider the roles (and potential contributions) of the various stakeholders and thus each stakeholder's responsibility for health improvement in the community.

3. *A focus on the origins of health creates multiple options for intervention.* A conceptual model of the determinants of health can serve as the starting point for communities to identify what is known about issues they wish to address. Options for intervening can reflect the unique characteristics of the community vis-à-vis available resources, cultural norms, and target populations. Per-

formance measures can then be developed as the basis for strategic actions.

The rationale for adopting a broad definition of health lies not only in its value to the population served by the health system and its usefulness in identifying measures of the origins of health. A broad definition of health also is appropriate for the changing nature of the "health care system," reflects the interconnectedness of health and social systems, and is consistent with current scientific evidence about how health is produced in communities (Aguirre-Molina, 1996; Warden, 1996).

Changing Nature of the "Health Care System"

Many Americans view health as a simple biomedical construct in which health is determined by the provision of health care (Lamarche, 1995). This perspective on health developed during this century, beginning in the 1930s with well-baby clinics and services for "crippled children" and expanding in the 1950s with national investments in biomedical research facilities such as the National Institutes of Health and construction and funding of hospitals through the Hill-Burton program (Guyer, 1990). With advances in medical science and increases in the number of hospitals, policymakers and health care providers became concerned about differential access to health care resources, especially for underserved and hard-to-reach populations. Poverty and geography were viewed as barriers to health care and thus to good health.

Beginning in the 1960s, programs designed to improve access to health services were created, including Medicare and Medicaid. These programs markedly reduced financial barriers for the poor and elderly, and they also ensured a supply of well-trained physicians by providing funds for medical school and residency training programs.

The biomedical model of health has fostered the development of a personal health care system centered around technologically advanced hospitals and highly trained medical specialists. However, the high cost of maintaining these resources is the subject of current public debate. In addition, questions have been raised about the overall contribution of the biomedical model to improvements in health status. Although important, health care has probably been overemphasized as a determinant of health. Of the 30-year increase in life expectancy achieved this century, only 5 years can be attributed to health care services (Bunker et al., 1995).

The roles of the public sector in managing the health care system and in providing clinical and personal preventive care services as well as public health services are undergoing dramatic changes. Historically, public health departments have provided population-based services and, together with public hospitals and community health centers, have delivered clinical and personal preventive services to poor and uninsured populations. For many public health departments located in the South and in large metropolitan areas, the delivery of clinical and personal preventive services is a primary focus. In the late 1980s, however, the activities of public health departments were reexamined, and the Institute of Medicine (IOM, 1988) recommended a focus on three core functions—assessment, policy development, and assurance. In this framework, the direct provision of clinical and personal preventive services is only a small portion of the assurance function of public health departments. In many states, this transition is in progress. Public hospitals and community health clinics, however, remain important providers of these services.

Currently, most local public health departments do not play a significant role in assuring the quality of personal health care services that they do not purchase or provide. The quality assurance roles of state agencies have also been limited. Private-sector organizations, however, have developed complex and sophisticated quality assurance systems, often more in response to market forces than to demands of the public sector. As more public health departments become involved in quality assurance activities, providers and health plans can be expected to experience the influence of more public-sector demands via standard setting and licensure requirements as well as market forces.

The recent surge in the growth of managed care organizations has taken place in an environment that seeks to continue the delivery of high-quality clinical and personal preventive health services while constraining the costs of care. Managed care organizations are viewed as more capable of responding to the demands of third-party payers for performance and accountability than are clinicians practicing independently. Market forces, which spurred the recent growth of managed care organizations, have influenced the structure of the health care system (Rodwin, 1996). The experience of the Pacific Business Group on Health illustrates the changing relationships in the health system vis-à-vis new roles for purchasers and providers (see Box 2-1).

BOX 2-1
THE PACIFIC BUSINESS GROUP ON HEALTH

The experience of the Pacific Business Group on Health, a private-sector employer purchasing coalition based in the San Francisco Bay Area, demonstrates how "purchasers can shift the focus of the health care system from managing the delivery of medical services to improving health" (Schauffler and Rodriguez, 1996). This alliance is using financial and market share incentives to influence health plans to provide access to high-quality health promotion and disease prevention services. By defining health improvement as the goal, purchasers hope to encourage health plans to look beyond clinical encounters and beyond patient–provider contacts to identify partners who can help improve the lifestyles of individuals and the health of communities (Schauffler and Rodriguez, 1996).

Interconnectedness of Health and Social Systems

It has long been recognized that the health of a community has a tremendous impact on the function of its social systems and that the condition of the social and economic systems has a significant impact on the health of all who live in a community (Patrick and Wickizer, 1995). For example, a healthy workforce is more productive, a healthy student body can master lessons more readily, and a healthy population is better able to make progress toward societal goals. Working conditions, economic well-being, school environments, the safety of neighborhoods, the educational level of residents, and a variety of other social conditions have a profound impact on health. Only recently, however, has substantial attention been devoted to understanding and acting upon the interdependence of health and social systems (Ashton and Seymour, 1988).

Health is a growing concern of employers, community-based organizations, schools, faith organizations, the media, local governmental bodies, and community residents, even though their roles are not viewed as part of the traditional domain of "health activities." As communities try to address their health issues in a comprehensive manner, all parties will have to sort out their roles and responsibilities. By reaching out to new partners in the community, traditional partners in health can ensure that all relevant sectors are engaged in efforts to improve health. A recent IOM report on primary care (IOM, 1996) also emphasizes the need for

BOX 2-2
ESCONDIDO HEALTH CARE AND COMMUNITY SERVICES PROJECT

The *Escondido Health Care and Community Services Project* aims to reduce the harmful effects of alcohol and other drug use in the community of Escondido, California (population, 120,000; county population, 2.6 million). The project coordinates a cross section of community services, including law enforcement, hospital emergency rooms, and community agencies. Integration of data systems, administrative coordination, financing, and training are other integral elements. The municipal government functions as a facilitator for the community collaboration but does not provide services directly. Its interest is to reduce the cost of alcohol and drug use to the city and to improve the city's health.

Unlike many related programs, which target individuals who are already dependent on alcohol or drugs, the Escondido project seeks to identify users who are at high risk of *becoming* dependent in the future. The objective is to influence drinking behavior before it reaches a critically destructive level, not to identify those already in need of specialized services (although such referrals are made when necessary). The program involves routine screening for alcohol or drug use in high-volume, high-risk situations. It includes a three- to five-minute screening interview and brief intervention, which is administered to all adults in hospital emergency rooms, health centers, and law enforcement settings. A new component of the program is the "Sobering Service," which assists individuals who would otherwise be sent to the police or to the emergency room for alcohol- or drug-related care.

Three important lessons have been learned. First, the ability to cross sectors and create an integrated program has made it possible to capture savings in one sector and make those resources available to the program. For example, the city is investing in the project the money that would normally be spent on booking people for alcohol-related offenses. The project may become self-sustaining because local private funds may soon be raised from managed care firms and combined with ongoing public funding for uninsured participants. (Initial funding for the project came from local city general funds, county government funds, and a matching grant from The Robert Wood Johnson Foundation.)

Second, the availability of data has helped to identify stakeholders for the project and to create a collaborative value system, based on community participation. Third, development of a data system will be important in monitoring and maintaining the integration of screening and brief intervention services within multiple collaborating agencies.

SOURCE: D. Kelso, workshop presentation (1995); see Appendix D.

better collaboration among the diverse groups that can influence health. The Health Care and Community Services Project in Escondido, California, illustrates this kind of collaboration among diverse groups and the interconnectedness of health and social systems (see Box 2-2).

A MODEL OF THE DETERMINANTS OF HEALTH

A resurgence of interest in broader definitions of health and its determinants is, in part, a response to the growing realization that investments in clinical care and personal preventive health services were not leading to commensurate gains in the health of populations (Evans and Stoddart, 1994). In the early 1970s, an ecologic or systems theory approach to understanding health and its determinants generated a multidimensional perspective. Some grouped the factors influencing health into four principal forces: (1) environment, (2) heredity, (3) lifestyles, and (4) health care services (Blum, 1981). A Canadian government white paper, often referred to as the Lalonde Report (Lalonde, 1974), brought wider attention to this "force-field" paradigm.

Initial responses tended to focus on individual behavior as the target of both responsibility and clinical and policy interventions. In the United States as well, the broadened emphasis on health promotion was aimed primarily at modifications of individual behavior that could be, and often were, undertaken as clinical and community interventions (USDHHS, 1991).

Responding, in part, to this focus on individuals largely to the exclusion of the communities in which they live, Evans and Stoddart (1994) proposed an expanded version of this model, illustrated in Figure 2-1, that identifies both the major influences on health and well-being and the dynamic relationships among them. In developing a model that is consistent with current knowledge about the determinants of health, they identified nine components of interest:

1. social environment,
2. physical environment,
3. genetic endowment,
4. individual response (behavior and biology),
5. health care,
6. disease,
7. health and function,
8. well-being, and
9. prosperity.

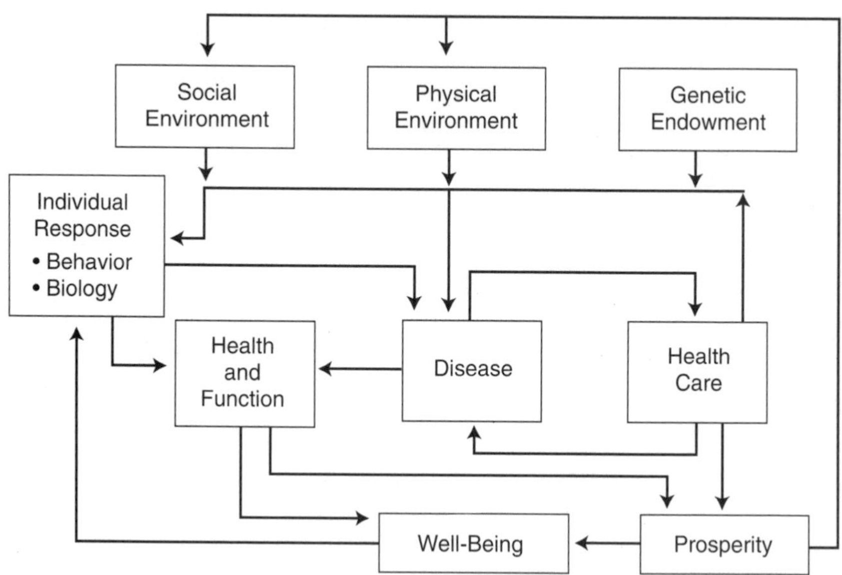

FIGURE 2-1 A model of the determinants of health. Source: Reprinted from R.G. Evans and G.L. Stoddart, 1990, Producing Health, Consuming Health Care, *Social Science and Medicine* 31:1347–1363, with permission from Elsevier Science Ltd, Kidlington, UK.

Unlike a biomedical model that views health as the absence of disease, this dynamic framework includes functional capacity and well-being as health outcomes of interest. It also presents the behavioral and biologic responses of individuals as factors that influence health but are themselves influenced by social, physical, and genetic factors that are beyond the control of the individual. The model emphasizes general factors that affect many diseases or the health of large segments of the population, rather than specific factors accounting for small changes in health at the individual level. It takes a multidisciplinary approach, uniting biomedical sciences, public health, psychology, statistics and epidemiology, economics, sociology, education, and other disciplines. Social, environmental, economic, and genetic factors are seen as contributing to differences in health status and, therefore, as presenting opportunities to intervene. It is important to note, as Evans and Stoddart (1994) have done, that each component of the model represents complex sets of factors that can be examined in greater detail (see Evans et al., 1994).

The committee found the model proposed by Evans and

Stoddart—which is referred to in this report as the *field model*—broad enough to encompass its vision. Although not yet widely tested, the model has been adapted for health policy and community planning in several Canadian provinces (Roos et al., 1995). Several features of the model were important to the committee. The model

- emphasizes the importance of considering the origins of health and the underlying causes of disease in individuals and populations;
- encourages explicit hypothesizing about the production of health in the community;
- underscores the interdisciplinary and multisectorial efforts often required to achieve health improvement in communities;
- makes explicit the possible trade-offs and benefits that occur across sectors; and
- encourages communities to identify possible performance and outcome measures from all of the categories.

In selecting indicators for performance monitoring, the determinants of health approach is useful in expanding the potential universe of indicators that should be considered. In addition to these practical reasons for adopting a model of the determinants of health such as that proposed by Evans and Stoddart, the field model provides an accurate representation of the complex contributions of physical environment, social environment, individual behavior, genetics, and health services to the well-being of communities.

Components of the Field Model: Some Examples

The components of the field model were discussed at the committee's second workshop.[1] The material below has been drawn from the summary of that workshop (see Appendix D).

Social Environment and Prosperity

Among the elements of the social environment that have been linked to health are family structure, the educational system, social networks, social class, work setting, and level of prosperity.

[1]The workshop discussion was based on a presentation by Jonathan Fielding.

Family structure, for example, is known to affect children's physical and mental health. On average, children in single-parent families do not do as well on measures of development, performance, and mental health as children in two-parent families. Children's relationships with their parents, social support, nurturance, and sense of self-efficacy have been shown to be related to their mental and physical health and even to their future economic productivity (Schor and Menaghan, 1995).

Education has an effect on health status separate from its influence on income. Years of formal education are strongly related to age-adjusted mortality in countries as disparate as Hungary, Norway, and England and Wales (Valkonen, 1989). Although most research is based on years of formal schooling, evidence suggests a broader relationship that includes the preschool period. An assessment at age 19 of participants in the Perry Preschool Study, which randomized children into a Head Start-like program, showed that participation in the preschool program was correlated with better school performance, attending college, and avoiding involvement with the criminal justice system (Weikart, 1989). Critical periods for education, particularly at young ages, may prove to be important in determining health. In addition, studies show that maternal educational attainment is a key determinant of child welfare and survival (Zill and Brim, 1983).

"Social networks" is a term that refers to an individual's integration into a self-defined community and the degree of connectedness to other individuals and to institutions. There is a strong inverse correlation between the number and frequency of close contacts and mortality from all causes, with odds ratios of 2:1 or higher and a clear "dose-response" relationship (Berkman and Syme, 1979). Other aspects of physical and mental functioning also appear to be influenced by the quantity and quality of social connections (Seeman, 1996). Although it is possible to see the impact of social networks on health, the pathways responsible for those effects are not yet known.

Social class is another well-described determinant of health, independent of income. Major studies have been done in Britain, where social class is defined more explicitly than in the United States. In the Whitehall study of British civil servants, Marmot and colleagues (1987) demonstrated a clear relationship between social class (based on job classification) and mortality. The relationship persists throughout the social hierarchy and is unchanged after adjusting for income and smoking. The effect of social class may raise uncomfortable issues in the United States but is important to consider in dealing with issues of health and equity.

The health effects of work-related factors are seen in studies of job decision latitude, autonomy, and cardiovascular mortality (Karasek and Theorell, 1990). Involuntary unemployment negatively affects both mental and physical health. Economic prosperity is also correlated with better health. Throughout history, the poor have, on average, died at younger ages than the rich. The relationship between prosperity and health holds across the economic spectrum. For every decile, quintile, or quartile of income, from lowest to highest, there is a decline in overall age-adjusted mortality. In international comparisons by the Organization for Economic Cooperation and Development, the difference in income between the highest and lowest deciles of income shows a stronger relationship with overall mortality rates than does median income (Wilkinson, 1992, 1994).

Physical Environment

The physical environment has long been recognized as an important determinant of health. The public health movement of 1840–1870 emphasized environmental changes as a successful strategy for reducing the epidemic rates of infectious diseases, which flourished in the overcrowded housing with poor sanitation in industrial cities in Europe and North America (Ashton and Seymour, 1988).

The physical environment affects health and disease in diverse ways. Examples include exposures to toxic substances, which can produce disorders such as lung disease or cancers; safety at home and work, which influences injury rates; the design of vehicles and roadways, which can alter crash survival rates; poor housing conditions and overcrowding, which can increase the likelihood of violence, transmission of infectious diseases, and mental health problems; and urban–rural differences in cancer rates.

Genetic Endowment

The contribution of genetic makeup to the health of an individual is a new and emerging area of scientific inquiry. As scientific knowledge about genetics increases, this component of the field model is likely to become increasingly important.

For the most part, genetic factors are currently understood as contributing to a greater or lesser *risk* for health outcomes, rather than determining them with certainty. One area of particular interest is the link seen between genetics and behavior. Studies of twins separated at birth demonstrate a high concordance rate in alcoholism, schizophrenia, and affective disorders (Baird, 1994). Even so-called voluntary behaviors such as smoking and eating habits may be subject to genetic predispositions (e.g., Carmelli et al., 1992; de Castro, 1993; Falciglia and Norton, 1994). Health behaviors are complex, and the influences that determine them are likely to be extremely complex.

Genetic factors also interact with social and environmental factors to influence health and disease. It will be important to understand these interactions to learn why certain individuals with similar environmental exposures develop diseases whereas others do not (e.g., why most smokers do not develop lung cancer).

Behavior

In the field model framework, behavior is seen as a response to other factors and can be treated as an *intermediate* determinant of health. Rather than a voluntary act only amenable to direct intervention, behavior is shaped by multiple forces, particularly the social and physical environments and genetic endowment. At the same time, behavior change remains a goal. Behaviors related to health care, such as adherence to treatment regimens, are influenced by these forces as are behaviors directly influencing health, such as smoking.

Health Care

Health care is an essential determinant of health. In the United States, however, its contribution has probably been overemphasized. As noted above, about 5 years of the 30-year increase in life expectancy achieved in this century can be attributed to health care (Bunker et al., 1995). The greatest share of this gain can be attributed to diagnosis and treatment of coronary heart disease, which contributes 1 to 2 of these additional years of life.

Linking the Determinants

The committee was impressed by several implications of the field model's theoretical perspective. First, the model clearly reinforces the interrelatedness of many factors. Health outcomes are the product of complex interactions of factors rather than of individual factors operating in isolation. Indeed, these interactions are probably as important as the actions of any single factor. Currently incomplete, however, are descriptions of mechanisms underlying the linkages among the various determinants and full characterizations of the interactions among factors. The committee encourages the continued research needed to gain a better understanding of these mechanisms.

Second, not all of the determinants, viewed as causes, act simultaneously. The effects of some determinants, in fact, may be necessary antecedents to others, and some may have their primary influence by modifying the effects of others. Some may also differ in their relationship to health according to when they are present in the life cycle. Evidence suggests that there are certain times in the human life cycle that are critical for future health and well-being. During infancy and early childhood, crucial neurologic, cognitive, and psychosocial patterns are established (Carnegie Task Force on Meeting the Needs of Young Children, 1994; Entwisle, 1995). Experiences in childhood and adolescence may also have a critical influence on adult health risk factors such as weight and smoking (Dietz, 1994; IOM, 1994).

Another Perspective

Patrick and Wickizer (1995) have extended the field model framework by focusing on factors in the social and physical environments that operate at the community rather than the individual level. These two components are seen as affected by cultural, political, policy, and economic systems. In turn, they influence elements such as community response, activation, and social support, and ultimately community outcomes including social behaviors, community health, and quality of life. For example, establishing a smoke-free workplace policy exerts an influence on exposure to tobacco smoke separate from the smoking practices of individuals. This perspective points both to the influence of community-level factors and to the opportunities for community-level interventions.

INTERVENTIONS TO IMPROVE HEALTH

Many factors can influence the impact of interventions to improve health. It is possible to target various determinants of health to produce change at an individual level, a community level, or both. All aspects of each broad determinant of health are not equally amenable to intervention, however. For example, the social environment of isolated senior citizens can be improved by increasing contact with others, but their genetic makeup is not amenable to change.

Time frames for measuring health changes vary widely, from days to decades. Some successful interventions will produce observable results within a year or two, but others may be followed by long latency periods before significant changes in health status can be observed. The impact of an intervention may also be influenced by when it reaches an individual because, as noted above, there appear to be "critical periods" in human development. Certain interventions in childhood may have long-delayed yet long-lasting results. In addition, the population effects of interventions are also important to consider. Small changes at the individual level may have important ramifications when applied to a whole community (Rose, 1992).

The traditional targets for intervention have been specific diseases or behaviors, and categorical funding streams for both research and the delivery of services encourage this approach. The field model of the determinants of health encourages consideration of a wider array of targets. For example, if adolescents' sense of well-being can be improved by reducing their feelings of alienation and hopelessness, can unintended pregnancies, alcohol and other drug use, crime, and the school dropout rate all be reduced? A multidimensional approach would be required, focusing on education, social and community involvement, family preservation, and improved social networks for teens and their parents. Community-level interventions might include after-school programs, athletics (e.g., midnight basketball), and church-based programs.

Whether focused on individuals or the community as a whole, health improvement efforts should be targeted at specific causal pathways or should employ interventions that have been proven effective. There is an obvious tension between what is now known and what we need to know to improve health. For example, the biologic pathways through which poverty or low social class influence health have not been adequately elucidated. A tension also exists between what is now measurable with valid and reliable indicators and what is not measurable, but may be important.

The multidimensional approach may be unfamiliar to health professionals because it is new and relies on partnerships with people from fields beyond those traditionally encompassed by a medical model. It is, however, consistent with the field model and may provide expanded opportunities for performance monitoring and improving the community's health.

IMPLICATIONS FOR COMMUNITIES

An examination of the field model points to the importance of considering both individual- and community-level data. Performance monitoring should include measures of inputs, process, and outcomes for health and health improvement activities. It may prove useful to monitor some key determinants, regardless of whether they are amenable to change at the local level, so that communities can understand the range of important factors. In addition, qualitative data may contribute important information about community needs. For example, information on social support, perceived barriers to service utilization, and attitudes toward the community and its resources are all relevant to performance monitoring and can be obtained from community surveys.

Performance monitoring provides an opportunity for a community to define and articulate expectations for organizations' contributions to the population's health. Although organizations might disagree with the appropriateness of the expectations, a useful dialogue may ensue. Communities may want to focus special attention on expectations regarding managed care organizations (MCOs) and the business sector. MCOs, for example, have generally defined "community" as their enrollees and not considered the entire community or public health as their area of concern. A community expectation that the health of the entire local population is part of an MCO's corporate and social responsibility could lead to their broader involvement in public health activities. Businesses, including MCOs, that have strong ties with a city or region may have a history of interest in local health issues. As corporations expand to multiple regions, however, they may require added encouragement to become involved and accountable in the local communities where they have a presence.

CONCLUSIONS

Contributing to the interest in health improvement and performance monitoring is a wider recognition that health embraces well-being as well as the absence of illness. For both individuals and populations, health can be seen to depend not only on medical care but also on other factors, including individual behavior and genetic makeup, and social and economic conditions for individuals and communities. The field model, as described by Evans and Stoddart (1994), presents these multiple determinants of health in a dynamic relationship. The model's feedback loops link social environment, physical environment, genetic endowment, an individual's behavioral and biologic responses, health care, disease, health and function, well-being, and prosperity. The committee found this model to be an effective basis for its work.

This multidimensional perspective reinforces the value of public health's traditional emphasis on a population-based approach to health issues. It also provides a basis for looking to segments of the community beyond those traditionally associated with health to address factors affecting health and well-being. Some of the additional parties who can be brought to the table as interested stakeholders and accountable partners include, among many others, schools, employers, community-based organizations, the media, foundations, and public safety agencies. A performance monitoring program can promote the articulation of roles and responsibilities among these participants.

The committee has concluded that entities engaged in performance monitoring for community health improvement should

- adopt a broad definition of health;
- adopt a comprehensive and conceptual model of the way in which health is produced within the community; the field model, as elaborated by Evans and Stoddart, is a good starting point; and
- develop a concrete and specific hypothesis of how the multiple sectors of the community and individual stakeholders in each sector can contribute to the solution of a health problem.

In addition, federal agencies and foundations should provide support for further research on the determinants of health to clarify pathways, to develop reliable and valid measures useful for performance monitoring related to these pathways, and to identify community programs and clinical and public health interventions that are successful in addressing the underlying causes of ill health in communities.

REFERENCES

Aguirre-Molina, M. 1996. Community-Based Approaches for the Prevention of Alcohol, Tobacco, and Other Drug Use. *Annual Review of Public Health* 17:337–358.

Ashton, J., and Seymour, H. 1988. *The New Public Health: The Liverpool Experience.* Philadelphia: Open University Press.

Baird, P.A. 1994. The Role of Genetics in Population Health. In *Why Are Some People Healthy and Others Not? The Determinants of Health of Populations.* R.G. Evans, M.L. Barer, and T.R. Marmor, eds. New York: Aldine de Gruyter.

Berkman, L.F., and Syme, S.L. 1979. Social Networks, Host Resistance, and Mortality: A Nine Year Follow-up Study of Alameda County Residents. *American Journal of Epidemiology* 109:186–204.

Blum, H. 1981. *Planning for Health: Generics for the Eighties.* 2nd ed. New York: Human Sciences Press.

Bunker, J.P., Frazier, H.S., and Mosteller, F. 1995. The Role of Medical Care in Determining Health: Creating an Inventory of Benefits. In *Society and Health.* B.C. Amick., S. Levine, A.R. Tarlov, and D.C. Walsh, eds. New York: Oxford University Press.

Carmelli, D., Swan, G.E., Robinette, D., and Fabsitz, R. 1992. Genetic Influence on Smoking: A Study of Male Twins. *New England Journal of Medicine* 327:829–833.

Carnegie Task Force on Meeting the Needs of Young Children. 1994. *Starting Points: Meeting the Needs of Our Youngest Children.* New York: Carnegie Corporation.

de Castro, J.M. 1993. Genetic Influences on Daily Intake and Meal Patterns of Humans. *Physiology and Behavior* 53:777–782.

Dietz, W.H. 1994. Critical Periods in Childhood for the Development of Obesity. *American Journal of Clinical Nutrition* 59:955–959.

Entwisle, D.R. 1995. The Role of Schools in Sustaining Early Childhood Program Benefits. *The Future of Children* 5(3):133–144.

Evans, R.G., and Stoddart, G.L. 1994. Producing Health, Consuming Health Care. In *Why Are Some People Healthy and Others Not? The Determinants of Health of Populations.* R.G. Evans, M.L. Barer, and T.R. Marmor, eds. New York: Aldine De Gruyter.

Evans, R.G., Barer, M.L., and Marmor, T.R., eds. 1994. *Why Are Some People Healthy and Others Not? The Determinants of Health of Populations.* New York: Aldine De Gruyter.

Falciglia, G.A., and Norton, P.A. 1994. Evidence for a Genetic Influence on Preference for Some Foods. *Journal of the American Dietetic Association* 94(2):154–158.

Guyer, B. 1990. The Evolution and Future Role of Title V. In *Children in a Changing Health System: Assessments and Proposals for Reform.* M. Schlesinger and L. Eisenberg, eds. Baltimore: Johns Hopkins University Press.

IOM (Institute of Medicine). 1988. *The Future of Public Health.* Washington, D.C.: National Academy Press.

IOM. 1994. *Growing Up Tobacco Free: Preventing Nicotine Addiction in Children and Youths.* B.S. Lynch and R.J. Bonnie, eds. Washington, D.C.: National Academy Press.

IOM. 1996. *Primary Care: America's Health in a New Era.* M.S. Donaldson, K.D. Yordy, K.N. Lohr, and N.A. Vanselow, eds. Washington, D.C.: National Academy Press.

Karasek, R.A., and Theorell, T. 1990. *Healthy Work: Stress, Productivity and the Reconstruction of Working Life.* New York: Basic Books.

Lalonde, M. 1974. *A New Perspective on the Health of Canadians.* Ottawa: Health and Welfare, Canada.

Lamarche, P.A. 1995. Our Health Paradigm in Peril. *Public Health Reports* 110:556–560.

Marmot, M.G., Kogevinas, M., and Elston, M.A. 1987. Social/Economic Status and Disease. *Annual Review of Public Health* 8:111–135.

Patrick, D.L., and Wickizer, T.M. 1995. Community and Health. In *Society and Health.* B.C. Amick., S. Levine, A.R. Tarlov, and D.C. Walsh, eds. New York: Oxford University Press.

Rodwin, M.A. 1996. Managed Care and the Elusive Quest for Accountable Health Care. *Widener Law Symposium Journal* 1(1):65–87.

Roos, N.P., Black, C.D., Frohlich, N., et al. 1995. A Population-Based Health Information System. *Medical Care* 33(12):DS13–20.

Rose, G. 1992. *The Strategy of Preventive Medicine.* New York: Oxford University Press.

Schauffler, H.H., and Rodriguez, T. 1996. Exercising Purchasing Power for Preventive Care. *Health Affairs* 15(1):73–85.

Schor, E.L., and Menaghan, E. 1995. Family Pathways to Child Health. In *Society and Health.* B.C. Amick, S. Levine, A.L. Tarlov, and D.C. Walsh, eds. New York: Oxford University Press.

Seeman, T.E. 1996. Social Ties and Health: The Benefits of Social Integration. *Annals of Epidemiology* 6:442–451.

Syme, S.L. 1996. Rethinking Disease: Where Do We Go from Here? *Annals of Epidemiology* 6:463–468.

USDHHS (U.S. Department of Health and Human Services). 1991. *Healthy People 2000: National Health Promotion and Disease Prevention Objectives.* DHHS Pub. No. (PHS) 91-50212. Washington, D.C.: Office of the Assistant Secretary for Health.

Valkonen, T. 1989. Adult Mortality and Level of Education: A Comparison of Six Countries. In *Health Inequalities in European Countries.* J. Fox, ed. Aldershot, England: Gower.

Warden, G. 1996. Key Factors in the Transition to IHCOs (Integrated Health Care Organizations). *Frontiers of Health Services Management* 12(4):53–56.

Weikart, D.P. 1989. Early Childhood Education and Primary Prevention. *Prevention in Human Services* 6(2):285–306.

WHO (World Health Organization). 1986. A Discussion Document on the Concept and Principles of Health Promotion. *Health Promotion* 1(1):73–78.

WHO. 1994. *Constitution of the World Health Organization.* Basic Documents, 40th ed. Geneva: WHO.

Wilkinson, R.G. 1992. Income Distribution and Life Expectancy. *British Medical Journal* 304(6820):165–168.

Wilkinson, R.G. 1994. The Epidemiological Transition: From Material Scarcity to Social Disadvantage? *Daedalus* 123(4):61–77.

Zill, N. II, and Brim, O.G., Jr. 1983. Development of Childhood Social Indicators. In *Children, Families, and Government: Perspectives on American Social Policy.* E.F. Zigler, S.L. Kagan, and E. Klugman, eds. New York: Cambridge University Press.

3

Managing a Shared Responsibility for the Health of a Community

The health of a community is a shared responsibility of all its members. Although the roles of many community members are not within the traditional domain of "health activities," each has an effect on and a stake in a community's health (Patrick and Wickizer, 1995). As communities try to address their health issues in a comprehensive manner, all parties—including individual health care providers, public health agencies, health care organizations, purchasers of health services, local governments, employers, schools, faith communities, community-based organizations, the media, policymakers, and the public—will need to sort out their roles and responsibilities, individually and collectively. These interdependent sectors must address issues of accountability and shared responsibility for various aspects of community health. They also must participate in the process of "community-wide social change" that is needed for performance monitoring to succeed in improving health. In most communities, there will be only limited experience with collaborative or coordinated efforts among these diverse groups. To work together effectively, they will need a common language and an understanding of the multidimensional nature of the determinants of health. They must also find a way to accommodate diversity in values and goals.

As noted in Chapter 1, the committee has adopted as a basis for its discussions of community a description offered by Labonte (1988): individuals with shared affinity, and perhaps a shared geography, who organize around an issue, with collective discussion, decision making, and action. Geography, however, emerged as a critical point of reference in the committee's discussions. Although geographic (or civic) boundaries cannot adequately capture all of the potentially meaningful community configurations, they are a practical starting point.

This chapter begins with a discussion of the social and political realities of engaging communities in performance monitoring activities to improve community health. It proposes an approach in which responsibility for health goals is shared among community stakeholders and accountability for specific accomplishments is ascribed to individual entities. Strategies for managing the process of community-wide change are presented in the final section.

SOCIAL AND POLITICAL CONTEXT FOR IMPROVING COMMUNITY HEALTH

As communities undertake health improvement efforts, they need to be informed about the social and political environments in which a health system operates at the local, state, and national levels; ways in which those environments influence the health system; and ways in which the health system influences those environments.

At the national level, health care emerged as a high-priority issue in 1992. This reflected several factors related to underlying conflicts in the needs, resources, and values of various sectors of American society. First, questions have been raised about the limit to which the country can invest in health care. No nation spends a greater share of its national income on health care than the United States (Levit et al., 1994), and concerns about the unbridled growth of health care spending are so widespread that they have become the subject of presidential political debates. Proposals to constrain spending in the public sector for services to vulnerable populations (e.g., Medicaid and Medicare) raise questions about economic disparity in the nation. In the private sector, employers are concerned about their ability to meet current and future financial obligations to provide health benefits for employees. Similar concerns extend to health care institutions, which continue to absorb losses for charity care.

A second factor in the emergence of health as a high priority national issue has been politics. Health care was viewed as an important issue in the senatorial and presidential elections of

1992. As the new administration took office, health care reform was a prominent initiative. Failure to reach consensus on national health care legislation in 1993–1994 indicates the level of conflict between stakeholders over needs, resources, and values. Conflicts were most striking with regard to balancing responsibility between federal and state levels of government. Federal legislators placed a higher value on the states' rights to determine health care policy for their populations than on having a uniform national health care policy. Conflicts also arose in balancing the needs of the uninsured and other vulnerable populations (served by programs such as Medicaid and Medicare) and the political goal of a balanced budget.

A third factor has been the pervasive and growing anxiety of individuals and families about health care coverage. Because health insurance in the United States is most often provided through employer-based programs, this concern reflects, in part, a growing sense of insecurity about employment. It also reflects an ambiguity about where the responsibility for health care insurance lies. Although considered an entitlement by some, there is a growing sense that responsibility for health care is being placed on the individual. After much negotiation and compromise, federal legislators have found common ground on certain aspects of this issue. Two years after the demise of comprehensive health care reform legislation, a bipartisan bill—the Health Insurance Portability and Accountability Act of 1996—addressing the portability of employment-based health insurance and prohibiting the denial of coverage for preexisting conditions was signed into law.

Conflicts at the national level over issues of accessibility, quality, and affordability of health care reflect the vastly different needs, resources, and values of stakeholders in the health system. Within communities, especially in a pluralistic society such as the United States, there also is considerable diversity among stakeholders in their perspectives, interests, needs, resources, values, influence, and access to power. For example, the public values health care that is affordable, places no limits on choice, provides comprehensive benefits, limits the financial risk to consumers, and offers open access. Group purchasers and payers attempt to balance the needs of their covered populations against the need for predictable and minimal financial liability, protection against legal and ethical dilemmas, and administrative simplicity. Health care providers want to optimize patient interests while maximizing revenues and minimizing intrusion from third parties. Policymakers serve to protect the perceived interests of the community regarding public health and personal health care services, thereby promoting the well-being of the population while also providing fiscal and legal oversight of public expenditures for health care. As communities try to address their health issues in a comprehensive manner, all relevant parties will have to be engaged so that their roles and responsibilities can be examined.

The field model (presented in Chapter 2) identifies the broad range of factors that influence a community's health, and these suggest a variety of public and private entities that, through their actions, can influence the health of the community. Such entities can include health care providers, public health agencies, and community-based organizations explicitly concerned with health. They can also include other government agencies, community organizations, private industry, and other entities that do not explicitly, or sometimes even consciously, see themselves as having a health-related role—for example, schools, employers, social service and housing agencies, transportation and justice departments, faith communities, and the media. Although many of the entities that play an essential role in determining local health status are based in and focus their attention on the community in question, others, such as state health departments, federal agencies, managed care organizations, foundations, and national corporations, have a broader scope than a single community.

For a performance monitoring effort to succeed, communities will have to do more than identify relevant parties; they will have to find effective ways to engage parties with varying needs, resources, and values; to set goals for the performance monitoring effort; to ascribe responsibility for meeting these goals; and to manage the complex process of community-wide change. Assessments of other initiatives (e.g., Newacheck et al., 1995) suggest that communities will have to overcome barriers such as the absence of performance monitoring models with demonstrated effectiveness, political difficulties in gaining cooperation and commitment from multiple parties, challenges in implementing a new program when the health care system itself is undergoing changes, and the complications of maneuvering through legislative and regulatory restrictions.

Growing Concerns About Accountability and Shared Responsibility

Currently, the health care system is accountable to numerous parties for a variety of activities. Accountability is promoted by ethics and professional norms, politics, and law. Regulatory agencies have a long history of holding the health care system accountable for meeting standards for the quality of care, access to care, and provision of certain data. Competition and enlightened self-interest also influence the health system to maintain high standards and to continually improve its standards. Yet, there is a growing public concern about accountability (Rodwin, 1996). Questions exist about the value the population receives for the money the nation spends on health and health care. Moreover, with the increasing complexity and changing nature of the health care system, the public wants to know which entities are responsible for specific tasks. In addition, the market forces that are restructuring the health care system demand accountability.

Given the pressure for accountability, there is surprisingly little evidence in the nation of coordinated efforts to examine the performance of the health care system as it relates to the overall health of a community's population, and there is little evidence of coordinated efforts to examine the performance of entities other than health care providers that influence health. During a workshop held in December 1995, the committee heard from representatives of community-based health improvement activities (see Appendix D). None of the programs assigned accountability for tasks and use of performance-related measurement was limited.

Communities need to meet this challenge. The committee has concluded that a coordinated effort to monitor the performance of the health system in communities, which involves a broad range of stakeholders, would yield tremendous benefits. Such efforts may improve the health of a community's population by providing a process for working toward health goals and a toolbox for measuring progress (see Chapter 4). It is likely that one of the most difficult tasks in implementing a community-wide and cooperative performance monitoring system will be developing an approach for ascribing accountability to stakeholders.

For the purposes of this report, the committee has distinguished stakeholders and "accountable entities" in relation to the roles they play in the process of improving community health.

- *Stakeholders* are organizations and individuals who have an interest in the health of a community's population. As a group, stakeholders should include consumers, providers, businesses, government, and other relevant sectors of the community. In a performance monitoring effort, stakeholders share responsibility for the community's health. The group of stakeholders may expand or contract in number, and membership may change during the performance monitoring activity. The changes in stakeholders may reflect changes in the health issues and strategies that are being considered.

• *Accountable entities* are stakeholders that are expected to achieve specific results as part of the community's strategy for addressing a health issue. The process of ascribing accountability for particular actions to specific accountable entities will differ from problem to problem, from strategy to strategy, from time to time, and from place to place. The basis for designating a stakeholder as an accountable entity may be voluntary assumption, enlightened self-interest, regulatory requirements, legislative mandate, court order, social pressure, market forces, lobbying, or other reasons. As with stakeholders, the entities that are to be accountable for specific tasks may change during the performance monitoring activity in response to progress or to changes in the issues being addressed and strategies being followed.

Changing Our Approach to Accountability

Traditionally, accountability in public health and medicine has been viewed from a managerial perspective as a vertical, or top-down, process. Federal funding agencies often place reporting demands on those receiving funds at state and local levels. States are required to submit reports indicating the number and types of services provided. At the community level, local health agencies and community-based organizations are required to report to a myriad of federal, state, and local government funding agencies. Reporting requirements often are not coordinated and the reports often are not shared with communities unless interested parties request them.

More recently, local organizations have become advocates of a different approach to accountability. For example, as part of a public health reengineering initiative in Illinois called Project Health, local health agencies suggested that they should be accountable to the communities that they serve (Illinois Local Health Liaison Committee, 1994). Although the committee acknowledges that some activities necessitate accountability to state and federal agencies, it applauds efforts to involve communities in the accountability process and to make accountability meaningful at the local level.

Similar changes are occurring in the private sector, especially among health care plans. The National Committee for Quality

Assurance (NCQA) focuses on quality in health care and on providing purchasers and consumers of health care services with information that helps them select among health plans offering those services (NCQA, 1993). It uses performance measurement to provide information that can be used to assess health plans' effectiveness in providing services and to identify areas for improvement. NCQA has begun to solicit consumer input, but the impact of this input has not yet been evaluated. More recently, a coalition of health care purchasers and consumer organizations established the Foundation for Accountability (FAcct, 1995), which is developing sets of measures that can be applied to care for specific health conditions.

The Promise of Accountability at the Community Level

As the committee considered ways in which to encourage, implement, and enforce accountability in the health system, it has embraced procedures that foster the promises of performance monitoring. It views these promises as (1) creating a process that encourages stakeholders to come to the table in a productive way; (2) influencing stakeholders and communities to adopt a broader model of health and to structure their health systems to reflect the model; (3) providing meaningful incentives for performing well; and (4) furnishing a set of measurement tools that will help communities examine changes in the health and well-being of their populations.

In order to fulfill its promise, accountability needs to be conceptualized as a collaborative and cooperative process as opposed to a punitive process imposed by outside forces. This approach can be viewed as moving from a vertical to a horizontal structure or from a "top-down" to a "roundtable" approach. Accountability for improving health should be an open process that involves stakeholder participation and negotiation.

The committee proposes a two-step approach to accountability. The first step involves the issue of shared responsibility. Communities should acknowledge that all stakeholders share responsibility for improving the health of a community's population. Stakeholders include a wide range of organizations and individuals who have an interest in the health of a community. As stated earlier, the group of stakeholders may expand or contract in number or change in membership in response to changes in the health issues and strategies being considered.

Sharing responsibility should not be viewed as an insurmountable barrier to establishing practical procedures for measuring accountability. Holding a dialogue about the shared responsibility of stakeholders for overall performance of the health system (e.g., meeting a specific health goal such as full immunization of all children by age 2) prompts stakeholders to recognize that they function as part of a larger system (Jencks, 1994).

The second step in accountability involves designating accountable entities. As mentioned above, accountable entities are the stakeholders who are responsible for accomplishing specific results as part of a community's strategy for addressing a health issue. The committee suggests that the process of ascribing accountability for particular actions to specific accountable entities will differ depending on the problem and the strategies being considered, and other circumstances specific to each community. The basis for designating a stakeholder as an accountable entity may vary, depending on the ways in which communities are organized and on the interests, values, and resources of their stakeholders. However, accountability may be ascribed for various reasons (voluntary assumption, enlightened self-interest, regulatory requirements, legislative mandate, court order, social pressures, market forces, lobbying, and so on).

The process of ascribing accountability should be open and should involve all relevant stakeholders. At its conclusion, the stakeholders will have established a social contract that identifies goals, areas of responsibility, and accountable entities. The committee suggests that successful performance should be rewarded. Failures to perform should trigger problem analysis and a reformulation of the stakeholder's approach to the health issue. However, penalties might also be considered, depending on the circumstances. Such decisions should be made by the stakeholders.

KEY CONCEPTS FOR MANAGING CHANGE

The development of performance monitoring systems will typically require change—changes in the roles played by different stakeholders, in the relationships among stakeholders, and often in the behaviors required or expected of certain participants. For example, health care providers and health plans may have to collect and make available new or different data. In most communities, there will be only limited experience with managing such change and with accommodating diversity in values and goals. This section provides key concepts for such activities.

Resistance to Change

Change is frequently resisted by those who are expected to do the changing. Similarly, those who perceive that others want to judge or monitor their performance, or hold them accountable for their performance, frequently resist. It is critical that *change agents* (i.e., those individuals who are leading the effort for change) recognize that such resistance is fairly normal; most individuals prefer to have greater control over their circumstances, value at least some elements of the status quo, and are anxious about the unknown.

Although Western cultures tend to place a positive value on change and progress, communities, organizations, groups, and individuals vary in their responses to change. The response to proposed changes will depend on the content and process of change. Even when the content of change is acceptable, change is likely to be resisted if the process and pace are not acceptable. Change agents can increase the likelihood that communities will be receptive if they consider the following principles from the literature:

- *Involve all relevant stakeholders in the change process as early as possible.* Responses to proposed changes are significantly mediated by the extent of involvement of a particular group in the process of deciding that change is needed, in designing the change to be implemented, and in determining the pace of change. Groups that are not involved frequently become barriers to change, even if the proposed change is arguably in their best interest. In the performance monitoring system that the committee envisions, multiple stakeholders should be involved in the change processes so that the process becomes jointly owned rather than controlled by a single or small set of stakeholders. The process should be inclusive and open to newcomers.
- *Understand what stakeholders value about the current system.* All change, even change for the better, involves some loss for someone. In the course of change, there is an inescapable but valuable tension between the desire to remain attached, committed, and loyal to circumstances and experiences that were important in the past and the desire to embrace and move into the future. Acceptance of change depends on the ability to identify what is most valuable from the past and find a way to bring it, albeit in a transformed manner, into the future. Often, stakeholders are stigmatized as "resistant to change" when the change agent

has failed to understand what those stakeholders value, and fear losing, in the current system (Marris, 1986). The incentives and motivations of stakeholders will vary. Change agents should model in their own behavior the ability and willingness to change. Thus, those who take the lead in performance monitoring efforts need to demonstrate that they can and will make difficult changes and adaptations themselves, even as they ask others to do the same.

- *Whenever possible, introduce new resources to ease the process of change.* Change typically involves making decisions that are difficult, especially when institutions and communities are operating in a context of limited resources. Change may be facilitated by the introduction of new resources; it is always made more difficult, and generates greater conflict, if it is accompanied by reductions in resources.

It may well be that change will require a redistribution of resources. This is among the most difficult kinds of change to achieve because there are always perceptions of "winners" and "losers." Performance monitoring systems may be designed explicitly to support the reallocation of resources to high performers and away from low performers (e.g., by providing report cards to consumers that encourage them to select health plans or obtain services from providers who give "value" for money). Even if performance monitoring systems are not explicitly designed in this way, experience indicates that those being monitored will presume that resources are at stake and that they may lose as well as win. Frequently, those who are most supportive of change, or least resistant to it, are those who have confidence in their ability to "win" (Marris, 1986).

Alternate Approaches to the Change Process

The process of change can be approached through two basic models, an authoritarian model and a willing compliance model. Although the authoritarian model has, in fact, been used to implement many changes, the committee suggests that it is an inappropriate approach to performance monitoring in communities. The authoritarian model creates circumstances in which important stakeholders must change to survive. This model presumes that one or more parties have sufficient power over the circumstances of those who are expected to change and that they also have the desire and the will to "drive change." Although there is considerable concentration of power in American society, there is no one single center of power. Therefore, those trying to drive change are facing others who may have less power than they do, but who do have some power. The use of power often results in the development and exercise of countervailing power. When resistance rises, it is possible for the balance of power to shift unexpectedly and dramatically, thereby overturning the change.

Change may be difficult to sustain when it is approached through the authoritarian model. When people comply unwillingly, they typically live up only to the letter, rarely to the spirit, of what they perceive is required. Given the complexity and subtlety of the behaviors that will be required to improve community health, it is unlikely that they will be elicited in a sustained manner from unwilling compliers. Even when only simple and easily observable behaviors are being pursued, forcing such behaviors from unwilling compliers is an expensive and probably never-ending proposition. In today's health care delivery system, much costly "micromanagement" is a consequence of presumptions that cooperation will not be forthcoming from those whose performance is being monitored.

Instead, the committee suggests that communities adopt the second model for approaching the change process, that of willing compliance with mutually established strategies. Founded on cooperation, collaboration, and negotiation, the willing compliance model is appropriate for community-based work and is more likely to result in sustainable changes. A good deal of the literature in organizational change emphasizes strategies that reduce (if not eliminate) resistance to the content, direction, process, and pace of change. The committee suggests that communities use the successful strategies and tactics for achieving change shown in Box 3-1.

Many of these "noncoercive" strategies can be used not only directly (i.e., with those who are being asked to change) but also indirectly, to convince additional parties to support the direction of change. However, it is unlikely that significant change will occur without some degree of conflict. Some who resist change may do so because they are uncomfortable with conflict. Among the common responses to conflict are avoidance, denial, acknowledgment, escalation, management, and resolution. It is possible that within an overall strategy of willing compliance, some parties will use authoritarian relationships to gain participation or change from others. This adds to the conflict that must be resolved. Those who pursue change must be prepared to encounter and

BOX 3-1
SUCCESSFUL STRATEGIES AND TACTICS FOR ACHIEVING CHANGE

- Using information and logic to make a convincing cognitive case for change
- Using persuasion to make a convincing case for change that typically has both a cognitive and a normative or affective component
- Using positive incentives to encourage parties to at least consider changes or try them out; similarly, using rewards for those who change in desired directions
- Involving all stakeholders who are likely to be asked to change in some or all aspects of the change process
- Encouraging a sense that all stakeholders, including the change agents, will have to change, not just a subset
- Supporting the development of consensus
- Identifying areas of differing opinion ("dissensus") and developing strategies for proceeding in the face of such differences
- Creating controlled experiments or health improvement projects to try out changes on a small scale before moving to their full-scale adoption
- Disaggregating changes so they can be pursued incrementally and in stages
- Creating fallback positions or protections if the consequences of change are especially burdensome for one or another party
- Focusing on the common mission and vision—to improve the health of the community

acknowledge conflicts and must have the resources necessary to support conflict management and resolution.

Lessons from Community Coalition Building

The committee's approach to using performance monitoring to improve community health assumes that a vehicle exists or will be created to bring together important stakeholders from multiple sectors, both to guide and to legitimate the process. Community coalitions, in their many forms, are one such vehicle. The capacity to mobilize multiparty groups such as community coalitions, and to support their ability to make decisions and take actions, is important to an effective performance monitoring system.

Community coalitions—defined as organizations of individuals representing diverse organizations, factions, or constituencies who agree to work together in order to achieve common goals (Feighery and Rogers, 1990)—have become a popular vehicle for addressing complex social issues. Coalitions in the area of health tend to have a long-term and multifaceted focus and to be directed toward substantive and seemingly intractable problems such as violence and drug abuse. These coalitions are often action oriented. They serve as vehicles for bringing together public agencies, interest groups, and community members for planning, coordinating, and advocating in areas of mutual interest on behalf of the community. Coalitions can be based in a public agency or a community setting (Butterfoss et al., 1993).

Research on coalition building is under way, and factors that influence the success of these entities are being investigated. Early findings indicate that the maturation of coalitions into entities that can successfully carry out activities requires time, effort, and resources. Coalitions progress through a series of developmental stages that include an early stage in which members form relationships; a middle stage in which members prepare to take action; a mature stage in which members take action; and a final stage in which members disband or restructure. Development through the stages is not always linear, and some coalitions never reach the mature stage (Sofaer, 1992). Preliminary findings from the Massachusetts Community Health Network Areas affirms these conclusions (D.K. Walker, personal communication, 1996).

The ability of a coalition to undertake activities will be determined by its key dimensions such as its stated purpose; whether it is mandated by law or a voluntary entity; and its jurisdictional scope, membership, representation, available resources, structure, leadership, and decision-making ability (Sofaer, 1992).

Foundation-supported research and demonstration efforts will provide new information about coalition building and maintenance. For example, support from The Robert Wood Johnson Foundation and the federal Center for Substance Abuse Prevention has helped in the formation of local community partnerships and coalitions that focus on the problems of alcohol, tobacco, and other drug abuse. The development of practical tools for program evaluation and other essential activities has also been supported by foundations and federal agencies (Linney and Wandersman, 1996).

More recently, a large research and demonstration effort called the Community Care Network (CCN) has begun with funding from the W.K. Kellogg Foundation and The Duke Endowment. The program is being led by the American Hospital Association Hospital Research and Educational Trust in collaboration with the Catholic Health Association and VHA Inc. Through the CCN program, 25 coalitions of local organizations received funding in 1995 to create healthier communities (AHA, 1995). Researchers will monitor and analyze the coalitions, with the goal of developing tools to aid other interested health organizations.

Public health agencies are also promoting coalition building. The examples in Boxes 3-2 and 3-3 illustrate different approaches.

IMPLICATIONS FOR PERFORMANCE MONITORING TO IMPROVE COMMUNITY HEALTH

Some of the attributes that are either desirable or essential for managing change as a performance monitoring system is implemented at the community level include:

- will, commitment, patience, persistence, and pacing;
- leadership, including the capacity to develop and include new leaders;
- skills in communicating (advocating) effectively to policymakers in all sectors;
- the ability to generate and mobilize existing resources;
- the ability not only to access, integrate, and interpret data on system performance and on community needs, values, and preferences, but to transform data into information;
- the ability to assess the value added by current resource allocations and to project future resource needs and levels;
- the ability to set priorities across competing interests, concerns, and structures that link priority setting to the allocation and reallocation of resources;
- cultural competence—the ability to recognize and work with organizations, groups, and individuals from multiple cultures (including not only "ethnic" cultures but "professional" or "organizational" cultures);
- a parallel competence—the ability to integrate and utilize analytic methods and solutions from multiple academic and professional disciplines (health is inherently multidimensional);
- the ability to involve consumers and lay persons and to build their capacity for intelligent and equal involvement with professionals, and to recognize that they have their own unique expertise; and
- formal and informal organizational structures to facilitate collaboration and interchange; there is a growing literature ad-

BOX 3-2
KING COUNTY, WASHINGTON

King County, Washington, has found that coalitions of community stakeholders (e.g., public health agencies, health plans, hospitals, providers, employers, and others) should be developed early in the health assessment process. Such groups can provide valuable guidance on selecting indicators, interpreting assessment results, and understanding their policy implications. Public meetings and advisory groups that include community leaders can involve an even broader segment of the community in health assessment and planning. This kind of participation promotes greater "ownership" of the process and the results. Facilitating access to assessment data has also increased support for these activities. Currently in Seattle–King County, data are available to a relatively limited technical audience, but there are hopes of providing broad community access.

In King County, the local health department is a resource for essential technical and organizational services for community health assessment. It provides the expertise and computing facilities needed to frame some indicators and to perform data management and analysis tasks. The health department also helps bring together the community stakeholders and helps build coalitions.

SOURCE: J. Krieger, workshop presentation (1995); see Appendix C.

dressed to the development of partnerships, coalitions, consortia, federations and other entities, and to their role in promoting change in general and improvements in health in particular.

CONCLUSIONS

Improving the health of a community will typically require change—changes in the roles played by different stakeholders, in the relationships among stakeholders, and often in the behaviors required or expected by certain participants. Performance monitoring is a tool for promoting such change. The committee suggests that communities adopt an approach to performance monitoring that is cooperative and collaborative. In addition, the committee suggests that communities use the successful change strategies and tactics described in this chapter.

The committee's approach to using performance monitoring to improve community health assumes that a vehicle exists or will

BOX 3-3
MASSACHUSETTS COMMUNITY HEALTH NETWORK AREAS

In Massachusetts, the Department of Public Health has divided the state into 27 Community Health Network Areas (CHNAs). In each area, those interested in the improvement of health for their community are invited to work together to design a health improvement project that responds to health needs and health disparities. Each agency that receives funds from the Department of Public Health is required to participate in the CHNA. In all CHNAs, consumers are encouraged to participate in the development of health improvement strategies.

Central to this effort is the systematic use of health status data to inform the development of improvement strategies. The Department of Public Health has developed a set of health status indicators for each of the 27 CHNAs that provide demographic information, birth and death statistics, incidence of infectious disease, perinatal and child health indicators, hospital discharge data, and substance abuse data in comparison with the state, the nation, and *Healthy People 2000* (USDHHS, 1991) objectives. The data are available in written profiles, and the Department of Public Health anticipates making data available electronically.

In each CHNA, the profile data provide a picture of health status but are only a starting point. Other data sets and qualitative analysis have been added to develop an even more comprehensive basis for identifying health issues in some CHNAs. Based on the initial data, each CHNA has selected at least one health indicator to focus on for its initial work; several CHNAs have more than one health improvement activity.

Although the structure and organization of each CHNA differ, each has been established based on a common set of guiding principles. CHNAs are

- committed to continuous improvement of health status;
- focused on tracking area health status indicators and eliminating identified disparities;
- consumer oriented;
- inclusive of key stakeholders in health improvement—consumers, local government and business, and providers of community-based health, education, and human services;
- reflective of the diversity of the area, including racial, ethnic, gender, age, sexual orientation, and linguistic diversity; and
- a working partnership among the Department of Public Health, consumers, and local service providers.

SOURCE: Massachusetts Department of Public Health (1995); D.K. Walker, personal communication (1996).

be created to bring together important stakeholders from multiple sectors both to guide and to legitimate the process. Community coalitions, in their many forms, are one such vehicle. Through these vehicles, communities can identify relevant parties; find effective ways to engage parties with varying needs, resources, and values; set goals for the performance monitoring effort; ascribe responsibility for meeting goals; and manage the complex process of community-wide change.

Communities need to identify a variety of public and private stakeholders that can influence the health of their populations. These stakeholders can include health care providers, public health agencies, and community-based organizations explicitly concerned with health. They can also include other government agencies, community organizations, private industry, and other entities that do not explicitly, or sometimes even consciously, see themselves as having a health-related role—for example, schools, employers, social service and housing agencies, transportation and justice departments, faith communities, and the media.

The committee proposes a two-step approach to accountability. The first step involves the issue of shared responsibility. Communities should acknowledge that all stakeholders share responsibility for improving the health of a community's population. The second step involves ascribing to specific stakeholders accountability for accomplishing specific results as part of the community's strategy for addressing a health issue. Accountability should be conceptualized as a collaborative and cooperative process rather than a punitive process imposed by outside forces. This approach can be viewed as moving from a vertical to a horizontal structure, or from a top-down approach to a roundtable approach.

A process for putting these concepts into action is described in Chapter 4.

REFERENCES

AHA (American Hospital Association). 1995. News Release. 25 Partnerships Named to Receive Grants in Community Network Competition. Washington, D.C. August 22.

Butterfoss, F.D., Goodman, R.M., and Wandersman, A. 1993. Community Coalitions for Prevention and Health Promotion. *Health Education Research* 8(3):315–330.

Feighery, E., and Rogers, T. 1990. *Building and Maintaining Effective Coalitions.* How-To Guides on Community Health Promotion, No. 12. Palo Alto, Calif.: Stanford Health Promotion Resource Center.

FAcct (Foundation for Accountability). 1995. Guidebook for Performance Measurement: Prototype. Portland, Ore.: FAcct. September 22.

Illinois Local Health Liaison Committee. 1994. *Project Health: The Reengineering of Public Health in Illinois.* Springfield: Illinois Department of Public Health.

Jencks, S.F. 1994. The Government's Role in Hospital Accountability for Quality of Care. *Joint Commission Journal of Quality Improvement* 20(7):364–369.

Labonte, R. 1988. Health Promotion: From Concepts to Strategies. *Health Care Management Forum* 1(3):24–30.

Levit, K.R., Cowan, C.A., Lazenby, H.C., et al. 1994. National Health Spending Trends, 1960–1993. *Health Affairs* 13(5):14–31.

Linney, J.A., and Wandersman, A. 1996. Empowering Community Groups with Evaluation Skills. In *Empowerment Evaluation Knowledge and Tools for Self-Assessment and Accountability.* D.M. Fetterman, S.J. Kaftarian, and A. Wandersman, eds. London: Sage Publications.

Marris, P. 1986. *Loss and Change.* Revised ed. London: Routledge and Kegan Paul.

Massachusetts Department of Public Health. 1995. Community Health Network Areas: A Guide to the Community Health Network Initiative. Boston: Massachusetts Department of Public Health. (brochure)

NCQA (National Committee for Quality Assurance). 1993. *Health Plan Employer Data and Information Set and User's Manual, Version 2.0 (HEDIS 2.0).* Washington, D.C.: NCQA.

Newacheck, P.W., Hughes, D.C., Brindis, C., and Halfon, N. 1995. Decategorizing Health Services: Interim Findings from the Robert Wood Johnson Foundation's Child Health Initiative. *Health Affairs* 14(3):232–242.

Patrick, D.L., and Wickizer, T.M. 1995. Community and Health. In *Society and Health.* B.C. Amick, S. Levine, A.R. Tarlov, and D.C. Walsh, eds. New York: Oxford University Press.

Rodwin, M.A. 1996. Managed Care and the Elusive Quest for Accountable Health Care. *Widener Law Symposium Journal* 1(1):65–87.

Sofaer, S. 1992. Coalitions and Public Health: A Program Manager's Guide to the Issues. Washington, D.C.: Academy for Educational Development.

USDHHS (U.S. Department of Health and Human Services). 1991. *Healthy People 2000: National Health Promotion and Disease Prevention Objectives.* DHHS Pub. No. (PHS) 91-50212. Washington, D.C.: Office of the Assistant Secretary for Health.

4

A Community Health Improvement Process

Many factors influence health and well-being in a community, and many entities and individuals in the community have a role to play in responding to community health needs. The committee sees a requirement for a framework within which a community can take a comprehensive approach to maintaining and improving health: assessing its health needs, determining its resources and assets for promoting health, developing and implementing a strategy for action, and establishing where responsibility should lie for specific results. This chapter describes a *community health improvement process* that provides such a framework. Critical to this process are performance monitoring activities to ensure that appropriate steps are being taken by responsible parties and that those actions are having the intended impact on health in the community. The chapter also includes a discussion of the capacities needed to support performance monitoring and health improvement activities.

In developing a health improvement program, every community will have to consider its own particular circumstances, including factors such as health concerns, resources and capacities, social and political perspectives, and competing needs. The committee cannot prescribe what actions a community should take to address its health concerns or who should be responsible for what, but it does believe that communities need to address these issues and that a systematic approach to health improvement that makes use of performance monitoring tools will help them achieve their goals.

PROPOSING A PROCESS FOR COMMUNITY HEALTH IMPROVEMENT

The committee proposes a community health improvement process (CHIP)[1] as a basis for accountable community collaboration in monitoring overall health matters and in addressing specific health issues. This process can support the development of shared community goals for health improvement and the implementation of a planned and integrated approach for achieving those goals.

A CHIP would operate through two primary interacting cycles, both of which rely on analysis, action, and measurement. The elements of a CHIP are illustrated in Figure 4-1. Briefly, an overarching *problem identification and prioritization cycle* focuses on bringing community stakeholders together in a coalition, monitoring community-level health indicators, and identifying specific health issues as community priorities. A community addresses its priority health issues in the second kind of CHIP cycle—an *analysis and implementation cycle.* The basic components of this cycle are analyzing a health issue, assessing resources, determining how to respond and who should respond, and selecting and using stakeholder-level performance measures together with community-level indicators to assess whether desired outcomes are being achieved. More than one analysis and implementation cycle may be operating at once if a community is responding to multiple health issues. The components of both cycles are discussed in greater detail below.

The actions undertaken for a CHIP should reflect a broad view of health and its determinants. The committee believes that the field model (Evans and Stoddart, 1994), discussed in Chapter 2, provides a good conceptual basis from which to trace the multifactorial influences on health in a community. A CHIP must also

---

[1]The CHIP acronym adopted for this report is not unique to the community health improvement process. In a health context, others use it to refer to community health information programs/partnerships/profiles. See, for example, the discussion of MassCHIP—the Massachusetts Community Health Information Profile—in Chapter 5. The committee anticipates that communities will adopt their own designations for their local community health improvement process.

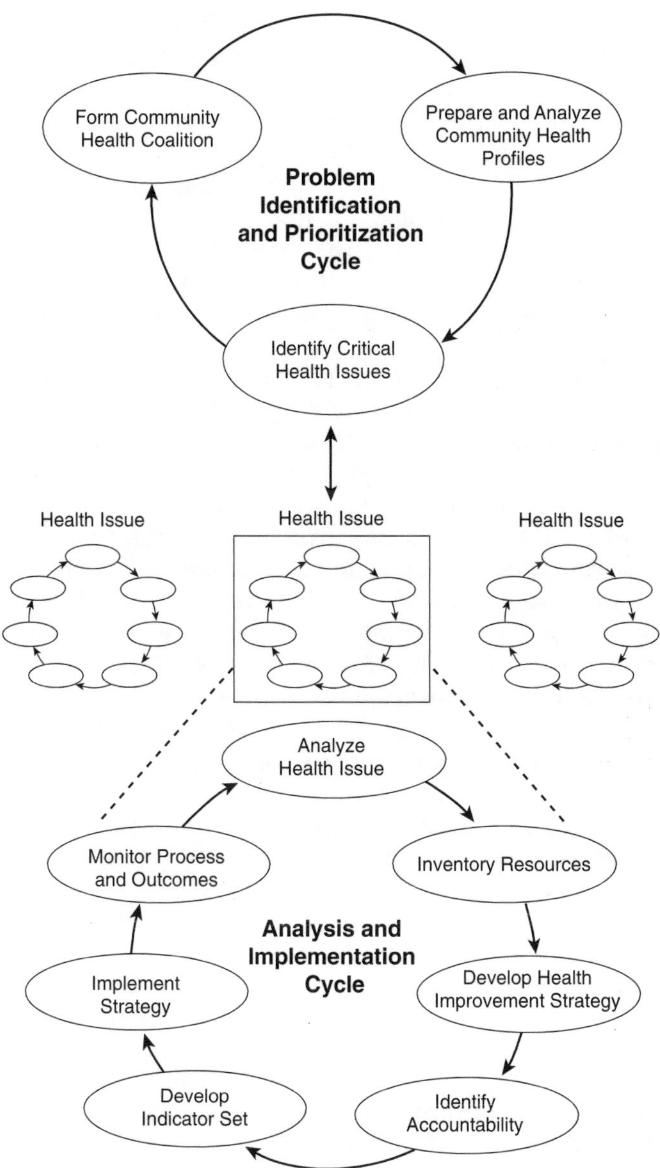

FIGURE 4-1 The community health improvement process (CHIP).

adopt an evidence-based approach to determining how to address a health issue. Evidence is needed not only to make an accurate assessment of the factors influencing health but also to select an appropriate process through which to make changes. For example, immunizations are an effective means of preventing some infectious diseases, but many children and older adults have not received recommended doses. Studies show that efforts to raise immunization rates should target *both* the barriers that keep people from using available immunization services *and* the provider practices that result in missed opportunities to administer vaccines (IOM, 1994b).

As envisioned by the committee, a CHIP can be implemented in a variety of community circumstances. Communities can begin working at various points in either cycle and with varying resources in place. The need to develop better data systems, for example, should not deter communities from using the CHIP framework. Using the process can focus attention on data needs and on finding ways in which they can be met. Participation from both the public and private sectors is needed, and leadership to initiate the process might emerge from either sector. The committee notes, however, that *The Future of Public Health* (IOM, 1988) suggests that public health agencies have a responsibility to assure that something like a health improvement process is in place. Thus, the committee recommends that local and state public health agencies assure that communities have an effective CHIP. At a minimum, these agencies should be CHIP participants, and in some communities they should provide leadership or an organizational home. Strong state-level leadership in places such as Illinois, Massachusetts, and Washington has helped promote progress at the community level.

The ongoing health improvement process must be seen as iterative and evolving rather than linear or short term. One-time activities, briefly assembled coalitions, and isolated solutions will not be adequate. A CHIP should not hinder effective and efficient operation of the accountable entities in the community that are expected to respond to specific health issues, and it must be able to accommodate the dynamic nature of communities and the interdependence of community activities. It should also facilitate the flow of information among accountable entities and other community groups and help them structure complementary efforts. Both community-level monitoring data and more detailed information related to specific health issues must feed back into the system on a continuing basis to guide subsequent analysis and planning. This information loop is also the means by which a CHIP links performance to accountable entities among the community stakeholders.

In emphasizing the community perspective, the committee does not want to overlook the broader state and national contexts for community efforts. For example, health policymakers at the federal and state levels could consider community-level performance indicators when planning and evaluating publicly funded health services programs such as managed care for Medicaid populations. Community performance measures could also contribute to state management of federal block grants (e.g., Maternal and Child Health Title V grants or those under the Community Mental Health Services Block Grant program) and the proposed federal Performance Partnership Grants (PPGs) (USDHHS, no date).

Some state health departments are prominent participants in community-level health improvement efforts. In Massachusetts, for example, which has only one county health department, the state has taken a lead by establishing 27 Community Health Network Areas (CHNAs; see Chapter 3) to serve as the base for local health improvement activities (Massachusetts Department of Public Health, 1995). Elsewhere, state-level accreditation for local health departments can stipulate measurable targets for performance at the community level and require accountability for achieving targets during the term of accreditation. Illinois, for example, has implemented performance-based state certification of local health departments (Roadmap Implementation Task Force, 1990). Similarly, state agencies that license private-sector health plans or design Medicaid managed care programs have the opportunity to specify performance measures to be used to evaluate the services provided.

Origins of the Community Health Improvement Process

The committee's proposal for a community-based process for health improvement builds on many other efforts in health care, public health, and public policy, some of which are noted below.

The Health Care Sector

In the United States, proposals for collaborative community-wide efforts to address health issues date back at least to the early 1930s (Sigmond, 1995). One activity that emerged at this time was comprehensive health planning (CHP), initially a voluntary effort to rationalize the configuration of personal health care facilities, services, and programs, often with a special emphasis on hospitals (Gottlieb, 1974). From the 1960s to the 1980s, the federal government supported formal programs for state- and community-level CHP as a strategy to improve the availability, accessibility, acceptability, cost, coordination, and quality of health care services and facilities (Benjamin and Downs, 1982; Lefkowitz, 1983). At the local level, however, CHP was hampered both by limited control over resource allocation and by its responsibilities to regulate the introduction of new health care facilities and programs (Sofaer, 1988). In addition, local "ownership" of these activities was weakened by strict federal requirements regarding their organization and operation.

Nevertheless, the governing bodies of local planning agencies brought together multiple constituencies, including health care professionals and other "experts," consumers, and in a few cases, private-sector health care purchasers (Sofaer, 1988). CHP efforts also combined data on a community's health care services, epidemiology, and socioeconomic characteristics to identify high priority health problems. Indeed, some planning theorists explicitly based their approach on a model of the determinants of health (Blum, 1981) that might be considered an early version of the field model.

Concerns about the quality of health care stimulated measurement and monitoring activities. Evidence of widespread variations in medical practice patterns (e.g., Wennberg and Gittelsohn, 1973; Connell et al., 1981; Wennberg, 1984; Chassin et al., 1986), inadequate information about the outcomes of common treatments (e.g., Wennberg et al., 1980; Eddy and Billings, 1988), and evidence of marked variations across providers in the outcomes of treatment (e.g., Bunker et al., 1969; Luft et al., 1979) prompted increased concern about the effectiveness of care (e.g., Brook and Lohr, 1985; Roper et al., 1988) and a recognition of the importance of monitoring health care practices (e.g., IOM, 1990). Continuous quality improvement (CQI) techniques have been adapted from their origins in industry for use in health care settings (e.g., Berwick et al., 1990; IOM, 1990; Batalden and Stoltz, 1993), and clinical practice guidelines are providing criteria for assessing quality of care (e.g., IOM, 1992; AHCPR, 1995). The basic Plan–Do–Check–Act cycle used in CQI is being applied to community health programs (Nolan and Knapp, 1996; Zablocki, 1996). Health departments are also exploring their role in promoting the quality of health care (Joint Council Committee on Quality in Public Health, 1996).

Community-oriented primary care (COPC), which gained increased attention in the 1970s and 1980s, starts from a health care provider perspective to bring together care for individuals with attention to the health of the community in which they live (Kark and Abramson, 1982; IOM, 1984). Although performance monitoring is not an explicit focus of COPC, this approach to health care emphasizes the importance of community-based data for understanding the origins of health problems.

The emergence of managed care and various forms of integrated health systems has been another factor that is broadening the health care focus from individual patient encounters to the health needs of a population. Enrolled members are generally the population of primary interest, but many of these organizations participate in activities serving the larger community such as violence prevention, immunization, AIDS prevention, and school-based health clinics. Some have formalized their commitment to community-wide efforts through mechanisms such as the Community Service Principles adopted by Group Health Cooperative of Puget Sound (1996). Nationally, organizations such as the Catholic Health Association (CHA, 1995) and the Voluntary Hospitals of America (VHA, 1992) have adopted community benefit standards that call for accountable participation in meeting the needs of the community. The attributes of a "socially responsible managed care system," proposed by Showstack and colleagues (1996), also support involvement in community-wide health improvement efforts.

More generally, financial incentives are encouraging health care organizations to consider community-wide health needs. Nonprofit hospitals and health plans, plus the foundations established by provider organizations and insurers, are responding to the "community benefit" requirements needed to preserve their tax status. In addition, managed care plans are serving an increasing proportion of Medicare and Medicaid beneficiaries (Armstead et al., 1995), whose health may be adversely affected by problems not easily resolved in the health care setting (e.g., violence, poverty, social isolation). Because limited periods of eligibility for Medicaid benefits mean frequent enrollment and disenrollment, health plans may increasing see value in services that improve the health of nonmembers who might be part of their enrolled population in the future.

The Public Health Sector

Renewed interest in the 1970s and 1980s in a population- and community-based approach to health improvement was also reflected in both national and international activities in the public health arena (Lalonde, 1974; Ashton and Seymour, 1988), including the World Health Organization's Health for All by the Year 2000 program (WHO, 1985). The Healthy Cities/Healthy Communities movement, an international activity that emerged from the WHO and related programs, emphasizes building broad community support for public policies that promote health by improving the quality of life (Hancock, 1993; Duhl and Drake, 1995; Flynn, 1996).

In the United States, the first *Healthy People* report in 1979 helped draw attention to issues of prevention and health promotion (USPHS, 1979). In the early 1980s, the Planned Approach to Community Health (PATCH), was developed to enhance the capacity of state and local health departments to plan, implement, and evaluate health promotion activities (Kreuter, 1992; CDC, 1995b). It emphasizes collaboration both within the community and across federal, state, and local levels. Among other tools that have been developed to guide community health assessment activities is the Model Standards program, which was initiated in 1976. The most recent report, *Healthy Communities 2000: Model Standards* (APHA et al., 1991), outlines an 11-step community-based process for assessing health department and other community resources, identifying health needs and priorities, selecting measurable objectives, and monitoring and evaluating results of interventions.

Another approach, described in *APEXPH: Assessment Protocol for Excellence in Public Health* (NACHO, 1991), provides an eight-step process for assessing community health, assembling a community-based group through which to work, identifying and prioritizing issues of concern, and formulating a plan for responding. The APEX*PH* process is designed to begin with action by a local health department, but initial steps can also be taken by others in the community. *The Healthy Communities Handbook* (National Civic League, 1993b), developed under the auspices of the Healthy Cities/Healthy Communities initiative in the United States, reviews a process divided into a planning phase and an implementation phase. Steps in the planning phase include assembling a stakeholder coalition, (re)defining "community health," assessing influences on health in and beyond the community, reviewing health indicators and community capacities, identifying key performance areas, and creating an implementation plan. The implementation phase includes monitoring activities and their outcomes.

In a recent survey of local health departments, 47 percent reported using Model Standards for planning activities, 32 percent reported using APEX*PH*, 12 percent reported using PATCH, and 6 percent reported using Healthy Cities (NACCHO, 1995). Many hospitals and health systems in the private sector also are using the APEX*PH* model to guide their health assessment activities (Gordon et al., 1996).

The interest in community-based health improvement activities also led to several major intervention trials targeting specific health problems. The National Heart, Lung, and Blood Institute (NHLBI), for example, sponsored projects in California (Farquhar et al., 1985), Minnesota (Mittelmark et al., 1986), and Rhode Island (Elder et al., 1986) to test a community-based approach to primary prevention of coronary heart disease. The National Cancer Institute initiated the Community Intervention Trial for Smoking Cessation (COMMIT) in 11 pairs of communities (COMMIT, 1991). Community-based approaches to health improvement also received support from foundations, as in the Henry J. Kaiser Family Foundation Community Health Promotion Grant Program (Tarlov et al., 1987).

Health Status and Performance Measurement

The committee's proposal draws from a variety of indicator development and performance measurement efforts. *Healthy People 2000* (USDHHS, 1991), one of the most prominent, provides more than 300 national health promotion and disease prevention objectives. A smaller set of related indicators was endorsed for use in monitoring key elements of community health status (CDC, 1991). Many states have assembled their own objectives for the year 2000, and *Healthy Communities 2000: Model Standards* (APHA et al., 1991) specifically addresses how communities can adapt these and other related objectives to their particular circumstances. With stated targets to be achieved, objectives such as these are not only measurement tools but also statements of intended performance. In addition, more specialized assessments are being made such as monitoring the status of children at the state and local levels (Annie E. Casey Foundation, 1996; Children Now, 1996).

Interest in performance-based assessments of health care has resulted in the development of "report cards" by some individual health plans and in a variety of nationally used and proposed health care indicator sets (e.g., Nadzam et al., 1993; NCQA, 1993, 1996a; AMBHA, 1995; FAcct, 1995). Individually, many health care organizations are monitoring performance for their internal quality improvement purposes and for tracking community benefit activities.

A focus on performance and outcomes also is central to ideas on "reinventing government" (Osborne and Gaebler, 1992; Gore, 1993; Hatry et al., 1994). The Government Performance and Results Act, for example, requires federal agencies to develop annual performance plans and to identify measures to assess progress (GAO, 1996). The proposals to implement PPGs for several health-related block grants would apply a similar approach to state grantees (USDHHS, no date). Some observers, however, caution against an overreliance on measurement in managing government activities, suggesting that many important tasks of government cannot be adequately quantified and that even if measurable may not be adequately insulated from political pressures (Mintzberg, 1996).

ADVANCING THE PROCESS

The process proposed by the committee reflects the need to combine features of these various activities to produce both a community-wide perspective and the performance measures that support accountability and inform further improvements. The current health planning and health assessment models provide a comprehensive community perspective but generally put less emphasis on the linkage between performance monitoring and stakeholder accountability than either the problem identification and prioritization cycle or the analysis and implementation cycle of the proposed CHIP. The quality improvement and performance measurement activities that have developed in the personal health care sector bring accountability for performance to the fore explicitly. They are, however, generally applied to specific institutions or health plan services for their members, not to activities of many entities responding to the needs of the entire population of a community.

Both community-wide and organization-specific performance measurement processes are needed to improve the health of the general population. Applying the field model perspective encourages consideration of the diversity of opportunities and agents, both inside and outside the usual "health" setting, that can contribute to health improvement efforts. Although the committee's recommendations for operationalizing a CHIP are based on a variety of theoretical and practical models for community health improvement and quality assurance or performance monitoring in health care, public health, and other settings, the complete set of components of the committee's proposal has not yet been tested in communities. That will be an essential step in validating and improving the process.

PROBLEM IDENTIFICATION AND PRIORITIZATION CYCLE

As proposed by the committee, the problem identification and prioritization cycle has three main phases:

- forming a community health coalition;
- collecting and analyzing data for a community health profile; and
- identifying high-priority health issues.

Community efforts can begin with *any* phase of the cycle. For example, the availability of data from the health department on various aspects of health status might spark action on a specific health issue before any community-wide coalition is established. Alternatively, efforts around a specific health issue might be the catalyst both for more broadly based activities and for the collection of additional health status data.

Form Coalitions

A long-term community coalition is an essential element in a CHIP. As noted in Chapter 3, a coalition is an organization of individuals representing diverse organizations, factions, or constituencies who agree to work together to achieve common goals (Feighery and Rogers, 1990). In the context of a CHIP, a coalition provides the mechanism for bringing together the community's stakeholders and accountable entities to develop a broad perspective on health needs and how they might be addressed.

Leadership is essential, both to initiate and to maintain a coalition. Many may look to the health department to play this role, but private-sector initiatives or public–private collaborations can also be the motivating force. The coalition's roles include obtaining and analyzing community health profiles, identifying critical issues for action, supporting the development of improvement strategies, fostering the allocation of responsibility for health improvement efforts among community stakeholders, and serving as a locus of accountability for performance by those stakeholders.

A CHIP coalition should operate in the configuration that best suits a community's particular circumstances. The organizational structure may be more or less formal, and the name applied to the group may vary (e.g., committee, alliance, network). Some communities will already have coalitions that can assume a role in a CHIP. In other communities, an existing group may need to expand or adapt to a new role. In some cases, a local board of health might provide a starting point. If several groups are already in place, perhaps to address specific health issues or to represent specific segments of the community, they should establish a workable forum for collaboration with a more broadly based coalition and with each other. Once a coalition is in place, continuing CHIP cycles should provide an opportunity to bring into the process community constituencies that are not yet represented.

Coalition participants should include a community's major stakeholders and accountable entities. Among these groups are health departments and other public agencies, individual and institutional health care providers in the public and private sectors, schools, employers, insurers, community groups, the media, and the general public. Participants should include not only those groups that implement health improvement activities but also those that will have to collect, analyze, and report data used in the health improvement process.

Efforts must also be made to ensure that the general public has opportunities to participate and that public- and private-sector entities that may not traditionally have assumed a role in health issues are brought to the table. Because community health and resources are influenced by factors such as federal and state programs and policies and by private-sector activities such as corporate practices and accreditation standards, communities should consider how those perspectives can be represented in a coalition.

In the committee's view, inclusiveness is an important principle for these coalitions, but it recognizes that some activities may warrant attention from a more strategically focused group of participants. For example, public schools might be expected to play a more limited role in examining the health needs of the elderly than in smoking prevention and cessation programs for adolescents.

In most cases a coalition will function on the basis of willing participation and acceptance of shared responsibility for improving health in the community, but incentives to participate may vary among stakeholders. For health departments, participation in a coalition may be an effective way to meet responsibilities to the community under the three "core functions" of assessment, policy development, and assurance (IOM, 1988).

For some, participation in health improvement activities reflects a basic commitment to the well-being of the community (e.g., CHA, 1995; Showstack et al., 1996). Good will may not always be sufficient, however, and financial responsibilities cannot be ignored. It was noted in discussions at the committee's workshops that despite a commitment to efforts on behalf of the community's health in an organization such as the Group Health Cooperative of Puget Sound, it will be difficult to sustain that commitment unless other health care organizations accept a similar responsibility, including public reporting on the extent to which their efforts are meeting expectations (see Appendix C). Sigmond (1995) proposes that the private sector use the influence of accreditation to encourage community involvement. Standards could be established for participation in community partnerships.

Self-interest can also be an effective motivation. Employers, for example, may expect to benefit from reduced health care costs if community efforts can improve the health status of the workforce. Some coalition participants may find that they can use resources more efficiently because they can coordinate their activities with others working on similar projects. For some hospitals and health plans, economic incentives to participate may exist because of "community benefit" requirements for nonprofit tax status or contract provisions for Medicaid and Medicare providers. Participants should not, however, allow a coalition to become a means of furthering a particular constituency's goals at the expense of the best interests of the community.

Missouri has assembled a Community Health Assessment and Resource Team (CHART) specifically to provide technical assistance to the state's communities in coalition formation and other steps in the health improvement process (see Box 4-1). Additional discussion of coalition building appears in Chapter 3.

Collect, Analyze, and Publicize Community Health Data

Another phase of the problem identification and prioritization cycle is assessing the community's health status and health needs

BOX 4-1
MISSOURI'S COMMUNITY HEALTH ASSESSMENT AND RESOURCE TEAM

Missouri has formed the Community Health Assessment and Resource Team (CHART) to provide resources and technical assistance to collaborative efforts to improve community health. CHART, based in the Missouri Department of Health, is itself a coalition, whose members are representatives of several health- and community-related agencies and organizations in the state. The members of the team bring expertise in community assessment and in development of strategies that improve community health. CHART also serves as a clearinghouse for information and resource materials for communities.

The CHART partners include the Joint Committee on Health Care Policy and Planning, the Missouri Alliance for Home Care, the Missouri Association of Osteopathic Physicians and Surgeons, the Missouri Chamber of Commerce, the Missouri Coalition for Primary Health Care, the Missouri Department of Health, the Missouri Department of Mental Health, the Missouri Department of Social Services, the Missouri Hospital Association, the Missouri Nurses Association, the Missouri Public Health Association, the Missouri State Medical Association, the Partnership Council, the Transition Advisory Team, and the University of Missouri–Columbia Health Services Management Department.

Five "how-to" manuals for implementing local health assessment and improvement programs have been developed. They emphasize collaboration at the local level and provide state-of-the-art information on community health. The manuals are intended to be used, not in a "cookbook" approach, but rather as resources that should be adapted and revised over time to meet the needs of a continuing health improvement process in individual communities. Each manual contains explanatory text, as well as specially designed tools and worksheets. The tools and worksheets are intended to help communities organize their members, assess community health status, prioritize community health issues, and develop effective interventions for improving community health.

Two of the manuals focus specifically on coalition issues. "Building a Community Health Coalition" includes recommendations for securing a project sponsor, developing a team, defining leadership for the project, determining how to get the project started, and deciding on an overall project time frame. "Establishing a Foundation for a Successful Community Health Strategy" addresses defining the community, identifying key relationships, establishing a shared vision, refining team members' roles and responsibilities, and determining how to coordinate and use project resources. The other three manuals cover data collection and analysis issues in community health assessment, prioritizing community health issues, and developing and implementing a community health strategy.

SOURCE: Missouri Department of Health (1996).

by collecting and analyzing data and making that information available to inform community decision making. The committee sees a need, at a minimum, for these health assessment activities to produce a *community health profile* that can provide basic information about a community's demographic and socioeconomic characteristics and its health status and health risks. This profile would provide background information that can help a community interpret other health data. Comparing these data over time or with data from other communities may help identify health issues that require more focused attention. The committee's proposal for a basic set of indicators for a community health profile appears in Chapter 5. Where resources permit, states and communities may choose to develop a more extensive set of indicators.

The community health coalition should oversee the development and use of a health profile, but responsibility for data collection and analysis may lie with particular coalition participants that have resources suited to specific tasks. Health departments, in particular, have health assessment as a core function (IOM, 1988) and should, in the committee's view, be expected to promote, facilitate, and where necessary, perform the periodic health assessments needed to produce a community health profile. Profile updates should be produced regularly, and profile data should be compiled over time, ideally in electronic format, to facilitate assessment of trends. Annual updates may be possible for some measures, but others may depend on specialized data collection, such as the census, that occurs less frequently. The committee urges that all measures be updated at least once every five years and that more frequent updates be a goal.

Although some communities will have the resources and technical expertise to assemble a health profile on their own, many will not. The committee recommends that responsibility for assuring the availability of these data lie with state health departments. The state role includes collecting and publishing data and providing technical assistance to communities to use data and to collect community-level data that are not available from other sources. Working together, states and communities should seek to develop the information resources and technical skills that can support annual updates of most health profile measures. Some states, including Illinois, Iowa, and Massachusetts, are already making data available to communities electronically. Other states (e.g., Florida, Missouri, and New York) are beginning to publish some county-level data on the World Wide Web, which not only facilitates access to this information for communities within the state but also allows other states and communities to use those data as points of comparison.

Data held in the private sector by health plans, indemnity insurers, employers, and others can also be valuable for community health assessments, and these organizations should provide appropriate data as part of their responsibility to the community, a position also taken by others (VHA, 1992; Showstack et al., 1996). To ensure access to essential data, however, the committee recommends that states and the federal government require that certain standard data be reported, including data on the characteristics and health status of enrolled populations, on services provided, and on outcomes of those services. In turn, these organizations should have access for their own decision-making purposes to other community data. This opportunity for mutual benefit should reinforce CHIP goals.

For all data collected and used for a community profile or other aspects of a CHIP, adequate safeguards for confidentiality will be essential. At the community level, ensuring that confidentiality is maintained will require special attention because of the small numbers of cases that many measures will produce. These issues are of continuing concern and have been discussed in the Institute of Medicine report *Health Data in the Information Age* (IOM, 1994a) and elsewhere (e.g., Gostin et al., 1993, 1996; Gostin and Lazzarini, 1995).

Discussions with the committee at its workshops emphasized the importance of involving both decision makers and community groups in assembling, reviewing, and responding to health data (see Appendixes C and D). A community coalition can undertake these collaborative assessments, but more extensive consultation with community constituencies may also be appropriate. The varied perspectives of these constituencies can produce a better understanding of points such as whether the results seem reasonable, whether there are gaps between findings and perceptions, and whether there are concerns that have not been identified through more quantitative approaches. The review can also identify areas of special interest to the community and generate guidance on how to treat sensitive issues. Involving the community and responding to its concerns may increase the community's interest in and support for health assessment activities. Experience in Seattle–King County, Washington, for example, suggests that making assessment data more readily available to the community can lead to increased support for these activities (see Appendix C).

Identify Critical Health Issues

The third phase of the problem identification and prioritization cycle is identifying those health issues that are of special concern to the community and determining which ones should be given the highest priority for additional attention. These priorities should reflect not only the judgment of public health agencies and health care providers but also the broader spectrum of community stakeholders, including the general public. A coalition should be able to bring many perspectives to these considerations, but views not represented within the coalition should not be neglected. A variety of specific techniques can be used for priority setting (e.g., see Krasny, 1980; Pickett and Hanlon, 1990; Vilnius and Dandoy, 1990; Chambers et al., 1996) and resources such as APEX*PH* (NACHO, 1991) can provide useful guidance to communities.

A health profile's standard epidemiologic data on morbidity, mortality, and health risk factors will influence but may not determine where a community's priorities lie. If a problem is of sufficient concern, small numbers of cases may be enough to motivate a community to respond (e.g., drug-resistant tuberculosis or adolescent suicides). Measures, from a community profile or other sources, that describe other aspects of the community's health-related environment, such as employment, housing, and transportation resources, can also be important in shaping priorities. The costs of possible interventions in relation to their potential benefits should be considered, and if available, formal economic analyses (e.g., cost-effectiveness studies) could help guide a community's priority setting.

A community may decide to respond to evidence that conditions have changed or that the community compares unfavorably with others or with a measure such as a *Healthy People 2000* target. Benchmarks such as this can provide a basis for assess-

---

A *benchmark* is a standard established for anticipated results, often reflecting an aim to improve over current levels.

---

ing the acceptability of a health status level or the outcome of a health intervention.

Qualitative information should be considered as well. Information on the "who, what, when, where, and how" of a community provides a context for interpreting quantitative measures. A community coalition should encourage the use of mechanisms such as meetings with neighborhood or community groups to give those who may not consider themselves part of a coalition an opportunity to learn about and contribute to discussions regarding the community's health issues. Skilled meeting facilitators can help ensure that these discussions are effective, and the discussions may benefit from efforts to inform the community about the field model and the framework it provides for thinking about the determinants of health.

Other factors may also be operating when a community coalition decides which health issues will be targeted. Opportunities for an early "success" may be valued as a way to strengthen the coalition and increase support for the health improvement process. The coalition may find that an issue already being addressed by many groups provides an opportunity to build on available resources, including experience and prior commitment. In other cases, an issue that represents "neutral ground" for the various members of the coalition, because it is not a focus of competition for funding or does not target conflicting values, will be given priority. In Massachusetts, the CHNAs have found that considerations such as these influenced the selection of priority issues (D.K. Walker, personal communication, 1996). As a community gains experience with a CHIP, it will be possible to take up more challenging issues. The committee urges community coalitions to begin addressing specific health issues even if initial efforts are directed to topics that might not be seen by all as the "most important" ones.

Communities should expect to develop, over time and as resources permit, a "portfolio" of health initiatives. The mix of initiatives in the community portfolio will change as a CHIP continues. Some may move ahead more quickly than others. If a community's circumstances change, issues once given a lower priority may assume greater importance. The community coalition must periodically review the health issue portfolio to ensure that appropriate issues are being addressed and that progress is being made or reasons for lack of progress are being examined.

A balance is needed between issues that lend themselves to quick, easily measurable success and those that require sustained effort to produce a longer-term health benefit. Focusing only on the most difficult issues could undermine support for the health improvement process if progress is difficult to measure or will be evident only after many years. Important benefits of interventions that target critical developmental periods for infants and young children, for example, may not be evident until adolescence or adulthood. Communities and their coalitions should, however, guard against overemphasizing issues that are visible but have limited impact on community health. For example, "special event" immunization clinics will reach some children who have not received needed vaccinations but cannot provide the continuity necessary to ensure proper care for overall health and will not resolve the underlying problems in access to services or provider practices that contribute to underimmunization.

ANALYSIS AND IMPLEMENTATION CYCLE

Once an issue has been targeted by a community, the health improvement process proposed by the committee moves on to another series of steps:

- analysis of the health issue;
- an inventory of health resources;
- development of a health improvement strategy;
- discussion and negotiation to establish where accountability lies;
- development of a set of performance indicators for accountable entities;
- implementation of the health improvement strategy; and
- measurement to monitor the outcome of efforts by accountable entities.

These steps are displayed and described as sequential (see Figure 4-1), but in practice they interact and are likely to be repeated varying numbers of times while a community is engaged in a particular initiative.

Analyze the Health Issue

A community, through its health coalition or a designated agent such as the health department, will have to articulate the specific issues of concern in the community and goals for a health improvement activity. An analysis of the health issue should examine the general underlying causes and contributing factors, how they operate in that specific community, and what interventions are likely to be effective in meeting health improvement goals. The committee encourages the use of a framework such as the field model (see Chapter 2) to guide the analysis so as to ensure that consideration is given not only to health care or health department issues but also to a broader array of factors, such as those in the social and physical environments. This approach is necessary to identify the strongest determinants of health or those that may present the most promising opportunities for strategic change. Sources such as APEX*PH* (NACHO, 1991) and PATCH (CDC, 1995b) can provide additional guidance and offer tools such as a "health problem analysis worksheet" that can be used with the field model framework.

Where the factors that influence health are well understood (e.g., disease protection provided by immunizations or the added risk of low-weight births from maternal smoking), the analysis should be able to help community stakeholders understand what kinds of health improvement activities may be useful and who in the community might be expected to assume responsibility for some aspect of health improvement. Expert advice can be especially valuable when the determinants of health status are less well understood. Such advice can help coalition participants, and the larger community, to interpret the available evidence and determine how the accepted "best practices" can be applied to meet the community's needs.

Inventory Health Resources

A community will also have to assess the resources that it can apply to a health issue. Within the community, these can include organizations, influence, expertise, and funding that can be applied to required tasks, as well as individuals willing to volunteer time and effort. Another type of community resource will be factors that operate (or could be developed to do so) as protective influences that can mitigate the impact of adverse conditions. For example, stable families appear to help overcome some of the health problems that might be expected in the lower-income immigrant population of New York City's Washington Heights/ Inwood neighborhood (see Appendix C). Funding, technical assistance, and other forms of support may also be available from public- and private-sector sources outside the community. Tools such as APEX*PH* (NACHO, 1991) and the Civic Index (National

Civic League, 1993a,b) are available to assess community resources. APEX*PH* focuses in particular on the capacity of the local health department to perform a variety of functions important for health improvement activities such as building community constituencies, collecting and analyzing data, and developing and implementing health policy.

The experience of McHenry County, Illinois, described briefly in Box 4-2, illustrates one community's approach to a specific health concern.

Develop a Health Improvement Strategy

A health improvement strategy should reflect an assessment of how available resources can be applied most effectively to address the specific concerns associated with a health issue in a community. Several considerations should shape such strategies. Some actions can achieve short-term changes but may not ensure more fundamental improvements in health that can be seen only over a longer period. Interim goals for major health problems, such as risk reduction strategies, may help sustain a health improvement effort. If a community were interested in reducing cancer mortality, for instance, strategies might focus on a reduction in smoking initiation among teenagers and the implementation of workplace smoking restrictions as initial goals. Strategy development should also include consideration of the consequences of not taking any action.

Priority should be given to actions for which evidence of effectiveness is available. Evidence is needed not only that an action can be expected to have the desired health impact (e.g., immunization to prevent measles) but also that an effective form of implementation has been identified (e.g., reminders to providers that an immunization is due; e.g., Rosser et al., 1992). A source such as the *Guide to Clinical Preventive Services* (U.S. Preventive Services Task Force, 1996) provides an authoritative review of evidence on specific clinical services. The Centers for Disease Control and Prevention (CDC) is assisting a newly established task force in developing a similar report on "what works" in community-based preventive services (see Novick et al., 1995, for preliminary work in this area). Evidence from economic analyses (e.g., cost-effectiveness or cost-benefit analysis) should be considered as well. For many health issues, however, evidence for effective interventions will be limited, and communities are unlikely to have the expertise, funding, or time needed to conduct their own outcomes

BOX 4-2
ASSESSMENT OF ENVIRONMENTAL HEALTH ISSUES, RESOURCES, AND RESPONSES IN McHENRY COUNTY, ILLINOIS

As part of the Illinois Project for Local Assessment of Need (IPLAN), McHenry County undertook a local health needs assessment and developed a community health plan, which was issued in 1994. Following the APEX*PH* process (NACHO, 1991), the Community Health Committee reviewed IPLAN data provided by the state health department on the county's sociodemographic characteristics, general health status, and specific health issues such as maternal and child health, chronic disease, infectious disease, environmental health, injury, and access to care. Additional data from other sources supplemented IPLAN information.

Environmental health issues emerged as one of the county's priorities, and four specific concerns were identified: protecting groundwater supplies, limiting exposure to radon, preventing foodborne illness, and reducing pesticide exposure. *Outcome objectives* were established for each of these issues, for example: by 1999, reduce the number of additional community wells contaminated with volatile organic chemicals to fewer than five (baseline: 9 wells currently contaminated). A set of *impact objectives* addresses how the county expects to achieve its desired outcomes. For reducing contamination of wells, the impact objective is to develop a water management plan by 1997. *Process objectives and intervention strategies* were also identified, for example: convening a technical advisory committee on groundwater protection.

A diverse collection of *resources* was identified as being available in the county to respond these environmental health concerns: schools, media, conservation agencies, the Farm Bureau, the Environmental Protection Agency, hospitals, master gardeners and garden clubs, local consulting agencies, physicians in private practice, the McHenry County Medical Society, the Mental Health Board, and the McHenry County Department of Health.

SOURCE: McHenry County Department of Health (1994).

studies or economic analyses. A community should not ignore these issues or the interventions under consideration, but it will have to consider carefully what actions can make the best use of its resources. Advice from experts can help a community coalition identify and interpret available evidence and design appropriate interventions.

The strategy development step should also include consideration of potential barriers to success that may arise in trying to implement a strategy. Issues to consider include whether an intervention can or will be implemented; whether it will reach all who need it; and whether intended beneficiaries can or will take advantage of health improvement efforts. Early consideration of these questions may make it possible to recast the strategy to overcome anticipated problems.

Work done on the evaluation of "comprehensive community initiatives" points to the value of a thoughtful articulation of the "theory of change" embodied in an intervention strategy—how and why an intervention is expected to work (Weiss, 1995; Connell and Kubisch, 1996). Specifying intended long-term and intermediate outcomes and how they would be achieved can help clarify assumptions about the purpose and operation of an intervention and guide the selection of performance indicators. Connell and Kubisch (1996) suggest that this process can promote collaboration and commitment to the intervention and help clarify pathways of accountability.

Establish Accountability for Health Improvement Activities

Establishing accountability is a key to using performance monitoring in the health improvement process proposed by the committee. Specific entities must be willing to be held accountable for undertaking activities, within an overall strategy for dealing with a health issue, that are expected to contribute to achieving desired outcomes. The committee sees a collective responsibility among all segments of a community to contribute to health improvements, but each entity must accept individual responsibility for performing those tasks that are consistent with its roles, resources, and capabilities. (See Chapter 3 for additional discussion of these issues.)

Depending on the health issue and the community stakeholders involved, different approaches may be necessary to reach agreement on who will be accountable for what. In some cases, community cooperation may be a sufficient basis for negotiating assignments of accountability. In other instances, incentives such as compliance with funding requirements or response to market pressures may make entities in the community willing to be held accountable. In some situations, however, accountability may result from regulatory or other legal requirements. Any combination of these factors may operate as a community resolves issues of accountability. For health departments, in particular, accountability under the "assurance" function (IOM, 1988) might be viewed as encompassing facilitation of the overall intervention strategy in addition to responsibilities for specific services or activities.

Develop a Set of Performance Indicators

Accountability is operationalized in a CHIP through the adoption of concrete, specific, and quantitative performance indicators linked to accountable entities in the community that can contribute to health improvement. In contrast to a community health profile, which provides an overview of health status and community characteristics, performance indicators focus on a specific health issue and the activities undertaken as part of a health improvement strategy.

Because health issues have many dimensions and can be addressed by various sectors in the community, *sets* of indicators will be needed to make a meaningful assessment of overall performance. A set should include enough indicators to cover critical features of a health improvement effort but should not be so extensive that the details overwhelm the broader picture. As "indicators," these measures should be more than one dimensional, representing performance in important related areas (Sofaer, 1995).

Selecting indicators requires careful consideration of how to gain insight into progress achieved in the health improvement process. A set of indicators should be a balanced mix of population-based measures of risk factors and health outcomes and of health systems-based measures of services performed. An indicator set should include measures for the various accountable entities in the community, including those whose primary mission is not health specific. A balance is also necessary among indicators that reflect short-term gains and those that measure more fundamental long-term changes in community health.

Communities may also want to consider indicators of cooperation among organizations. The success of multiple organizations serving a particular community may depend on how well their services are coordinated. For example, senior citizens may be served by separate programs providing meals, transportation, outreach, and mental health services. Each program may be meeting its own goals, but if they are not working together, their overall impact may be diminished.

Communities will need criteria to guide the selection of indicators. In the committee's view, such criteria should include consistency with a conceptual framework such as the field model for understanding factors that contribute to the production of health, salience to community stakeholders, and support for the social change processes needed to achieve health improvements. Indicators should also be assessed against criteria of validity and reliability, evidence linking performance and health improvement, sensitivity to changes in community health status, and availability of timely data at a reasonable cost. It is also essential to develop an operational definition for each measure to determine what data are needed and how (or if) they can be obtained. A review of existing indicator sets may suggest measures that could be adopted for community use and may be a source of tested operational definitions.[2]

The development of indicator sets and the selection of indicators are discussed in greater detail in Chapter 5. Appendix A illustrates the application of the committee's proposals with prototypical sets of *community-level* performance indicators for several specific health issues.

Implement the Improvement Strategy

Implementation of health improvement strategies and interventions requires action by many segments of a community. The particular mix of activities and actors will depend on the health issue being addressed and on a community's organization and resources. In most instances, these activities will require participation by public- *and* private-sector entities and often by entities that may not traditionally be seen as part of the health system. Finding ways to pool and redirect resources so that they can be

[2]Several collections of indicators are mentioned throughout this report. Some of the broadest are *Healthy People 2000* (USDHHS, 1991), *Healthy Communities 2000: Model Standards* (APHA et al., 1991), and versions of the Health Plan Employer Data and Information Set (HEDIS) (NCQA, 1993, 1996a). Many other indicators have been developed by states, professional organizations, and individual health care organizations. As has been noted, indicators are included in federal block grant reporting requirements (e.g., CDC, 1994; MCHB, 1995). Communities might benefit from easy access to catalogs of such indicator sets. Recent reviews of indicators in use or being developed might provide a starting point (e.g., see Center for the Advancement of Health and Western Consortium for Public Health, 1995; Lewin–VHI, 1995). A detailed compilation of clinical performance measures is available (Center for Quality of Care Research and Education and Mikalix & Company, 1996), and the Joint Commission on the Accreditation of Healthcare Organizations (JCAHO, 1996b) is assembling a catalog of indicators that a broad range of health care organizations can use in their quality improvement efforts.

used as efficiently and effectively as possible is likely to be a considerable challenge. For example, official waivers may be needed to remove restrictions on the use of categorical state and federal funding.

The tools of continuous quality improvement may be useful to some accountable entities as they determine how to meet the performance expectations of the health improvement process (e.g., see Worrall and Chambers, 1989; Nolan and Knapp, 1996). The community as a whole must also be able to respond successfully to the change processes that are set in motion. Some of the challenges and keys for success in social change have been examined in Chapter 3.

Monitor Process and Outcomes of the Improvement Strategy

Once a health improvement program is under way, performance monitoring becomes an essential guide. Information provided by the selected performance indicators should be reviewed regularly and used to inform further action. In assessing progress, a community coalition or other designated agent should consider whether accountable entities are taking appropriate actions and whether appropriate strategies and interventions have been adopted. As current goals are achieved and new ones adopted, the analysis and implementation cycle described by the committee should lead to other activities and the adoption of new performance indicators. Over time, a community, through its health coalition and the broader aspects of a CHIP, should reexamine its priorities and determine whether other health issues can be added to the health improvement portfolio or can replace issues on which good progress has been made.

The monitoring process will require access to comparable data from multiple sources that can be combined to produce a community-wide information resource. Comparability is affected by factors such as consistency over time and among community stakeholders in data definitions and measurement techniques. Efforts are needed to improve both the comparability of data from separate sources and the techniques for pooling these data. Further discussion of technical concerns related to data and data collection appears in Chapter 5 and Appendix B.

As for the community health profile, it will be important to examine these quantitative indicators in conjunction with qualitative information that can contribute to a more complete picture of the community context. Valuable information about the implementation of a health improvement strategy and the interpretation of indicator data (e.g., what is and is not working, alternative approaches that could be considered) can be gained from sources such as focus groups, key informant interviews, and town meetings.

In regard to access to data, health departments and other public agencies are generally expected to support the collection, analysis, and publication of data (e.g., IOM, 1988; Roper et al., 1992; NACHO and CDC, 1994; Turnock et al., 1994), although new approaches and new skills may be needed for performance monitoring programs. Data collection and analysis are also well established in various parts of the private sector, but those data have not always been shared with the community on a routine basis.[3]

Because data on all accountable entities are essential for effective performance monitoring, the committee has recommended that states and the federal government (in their policy development and regulatory roles) facilitate access to relevant data held by the private sector. As noted above in the discussion of community profiles, the committee recommends requiring that health plans, indemnity insurers, and other private-sector entities report standard types of data. The principle of helping meet the community's information needs should extend to providing more specialized data in support of performance monitoring focused on a specific health issue.

LEARNING FROM AND ABOUT HEALTH IMPROVEMENT PROCESSES

The cooperative and collaborative arrangements that are essential features of the health improvement process outlined by the committee are based on shared responsibility and mutual accountability among peers within a community rather than hierar-

[3]One information resource has been federal and state Medicare and Medicaid databases for health care provider claims for fee-for-service payment. Increasingly, however, these services are being provided through capitated managed care programs, which eliminates the need to file claims. Because those beneficiaries who continue to receive care under fee-for-service arrangements will probably be sicker or more rural than the overall beneficiary population, their claims will not be representative of the Medicare or Medicaid population (Welch and Welch, 1995). A "fee-for-data" arrangement—that is, payment to a managed care provider for filing the equivalent of a claim—has been proposed as a way to overcome the loss of this data source (Welch and Welch, 1995).

chical relationships inside or outside a community. They will depend on goodwill and respect for diverse participants in the process. Experience suggests that using performance monitoring as a form of inspection and a basis for punishing those who are not producing as expected is not an effective way to alter behavior to improve outcomes (Berwick, 1989; Osborne and Gaebler, 1992). The monitoring process can become distorted by efforts to demonstrate adequate performance and thus lose its value as a tool to identify opportunities for improvement. Furthermore, in a voluntary collaboration, some participants may choose to leave rather than to change.

Instead, a CHIP should use performance monitoring to encourage productive action and broad collaboration. Because the health improvement process outlined by the committee is new, participants should see themselves as part of "learning organizations" (e.g., Senge, 1990a,b; Ulrich et al., 1993) that can examine their own experience and use that knowledge to improve their operations. Thus, CHIP activities should include periodic examination of past health improvement efforts in the community. Valuable insight can be gained from both successful and unsuccessful experiences. Efforts to improve the CHIP itself can serve as a model for the improvement process being applied to community health issues.

A learning approach should be applied not only to the process but also to the science base for health improvement activities. Communities should draw on sources such as program reports and evaluations for local activities and on findings in the published research and evaluation literature that can help them identify the most promising opportunities. Evaluations of several major community health intervention projects are producing findings on specific interventions to address health problems, on the community intervention process itself, and on the analytic techniques to apply to community studies.

For example, the NHLBI programs to reduce coronary heart disease can provide both practical guidance on a variety of community-based approaches and cautionary lessons about their limitations (e.g., Elder et al., 1993; Fortmann et al., 1995; Murray, 1995; Luepker et al., 1996). Although interventions were often successful in reducing disease risk at the individual level, they generally were not able to reach a sufficiently large proportion of the population to alter community-level health outcomes. In addition, the unanticipated strength of other influences that were reducing risks for heart disease largely overwhelmed the community-level impact of the interventions. Among the contributions of the studies of the Kaiser Family Foundation's Community Health Promotion Grant Program are methodological developments such as approaches to examine the element of "community activation" in health promotion efforts (Wickizer et al., 1993) and determining that community-level indicators (e.g., grocery store shelf space, amount of nonsmoking seating in restaurants) can be effective and less costly alternatives to individual-level measures for monitoring the impact of interventions (e.g., Cheadle et al., 1992).

The recently established Task Force on Community Preventive Services, organized by the CDC, is expected to compile evidence on the effectiveness of many kinds of community interventions. CDC has also collaborated with the University of Kansas to develop a handbook for evaluating community efforts to control and prevent cardiovascular disease (Fawcett et al., 1995). The handbook, which outlines an evaluation process and proposes many indicators that might be used, is being tested in a community setting. Additional guidance can be expected to emerge from the work of the 25 community coalitions participating in the Community Care Network research and demonstration grant program (AHA, 1995). Evaluation of Healthy Cities/Healthy Communities activities is just beginning and will require establishing a basis for assessing health impact. The diversity of the participating communities and their approaches to health promotion in the absence of a formal theoretical framework will, however, pose a challenge (Hancock, 1993).

The health improvement process and performance monitoring components presented by the committee in this report must be examined systematically from a broader perspective. The committee's proposal should be seen as a part of an evolving body of knowledge and expertise, but both the CHIP and the performance monitoring indicators discussed in Chapter 5 need to be tested and improved over time. The committee recommends implementing and assessing the proposed CHIP in a variety of communities across the country. These communities should differ in terms of size, political structure, socioeconomic and racial composition, region of the country, and specific health issues addressed. There should also be differences in how the health improvement process is operationalized in terms of the composition of the community coalition, how health issues are identified, the way in which performance indicators are selected and monitored, and the role played by state and local health departments.

An assessment will require documenting that the many aspects of the process have been implemented and examining its impact on a community in terms of structure, process, and outcomes. Points to be examined will include the sustainability of the health improvement process overall, the participation of various stakeholders (do most continue to participate?), the ability to obtain and use data for community profiles and performance indicators, and the impact on targeted health issues. Evaluation of the CHIP and other research on community health improvement should include consideration of the effectiveness of various approaches to the selection, collection, and presentation of data. Also needed is an assessment of the full range of public and private costs of carrying out the CHIP and of ways to achieve efficiencies in these efforts. Any examination of the impact on health outcomes must take into account the time needed to achieve desired changes; assessments conducted too soon may produce misleading results. Methodological issues addressed in other evaluation activities (e.g., Koepsell et al., 1992; Green et al., 1995) should be considered in developing a framework for an assessment of the community health improvement process. In addition, experience gained in evaluating multisectorial community programs that target social issues other than health can also help inform these assessment efforts (Connell et al., 1995).

Lessons drawn from the experiences of nine communities participating in the Community-wide Health Improvement Learning Collaborative, which was organized to demonstrate the application of CQI methods to community health issues, illustrate the potential value of looking back over a community's own experience and of looking at the experiences of others (see Box 4-3). Lessons such as these can be used by a CHIP already in operation or by a community that is just starting the process.

ENHANCING THE CAPACITY FOR COMMUNITY HEALTH IMPROVEMENT

To undertake activities aimed at maintaining and enhancing health, communities need certain basic capacities and resources to anticipate, prevent, and respond to health risks and to promote those community assets and protective factors that maintain and enhance the health of individuals, families, and populations. Some of these capacities include the authority to act, sufficient funds, access to data or data collection systems, varied expertise (coalition building, program management, data collection and

BOX 4-3
LESSONS FROM THE COMMUNITY-WIDE HEALTH IMPROVEMENT COLLABORATIVE

In 1993, the Institute for Health Improvement and GOAL/QPC organized projects in nine communities, generally under the leadership of a health care organization, to demonstrate the application of continuous quality improvement techniques to respond to community health issues. The issues addressed were postneonatal mortality in Anchorage, Alaska; teen violence in Baton Rouge, Louisiana; health of women of childbearing age in Camden, New Jersey; child abuse and neglect in Edmonton, Alberta; motor vehicle injuries to children and adolescents in Kingsport, Tennessee; falls among the elderly in London, Ontario; cardiovascular health in Monroe, Louisiana; preventive cardiovascular care in Rochester, New York; and teen traffic injuries and deaths in Twin Falls, Idaho.

The projects began with basic questions on what was to be accomplished, how to know that a change was an improvement, and what changes to make to achieve improvements. Once those questions had been answered, a second set of questions guided the planning process: how to choose a topic; how to set up a measurement system; and how to select interventions.

A review of experiences in planning and implementing these projects suggests several opportunities to move the health improvement process ahead more quickly:

- a large-scale community assessment need not be a prerequisite for initiatives on specific health issues;
- more than one approach can be followed in addressing a health issue;
- the overall goal of the intervention should be clear but a single point of control for activities undertaken by separate groups is not essential;
- implementation plans should include at least one step expected to produce a change within the first few months of a project;
- planned interventions should be tested on a small scale and revised as needed before pursuing community-wide implementation;
- once a test shows that an intervention can lead to improvements, support should be sought for more widespread implementation;
- participation by subject matter experts can help planning and implementation move more quickly; and
- information on similar efforts in other communities can suggest both opportunities and potential problems.

SOURCE: Knapp and Hotopp (1995); Nolan and Knapp (1996).

analysis, and so on), and the support of an array of community stakeholders. This section reviews capacities needed at the community level for health improvement efforts and performance monitoring and ways that activities in a broader context can improve the resources available to communities.

Community Capacities

"Capacity" includes those processes, products, and abilities that enable the entities contributing to the production of community health to perform varied functions. For example, the public health system should be able to maintain the readiness to respond to emerging health problems while operating population-based prevention and health protection programs on a routine basis. Similarly, health plans need the ability to provide high-quality clinical services and to maintain reliable administrative systems that support efficient operation of the organization. The ability of an individual or organization to perform according to expectations depends on motivation, capability, and preparedness to create the necessary infrastructure to carry out critical processes and thus achieve desired outcomes.

For the public health system, both core functions (IOM, 1988; see Box 4-4) and essential services (Baker et al., 1994)[4] have been specified. These functions and the activities required to carry them out point to needed capacities. One source, *Blueprint for a Healthy Community: A Guide for Local Health Departments* (NACHO and CDC, 1994), proposes the following set of capacities: health assessment, including data monitoring and analysis; policy development; administration; health promotion; health protection; quality assurance; training and education for competent staff; and

[4]The essential public health services have been defined as (1) monitor health status to identify and solve community health problems; (2) diagnose and investigate health problems and health hazards in the community; (3) inform, educate, and empower people about health issues; (4) mobilize community partnerships and action to identify and solve health problems; (5) develop policies and plans that support individual and community health efforts; (6) enforce laws and regulations that protect health and assure safety; (7) link people to needed personal health services and assure provision of health care when otherwise unavailable; (8) assure a competent workforce—public health and personal care; (9) evaluate effectiveness, accessibility, and quality of personal and population-based health services; and (10) research for new insights and innovative solutions to health problems (Baker et al., 1994).

BOX 4-4
CORE FUNCTIONS OF PUBLIC HEALTH

- *Assessment:* Regular collection, analysis, interpretation, and communication of information about health conditions, risks, and assets in a community
- *Policy development:* Development, implementation, and evaluation of plans and policies, for public health in general and priority health needs in particular, in a manner that incorporates scientific information and community values
- *Assurance:* Ensuring—by encouragement, regulation, or direct action—that programs and interventions that maintain and improve health are carried out

SOURCE: IOM (1988); Washington State Department of Health (1994).

community empowerment. Adequate funding is also cited as an essential resource.

Other entities in a community also have specific functions that guide their participation in health improvement. These functions have been articulated in varying ways. For example, accreditation standards for hospitals and health plans point to clinical, organizational, and administrative functions that are deemed important (e.g., see JCAHO, 1996a; NCQA, 1996b). The NCQA (1996b) standards, for example, address quality improvement, physician credentials, member's rights and responsibilities, preventive health services, utilization management, and medical records.

Looking to the future, the Pew Health Professions Commission (1995) has proposed a set of "competencies" that the health professions should develop and enhance over the next decade (e.g., care for the community's health, clinical competence, prevention and health promotion, appropriate use of technology).

It is also possible to consider the capacities of a community as a whole—what the National Civic League (1993a) has called the *civic infrastructure.* The specific elements identified are citizen participation, community leadership, government performance, volunteerism and philanthropy, intergroup relations, civic education, community information sharing, capacity for cooperation and consensus building, community vision and pride, and inter-community cooperation. Various resources related to each of these areas have been identified (National Civic League, 1993a).

Capacities for the Community Health Improvement Process

The collaborative health improvement process described by the committee requires capacity in at least three interacting contexts: the community as a whole, a community health coalition, and a variety of individual community stakeholders. For the community, critical capacities for initiating a CHIP include an interest in protecting and improving health and a willingness to participate in a collective process toward that end. This support for health improvement can derive from individuals, organizations, or both and might develop from perceptions of unmet needs or promising opportunities. Valuable health-enhancing activities can, of course, be undertaken without a CHIP and bring considerable benefit to the community. Such efforts, however, may not reflect broad community priorities and may end up duplicating work being done on other projects or by other entities in the community. Part of the challenge a community will face is organizing the CHIP so that it can successfully blend these capacities and resources.

Where a CHIP can be instituted, the community coalition, or other agents of the process, will require a varied set of capacities to carry out all phases of the process. The ability to organize and sustain a CHIP, including the performance monitoring elements, is key. For some tasks, such as data collection or service delivery, a coalition may want or have to rely on the resources of individual participants. These participants must be able to support the CHIP and carry out the activities that implement a coalition's health improvement strategy. (The relationships among a community, a CHIP, and CHIP participants are presented here in a generic form that does not reflect the complexity and diversity of specific community settings.)

By examining the steps in a CHIP, it is possible to identify several capacities that will have to be available to the overall process.

• *Leadership:* As proposed by the committee, a CHIP rests heavily on the willing collaboration of many community stakeholders and less on obligations created by law and regulation. Thus, a source of leadership is critical to initiate and sustain the process, particularly in reaching agreement among stakeholders regarding areas of accountable performance. In many communities, the health department is likely to lead a CHIP, but effective leadership may also come from others, in either the public or the private sector. Communities may be able to draw on a variety of resources in the public and private sectors to enhance leadership capacity (e.g., Chamber of Commerce programs, regional and state-based public health leadership programs; also see resources identified by the National Civic League [1994]).

• *Community empowerment:* This capacity, which complements leadership, is necessary to help bring a broad spectrum of the community into all phases of a CHIP. A broad characterization suggests that community empowerment promotes participation by individuals, organizations, and communities in a process that aims at achieving increased individual and community control, political efficacy, improved quality of community life, and social justice (Wallerstein, 1992). Based on the health department role described in *Blueprint for a Healthy Community* (NACHO and CDC, 1994), community empowerment encompasses the ability to establish and maintain a community (versus an "expert") perspective on health priorities and activities and to establish an environment in which many stakeholders can work together. The ability to facilitate priority setting might also be included here.

• *Authority to act:* Even though much of a CHIP depends on cooperative efforts, the need remains for formal authority to carry out some essential activities. Certain forms of data collection, for example, must have official sanction and must meet requirements for adequate protection of privacy and confidentiality. The implementation of specific health improvement strategies might also depend on having formal authority to act in the community at large or within a specific setting (e.g., to enforce environmental regulations, change a workplace smoking policy, or co-locate an immunization clinic with a public assistance office).

• *Expertise and skills*: A CHIP will require access to diverse expertise and skills through its own staff (if one is created) and through the individuals and organizations from the community who participate in the process. Two specific areas are noted here:

1. *Subject matter expertise:* A CHIP is likely to benefit from access to advice from subject matter experts to identify factors contributing to health problems, develop health improvement strategies that reflect evidence for the effectiveness of specific interventions, select performance indicators, and assess performance results. Academic health centers, schools of public health, and similar scholarly institutions could be particularly valuable sources of such assistance.

2. *Technical expertise:* Data collection and analysis along with the design and operation of information systems will be important for the success of the kind of health improvement and performance monitoring processes proposed by the committee. Expertise in these areas can be applied to health problems of all types. The need for such expertise is well recognized, if not always available, in state and local health departments. In addition, other public agencies as well as health plans and a variety of other organizations in the private sector could be resources for a CHIP.

• *Information systems:* Information systems reflect an operational capacity to receive, process, and communicate information, data, and reports to the community (e.g., vital statistics, population-based surveys, health services records, qualitative information). A CHIP is likely to rely on a variety of information systems in a community (e.g., the health department, other public agencies, hospitals, health plans) but will also need a means of drawing together the information from separate sources in a meaningful way. Support from CHIP participants could include funding, personnel, data, and data processing and analysis.

• *Implementation resources:* Successful implementation of a health improvement strategy will depend on the ability of various accountable entities in the community to provide needed services and take other actions as appropriate. The specific functions will vary depending on the health problem and the particular role of a specific entity.

• *Administrative skills and resources:* Administrative abilities and resources will be a critical element to support the operation of all CHIP activities. Among the elements that might be included are financial and organizational management, physical resources (e.g., computers, software, office space), and personnel (e.g., with skills in areas such as community development, analysis, report production). Some of these resources might reside in a CHIP-specific setting, but a CHIP might also rely on resources available among participants or through donated time and materials.

• *Funding:* Financial resources are an essential underpinning for almost any activity. A CHIP will benefit from access to an established and predictable source of funds, such as a yearly allocation from state or local government or from sources in the private sector. Alternatively, resources provided "in-kind" (e.g., staff time, materials, equipment) could limit but probably not eliminate the need for direct funding.

Capacity Assessment

Since publication of *The Future of Public Health* (IOM, 1988), ensuring the capacity of state and local health departments to carry out the core functions has been a concern in the public health sector. *APEXPH* process, for example, includes as one of its first steps an assessment of local health department capacity (NACHO, 1991). There is also a growing appreciation that the core functions include a range of activities that can be performed in partnership with the private sector and community-based organizations, a view that supports the CHIP's collaborative approach (Richards et al., 1995). Several state health departments (e.g., Illinois, Massachusetts, Minnesota, and Washington) have made capacity assessment and development a priority at both the state and the local levels. The approach taken by the Washington State Department of Health is described in Box 4-5. These efforts to address capacity in the public health system might serve as models for broader efforts to assess community capacity for health improvement activities. Also available are materials developed by the National Civic League (1993a) that can help communities evaluate their civic infrastructure.

National Opportunities for Capacity Development

Individual communities can benefit from lessons learned elsewhere, but they need a way to obtain such information and, perhaps, guidance on how to apply it. National organizations are well placed to produce or support the development of such information resources.

Better Tools

Professional expertise and community experience with the health improvement process need to be captured and shared. Although a wide variety of excellent resources on community health assessment and CQI currently exist, those materials generally do not link assessment and CQI concepts and techniques in the way that is envisioned for a CHIP. Therefore, in the committee's view, federal agencies, national professional organizations, and foundations should provide leadership to promote the development of new and better tools that can help communities achieve success with the proposed health improvement process. These tools might take the form of workbooks, seminars, or other materials that can

BOX 4-5
WASHINGTON STATE'S PUBLIC HEALTH IMPROVEMENT PLAN

In 1993, the Washington State Department of Health, in collaboration with multiple partners, undertook the design and implementation of a new paradigm for the public health system. Improving the health status of the state's population through prevention, health protection, and health promotion is the goal. The primary mission of state and local public health jurisdictions, in partnership with various community and health-related organizations, is providing population-based services through the core functions of public health. Part of this mission includes monitoring health system performance.

The core functions have been articulated as standards in the *Public Health Improvement Plan* (Washington State Department of Health, 1994), with accountability assigned to public health agencies, and indicators have been developed to monitor the public health capacities required to carry out those functions. The Public Health Improvement Plan also presents indicators for monitoring health outcomes and interventions for improving the health status of Washington's populations. In addition, it presents principles for structuring the governance and financing of the public health system.

Monitoring the performance of the public health system begins with a large-scale collaboration on a statewide health status report, *The Health of Washington*. The report covers the causes of most deaths, critical health risks, many serious illnesses, major injury categories, environmental indicators, and health system indicators. It provides data for comparisons across local, state, and national levels; time trends; indicator-to-indicator comparisons; examination of risk and protective factors; and guidance on possible interventions. It will be used, along with community assessments and other data tools, to make information-based policy decisions.

In addition, each of the state's 33 local health jurisdictions is expected to facilitate a comprehensive community health assessment process and the development of a report that presents locally derived health indicators as well as community risk and protective factors for a defined geographic area. These assessments are used to set community priorities for population-based activities through the public health system and its many partners.

Public health performance is monitored through performance-based contracts and a self-evaluation tool, which collects data on the capacity developed and maintained within public health and the performance of the core functions. Performance measurement indicators are based on the clusters of standards set by the Public Health Improvement Plan. Several demonstration pilot projects in the state are working on the development of tools for assessing health care system performance. One in particular is designed to demonstrate in real practice settings the practicability, utility, and value of implementing the Clinical Outcome Measure Amended HEDIS (COMAH) strategy.

catalog and convey to communities information on best CHIP practices, specific model performance measures for a variety of health issues, the interpretation of changes in these measures, and available data resources. States and academic institutions should assume a role in using these materials to provide technical assistance to communities. The committee believes that states have a special responsibility to assist communities in obtaining data for community health profiles.

There is also a need for further development of performance measurement tools to make the health improvement process more effective. Work is needed on standard measures for both community health profiles and model indicator sets for specific health issues. These measures should be able to perform well in individual communities and be suitable for cross-community comparison. Also necessary are efforts to address both the enhancement of existing measures and the development of valid measures in areas for which they do not currently exist. Measures of quality of life and consumer satisfaction that are suitable for use in community surveys are particularly important. For some health issues, the development of measurement tools cannot proceed until additional research has provided a suitable evidence base. Support should also be given to research to develop and improve the techniques of measurement and analysis that can be applied to community-level performance monitoring (e.g., small area analysis). Technical assistance from federal agencies with health data expertise could be particularly helpful to states and localities in testing and improving the quality of vital statistics and other health data.

As with work on other resource materials, this process should bring together federal agencies, national professional organizations, and foundations, in conjunction with state and local health agencies and other community stakeholders. Individuals and organizations with expertise in specific health issues (e.g., injury, reproductive health, environmental and occupational health) might assume leadership for the development of performance measures for those health issues. The indicators proposed by the committee (see Chapter 5 and Appendix A) should be viewed as an *initial* step in what must be a more extensive indicator development process.

Electronic systems have the potential to provide rapid and interactive access to such data, and as has been noted, some states (e.g., Massachusetts) have assigned a high priority to the development of broader electronic health information systems.

National leadership and resource support could also be helpful. Some states and communities are using the Information Network for Public Health Officials (INPHO) developed by the CDC (1995a) as a basis for electronic communication and data exchange. Support from foundations and from the CDC is also playing an important role in the development of computerized immunization registries in some states and communities (Faherty et al., 1996). Enhanced public health information resources are also being pursued through the National Information Infrastructure project, which is aimed at enhancing the nation's overall framework for telecommunications and computer technology (Lasker et al., 1995).

Work being done to develop more effective and extensive health *care* information systems is also relevant to the data collection and analysis tasks facing community health coalitions in a CHIP. The IOM report *Health Data in the Information Age* (IOM, 1994a) outlines the roles and obligations of what it generically calls "health data organizations" (HDOs), entities that are an anticipated product of the evolution of health and health care information systems. Discussions also refer to "community health information networks" (e.g., see Duncan, 1995). The prototypical HDO is described as operating under a single common authority; serving a specific, defined geographic area; having inclusive population files; having files with person-identified (or identifiable) data; having data covering administrative, clinical, and health status information and on satisfaction with services; acquiring and maintaining information from a variety of sources for multiple uses; having the capability to manipulate data electronically; and supporting electronic access for real-time use (IOM, 1994a). Although this work currently relies primarily on a health care provider perspective, the potential would seem to exist to adopt a broader approach that can support community health improvement activities (Milio, 1995)

Professional Training

In the long run, effective dissemination of CHIP practices and successful performance monitoring techniques will depend on the development of educational programs that can train a variety of professionals. Because health departments have a responsibility to assure that processes to protect and improve health are available to communities (IOM, 1988), schools of public health should be one of the starting points for such programs. The field model's multidimensional concept of the production of health, which is embedded in the committee's approach to the health improvement process and performance monitoring, suggests that an academic program should introduce CHIP as a way to think about the application of public health as a group of interrelated academic disciplines (epidemiology, biostatistics, environmental health, health behavior, and so on) to the practice of community health improvement (e.g., see Bor et al., 1995).

Public health is, however, only one of many fields that can contribute expertise to a community health improvement process and to performance monitoring components. Thus, the committee recommends that educational programs for professionals in fields including, but not limited to, public health, community medicine, nursing, health care administration, public policy, and public administration include CHIP and performance monitoring concepts and practices in their curricula for preservice and midcareer students. Other fields in which CHIP might be addressed include environmental health, mental health and substance abuse counseling and program administration, maternal and child health, and the behavioral sciences.

CONCLUSIONS

In this chapter, the committee has laid out the framework for an iterative and evolving community health improvement process that relies on collaboration among a diversity of stakeholders and uses measurement as a tool for establishing stakeholder accountability for contributions to that process. The broad perspective that the field model provides on health and the factors contributing to it gives a CHIP a basis for seeking opportunities for health improvement throughout the community, not just within the health department or the health care provider's office.

The committee's proposal for a CHIP builds on much other work that has been done in health assessment, community health planning, and performance measurement, but it advances these past efforts in two ways. First, it looks beyond assessments of community health status to accountability for measurable health improvement. Second, it looks beyond performance within an individual organization serving a specific segment of a community to the way in which the activities of many organizations contribute to health improvement throughout the community.

The proposed process reflects the committee's judgment based on experience and available evidence, but the CHIP needs to be tested and assessed so that it can be refined and enhanced. Individual communities should look to the national and state levels for these assessments and for the development of tools that can help them use a CHIP. Although the committee views the health improvement process it has described as an essential tool for communities, it emphasizes that attention to using and enhancing this process should not obscure the primary goal of health improvement.

REFERENCES

AHA (American Hospital Association). 1995. News Release. 25 Partnerships Named to Receive Grants in Community Network Competition. Washington, D.C. August 22.

AHCPR (Agency for Health Care Policy and Research). 1995. *Using Clinical Practice Guidelines to Evaluate Quality of Care.* Vol. 1. AHCPR Pub. No. 95-0045. Rockville, Md.: U.S. Department of Health and Human Services.

AMBHA (American Managed Behavioral Healthcare Association). 1995. *Performance Measures for Managed Behavioral Healthcare Programs.* Washington, D.C.: AMBHA Quality Improvement and Clinical Services Committee.

Annie E. Casey Foundation. 1996. *KIDS COUNT Data Book: State Profiles of Child Well-Being.* Baltimore: Annie E. Casey Foundation.

APHA (American Public Health Association), Association of Schools of Public Health, Association of State and Territorial Health Officials, National Association of County Health Officials, United States Conference of Local Health Officers, Department of Health and Human Services, Public Health Service, Centers for Disease Control. 1991. *Healthy Communities 2000: Model Standards.* 3rd ed. Washington, D.C.: APHA.

Armstead, R.C., Elstein, P., and Gorman, J. 1995. Toward a 21st Century Quality-Measurement System for Managed-Care Organizations. *Health Care Financing Review* 16(4):25–37.

Ashton, J., and Seymour, H. 1988. *The New Public Health: The Liverpool Experience.* Philadelphia: Open University Press.

Baker, E.L., Melton, R.J., Stange, P.V., et al. 1994. Health Reform and the Health of the Public: Forging Community Health Partnerships. *Journal of the American Medical Association* 272:1276–1282.

Batalden, P.B., and Stoltz, P.A. 1993. A Framework for the Continual Improvement of Health Care: Building and Applying Professional and Improvement Knowledge to Test Changes in Daily Work. *Journal on Quality Improvement* 19:424–447.

Benjamin, A.E., and Downs, G.W. 1982. Evaluating the National Health Planning and Resource Development Act: Learning from Experience? *Journal of Health Policy, Politics and Law* 7:707–722.

Berwick, D.M. 1989. Continuous Improvement as an Ideal in Health Care. *New England Journal of Medicine* 320:53–56.

Berwick, D.M., Godfrey, A.B., and Roessner, J. 1990. *Curing Health Care: New Strategies for Quality Improvement.* San Francisco: Jossey-Bass.

Blum, H.L. 1981. *Planning for Health.* 2nd ed. New York: Human Sciences Press.

Bor, D., Chambers, L.W., Dessau, L., Larson, T., and Wold, C., eds. 1995. *Community Health Improvement Through Information and Action.* San Francisco: University of California, Health of the Public Program.

Brook, R.H., and Lohr, K.N. 1985. Efficacy, Effectiveness, Variations, and Quality: Boundary-Crossing Research. *Medical Care* 23:710–722.

Bunker, J.P., Forrest, W.H., Mosteller, F., and Vandam, L.D., eds. 1969. *The National Halothane Study.* Bethesda, Md.: National Institute of General Medical Sciences.

CDC (Centers for Disease Control and Prevention). 1991. Consensus Set of Health Status Indicators for the General Assessment of Community Health Status—United States. *Morbidity and Mortality Weekly Report* 40:449–451.

CDC. 1994. Organization and Implementation of the Uniform Data Sets (Preventive Health and Health Services Block Grant). November 1. Atlanta, Ga.: U.S. Department of Health and Human Services. (mimeo)

CDC. 1995a. *CDC INPHO Fact Sheet* [WWW document]. URL http://www.cdc.gov

CDC. 1995b. *Planned Approach to Community Health: Guide for the Local Coordinator.* Atlanta, Ga.: CDC, National Center for Chronic Disease Prevention and Health Promotion.

Center for the Advancement of Health and Western Consortium for Public Health. 1995. *Performance Indicators: An Overview of Private Sector, State, and Federal Efforts to Assess and Document the Characteristics, Performance, and Value of Health Care Delivery.* Washington, D.C.: Center for the Advancement of Health.

Center for Quality of Care Research and Education and Mikalix & Company. 1996. *A COmputerized Needs-oriented QUality measurement Evaluation SysTem.* Final Report. Boston: Harvard School of Public Health.

CHA (Catholic Health Association). 1995. *A Workbook on Community Accountability in Integrated Delivery.* St. Louis: CHA.

Chambers, L.W., Bourns, E., and Underwood, J. 1996. *Setting Public Health Priorities: A Guide to Resource Allocation.* Regional Municipality of Hamilton–Wentworth, Ontario: Regional Public Health Department.

Chassin, M.R., Brook, R.H., Park, R.E., et al. 1986. Variations in the Use of Medical and Surgical Practices by the Medicare Population. *New England Journal of Medicine* 314:285–290.

Cheadle, A., Wagner, E., Koepsell, T., Kristal, A., and Patrick, D. 1992. Environmental Indicators: A Tool for Evaluating Community-Based Health Promotion Programs. *American Journal of Preventive Medicine* 8:345–350.

Children Now. 1996. *The Report Card Guide: A Step-by-Step Guide to Producing a Report Card on the Conditions of Children in Your Community* [WWW document]. URL http://www.dnai.com/~children/report_guide.html

COMMIT (Community Intervention Trial for Smoking Cessation). 1991. COMMIT: Summary of Design and Intervention. *Journal of the National Cancer Institute* 83:1620–1628.

Connell, J.P., and Kubisch, A.C. 1996. Applying a Theories of Change Approach to the Evaluation of Comprehensive Community Initiatives: Progress, Prospects, and Problems. Draft.

Connell, F.A., Day, R.W., and LoGerfo, J.P. 1981. Hospitalization of Medicaid Children: Analysis of Small Area Variations in Admission Rates. *American Journal of Public Health* 71:606–613.

Connell, J.P., Kubisch, A.C., Schorr, L.B., and Weiss, C.H. 1995. *New Approaches to Evaluating Community Initiatives: Concepts, Methods, and Contexts.* Washington, D.C.: Aspen Institute.

Duhl, L.J., and Drake, J.E. 1995. Healthy Cities: A Systematic View of Health. *Current Issues in Public Health* 1:105–109.

Duncan, K. 1995. Evolving Community Health Information Networks. *Frontiers of Health Services Management* 12(1):5–41.

Eddy, D., and Billings, J. 1988. The Quality of Medical Evidence: Implications for Quality of Care. *Health Affairs* 7(1):19–32.

Elder, J.P., McGraw, S.A., Abrams, D.B., et al. 1986. Organizational and Community Approaches to Community-Wide Prevention of Heart Disease: The First Two Years of the Pawtucket Heart Health Program. *Preventive Medicine* 15:107–117.

Elder, J.P., Schmid, T.L, Dower, P., and Hedlund, S. 1993. Community Heart Health Programs: Components, Rationale, and Strategies. *Journal of Public Health Policy* 14:463–479.

Evans, R.G., and Stoddart, G.L. 1994. Producing Health, Consuming Health Care. In *Why Are Some People Healthy and Others Not? The Determinants of Health of Populations.* R.G. Evans, M.L. Barer, and T.R. Marmor, eds. New York: Aldine De Gruyter.

FAcct (Foundation for Accountability). 1995. Guidebook for Performance Measurement: Prototype. Portland, Ore.: FAcct. September 22.

Faherty, K.M., Waller, C.J., DeFriese, G.H., et al. 1996. Prospects for Childhood Immunization Registries in Public Health Assessment and Assurance: Initial Observations from the All Kids Count Initiative Projects. *Journal of Public Health Management and Practice* 2(1):1–11.

Farquhar, J.W., Fortmann, S.P., Maccoby, N., et al. 1985. The Stanford Five-City Project: Design and Methods. *American Journal of Epidemiology* 122:323–334.

Fawcett, S.B., Sterling, T.D., Paine-Andrews, A., et al. 1995. *Evaluating Community Efforts to Prevent Cardiovascular Diseases.* Atlanta, Ga.: CDC, National Center for Chronic Disease Prevention and Health Promotion.

Feighery, E., and Rogers, T. 1990. *Building and Maintaining Effective Coalitions.* How-to Guides on Community Health Promotion, No. 12. Palo Alto, Calif.: Stanford Health Promotion Resource Center.

Flynn, B.C. 1996. Healthy Cities: Toward Worldwide Health Promotion. *Annual Review of Public Health* 17:299–309.

Fortmann, S.P., Flora, J.A., Winkleby, M.A., Schooler, C., Taylor, C.B., and Farquhar, J.W. 1995. Community Intervention Trials: Reflections on the Stanford Five-City Project Experience. *American Journal of Epidemiology* 142:576–586.

GAO (General Accounting Office). 1996. *Executive Guide: Effectively Implementing the Government Performance and Results Act.* GAO/GGD-96-118. Washington, D.C.: U.S. Government Printing Office.

Gordon, R.L., Baker, E.L., Roper, W.L., and Omenn, G.S. 1996. Prevention and the Reforming U.S. Health Care System: Changing Roles and Responsibilities for Public Health. *Annual Review of Public Health* 17:489–509.

Gore, A. 1993. *From Red Tape to Results: Creating a Government That Works Better and Costs Less.* Report of the National Performance Review. Washington, D.C.: U.S. Government Printing Office.

Gostin, L.O., and Lazzarini, Z. 1995. Childhood Immunization Registries: A National Review of Public Health Information Systems and the Protection of Privacy. *Journal of the American Medical Association* 274:1793–1799.

Gostin, L.O., Turek-Brezina, J., Powers, M., Kozloff, R., Faden, R., and Steinauer, D.D. 1993. Privacy and Security of Personal Information in a New Health Care System. *Journal of the American Medical Association* 270:2487–2493.

Gostin, L.O., Lazzarini, Z., Neslund, V.S., and Osterholm, M.T. 1996. The Public Health Information Infrastructure: A National Review of the Law on Health Information Privacy. *Journal of the American Medical Association* 275:1921–1927.

Gottlieb, S.R. 1974. A Brief History of Health Planning the United States. In *Regulating Health Facilities Construction.* C. Havighurst, ed. Washington, D.C.: American Enterprise Institute for Public Policy Research.

Green, S.B., Corle, D.K., Gail, M.H., et al. 1995. Interplay Between Design and Analysis for Behavioral Intervention Trials with Community as the Unit of Randomization. *American Journal of Epidemiology* 142:587–593.

Group Health Cooperative of Puget Sound. 1996. *Community Services Initiatives* [WWW document]. URL http://www.ghc.org/about_gh/comserv.html

Hancock, T. 1993. The Evolution, Impact and Significance of the Healthy Cities/Healthy Communities Movement. *Journal of Public Health Policy* 14:5–18.

Hatry, H., Wholey, J.S., Anderson, W.F., et al. 1994. *Toward Useful Performance Measurement: Lessons Learned From Initial Pilot Performance Plans Prepared Under the Government Performance and Results Act.* Washington, D.C.: National Academy of Public Administration.

IOM (Institute of Medicine). 1984. *Community Oriented Primary Care: A Practical Assessment.* Washington, D.C.: National Academy Press.

IOM. 1988. *The Future of Public Health.* Washington, D.C.: National Academy Press.

IOM. 1990. *Medicare: A Strategy for Quality Assurance.* Vol. I. K.N. Lohr, ed. Washington, D.C.: National Academy Press.

IOM. 1992. *Guidelines for Clinical Practice: From Development to Use.* M.J. Field and K.N. Lohr, eds. Washington, D.C.: National Academy Press.

IOM. 1994a. *Health Data in the Information Age: Use Disclosure and Privacy.* M.S. Donaldson and K.N. Lohr, eds. Washington, D.C.: National Academy Press.

IOM. 1994b. *Overcoming Barriers to Immunization: A Workshop Summary.* J.S. Durch, ed. Washington, D.C.: National Academy Press.

JCAHO (Joint Commission on Accreditation of Healthcare Organizations). 1996a. *Joint Commission Standards* [WWW document]. URL http://www.jcaho.org/stds.html

JCAHO. 1996b. Joint Commission to Create National Library of Healthcare Indicators. *Joint Commission Perspectives* 16(2):1,4.

Joint Council Committee on Quality in Public Health. 1996. *Promoting Quality Care for Communities: The Role of Health Departments in an Era of Managed Care.* Washington, D.C.: National Association of County and City Health Officials.

Kark, S.L., and Abramson, J.H. 1982. Community Oriented Primary Care: Meaning and Scope. In *Community Oriented Primary Care: Conference Proceedings.* E. Connor and F. Mullan, eds. Washington, D.C.: National Academy Press.

Knapp, M., and Hotopp, D. 1995. Applying TQM to Community Health Improvement: Nine Works in Progress. *The Quality Letter for Healthcare Leaders* 7(July–August):23–29.

Koepsell, T.D., Wagner, E.H., Cheadle, A.C., et al. 1992. Selected Methodological Issues in Evaluating Community-Based Health Promotion and Disease Prevention Programs. *Annual Review of Public Health* 13:31–57.

Krasny, J. 1980. A New Approach to Decision Making for Health Care Managers. *Health Management Forum* 1:71–87.

Kreuter, M.W. 1992. PATCH: Its Origin, Basic Concepts, and Links to Contemporary Public Health Policy. *Journal of Health Education* 23:135–139.

Lalonde, M. 1974. *A New Perspective on the Health of Canadians.* Ottawa: Health and Welfare, Canada.

Lasker, R.D., Humphreys, B.L., and Braithwaite, W.R. 1995. Making a Powerful Connection: The Health of the Public and the National Information Infrastructure. Report of the U.S. Public Health Service Public Health Data Policy Coordinating Committee. Washington, D.C. July 6.

Lefkowitz, B. 1983. *Health Planning: Lessons for the Future.* Rockville, Md.: Aspen Systems Corporation.

Lewin-VHI, Inc. 1995. *Key Monitoring Indicators of the Nation's Health and Health Care and Their Support by NCHS Data Systems.* Fairfax, Va.: Lewin-VHI.

Luepker, R.V., Rastam, L., Hannan, P.J., et al. 1996. Community Education for Cardiovascular Disease Prevention: Morbidity and Mortality Results from the Minnesota Heart Health Program. *American Journal of Epidemiology* 144:351–362.

Luft, H.S., Bunker, J.P., and Enthoven, A.C. 1979. Should Operations Be Regionalized? An Empirical Study of the Relationship Between Surgical Volume and Mortality. *New England Journal of Medicine* 301:1364–1369.

Massachusetts Department of Public Health. 1995. Community Health Network Areas: A Guide to the Community Health Network Initiative. Boston: Massachusetts Department of Public Health. (brochure)

MCHB (Maternal and Child Health Bureau). 1995. Annual Report Guidance for the Maternal and Child Health Services Block Grant Program. OMB No. 0915-0172. Rockville, Md.: U.S. Department of Health and Human Services/ PHS/HRSA.

McHenry County Department of Health. 1994. *McHenry County Project for Local Assessment of Need: Community Health Plan.* Woodstock, Ill.: McHenry County Department of Health.

Milio, N. 1995. Creating Community Information Networks for Healthy Communities. *Frontiers of Health Services Management* 12(1):53–59.

Mintzberg, H. 1996. Managing Government; Governing Management. *Harvard Business Review* 74(3):75–83.

Missouri Department of Health. 1996. *CHART: Community Health Assessment Resource Team* [WWW document]. URL http://health.state.mo.us

Mittelmark, M.B., Luepker, R.V., Jacobs, D.R., et al. 1986. Community-wide Prevention of Cardiovascular Disease: Education Strategies of the Minnesota Heart Health Program. *Preventive Medicine* 15:1–17.

Murray, D.M. 1995. Design and Analysis of Community Trials: Lessons from the Minnesota Heart Health Program. *American Journal of Epidemiology* 142:569–575.

NACCHO (National Association of County and City Health Officials). 1995. *1992–1993 National Profile of Local Health Departments.* Washington, D.C.: NACCHO.

NACHO (National Association of County Health Officials). 1991. *APEXPH: Assessment Protocol for Excellence in Public Health.* Washington, D.C.: NACHO.

NACHO and CDC. 1994. *Blueprint for a Healthy Community: A Guide for Local Health Departments.* Washington, D.C.: NACHO.

Nadzam, D.M., Turpin, R., Hanold, L.S., and White, R.E. 1993. Data-Driven Performance Improvement in Health Care: The Joint Commission's Indicator Measurement System (IMSystem). *Joint Commission Journal of Quality Improvement* 19:492–500.

National Civic League. 1993a. *The Civic Index: A New Approach to Improving Community Life.* Denver: National Civic League.

National Civic League. 1993b. *The Healthy Communities Handbook.* Denver: National Civic League.

National Civic League. 1994. *Healthy Communities Resource Guide.* Denver: National Civic League Press.

NCQA (National Committee for Quality Assurance). 1993. *Health Plan Employer Data and Information Set and Users Manual, Version 2.0 (HEDIS 2.0).* Washington, D.C.: NCQA.

NCQA. 1996a. HEDIS 3.0 Draft for Public Comment. Washington, D.C.: NCQA.

NCQA. 1996b. *What Is NCQA Accreditation?* [WWW document] URL http://www.ncqa.org

Nolan, T.W., and Knapp, M. 1996. Community-wide Health Improvement: Lessons from the IHI-GOAL/QPC Learning Cooperative. *The Quality Letter for Healthcare Leaders* 8(1):13–20.

Novick, L.F., Bialek, R., and Flake, M. 1995. *Practice Guidelines for Public Health: Assessment of Scientific Evidence, Feasibility, and Benefits.* Baltimore: Council on Linkages Between Academia and Public Health Practice.

Osborne, D., and Gaebler, T. 1992. *Reinventing Government: How the Entrepreneurial Spirit Is Transforming the Public Sector.* Reading, Mass.: Addison-Wesley.

Pew Health Professions Commission. 1995. *Critical Challenges: Revitalizing the Health Professions for the Twenty-First Century.* San Francisco: University of California at San Francisco Center for the Health Professions.

Pickett, G.E., and Hanlon, J.J. 1990. *Public Health Administration and Practice.* 9th ed. St. Louis: C.V. Mosby.

Richards, T.B., Rogers, J.J., Christenson, G.M., Miller, C.A., Taylor, M.S., and Cooper, A.D. 1995. Evaluating Local Public Health Performance at a Community Level on a Statewide Basis. *Journal of Public Health Management and Practice* 1(4):70–83.

Roadmap Implementation Task Force. 1990. *The Road to Better Health for All of Illinois: Improving the Public Health System.* Springfield: Illinois Department of Public Health.

Roper, W., Winkewerder, W., Hackbarth, G., and Krakauer, H. 1988. Effectiveness in Health Care: An Initiative to Evaluate and Improve Medical Practice. *New England Journal of Medicine* 319:1197–1202.

Roper, W.L., Baker, E.L., Jr., Dyal, W.W., and Nicola, R.M. 1992. Strengthening the Public Health System. *Public Health Reports* 107:609–615.

Rosser, W.W., Hutchison, B.G., McDowell, I., and Newell, C. 1992. Use of Reminders to Increase Compliance with Tetanus Booster Vaccination. *Canadian Medical Association Journal* 146:911–917.

Senge, P.M. 1990a. *The Fifth Discipline: The Art and Practice of the Learning Organization.* New York: Doubleday/Currency.

Senge, P.M. 1990b. The Leader's New Work: Building Learning Organizations. *Sloan Management Review* 32(1):7–23.

Showstack, J., Lurie, N., Leatherman, S., Fisher, E., and Inui, T. 1996. Health of the Public: The Private-Sector Challenge. *Journal of the American Medical Association* 276:1071–1074.

Sigmond, R.M. 1995. Back to the Future: Partnerships and Coordination for Community Health. *Frontiers of Health Services Management* 11(4):5–36.

Sofaer, S. 1988. Community Health Planning in the United States: A Post-Mortem. *Family and Community Health* 10(4):1–12.

Sofaer, S. 1995. *Performance Indicators: A Commentary from the Perspective of an Expanded View of Health.* Washington, D.C.: Center for the Advancement of Health.

Tarlov, A.R., Kehrer, B.H., Hall, D.P., et al. 1987. Foundation Work: The Health Promotion Program of the Henry J. Kaiser Family Foundation. *American Journal of Health Promotion* 2:74–80.

Turnock, B.J., Handler, A., Dyal, W.W., et al. 1994. Implementing and Assessing Organizational Practices in Local Health Departments. *Public Health Reports* 109:478–484.

Ulrich, D., Jick, T., and Von Glinow, M.A. 1993. High-Impact Learning: Building and Diffusing Learning Capability. *Organizational Dynamics* 22(2):52–66.

USDHHS (U.S. Department of Health and Human Services). 1991. *Healthy People 2000: National Health Promotion and Disease Prevention Objectives.* DHHS Pub. No. (PHS) 91-50212. Washington, D.C.: Office of the Assistant Secretary for Health.

USDHHS. No date. Performance Measurement in Selected Public Health Programs: 1995–1996 Regional Meetings. Washington, D.C.: Office of the Assistant Secretary for Health.

USPHS (U.S. Public Health Service). 1979. *Healthy People: Surgeon General's Report on Health Promotion and Disease Prevention.* DHEW (PHS) Pub. No. 79-55071. Washington, D.C.: U.S. Department of Health, Education, and Welfare.

U.S. Preventive Services Task Force. 1996. *Guide to Clinical Preventive Services.* 2nd ed. Baltimore: Williams and Wilkins.

VHA (Voluntary Hospitals of America). 1992. *Voluntary Standards: A Framework for Meeting Community Needs.* Irving, Texas: VHA, Inc.

Vilnius, D., and Dandoy, S. 1990. A Priority Rating System for Public Health Programs. *Public Health Reports* 105:463–470.

Wallerstein, N. 1992. Powerlessness, Empowerment, and Health: Implications for Health Promotion Programs. *American Journal of Health Promotion* 6(3):197–205.

Washington State Department of Health. 1994. *Public Health Improvement Plan.* Olympia: Washington State Department of Health.

Weiss, C.H. 1995. Nothing as Practical as Good Theory: Exploring Theory-Based Evaluation for Comprehensive Community Initiatives for Children and Families. In *New Approaches to Evaluating Community Initiatives: Concepts, Methods, and Contexts.* J.P. Connell, A.C. Kubisch, L.B. Schorr, and C.H. Weiss, eds. Washington, D.C.: Aspen Institute.

Welch, W.P., and Welch, H.G. 1995. Fee-for-Data: A Strategy to Open the HMO Black Box. *Health Affairs* 14(4):104–116.

Wennberg, J.E. 1984. Dealing with Medical Practice Variations: A Proposal for Action. *Health Affairs* 3(2):6–32.

Wennberg, J., and Gittelsohn, A. 1973. Small Area Variations in Health Care Delivery. *Science* 142:1102–1108.

Wennberg, J.E., Bunker, J.P., and Barnes, B. 1980. The Need for Assessing the Outcome of Common Medical Practices. *Annual Review of Public Health* 1:277–295.

WHO (World Health Organization). 1985. *Targets for Health for All.* Copenhagen: WHO, Regional Office for Europe.

Wickizer, T.M., Von Korff, M., Cheadle, A., et al. 1993. Activating Communities for Health Promotion: A Process Evaluation Method. *American Journal of Public Health* 83:561–567.

Worrall, G., and Chambers, L.W. 1989. Can We Afford Not to Evaluate Services for Persons with Dementia? *Canadian Family Physician* 35:573–580.

Zablocki, E. 1996. Improving Community Health Status: Strategies for Success. *The Quality Letter for Healthcare Leaders* 8(1):2–12.

5

Measurement Tools for a Community Health Improvement Process

Chapter 4 has outlined a community health improvement process (CHIP) through which communities can assess health needs and priorities, formulate a health improvement strategy, and use performance indicators as part of a continuing and accountable process. This chapter reviews in more detail the two kinds of indicators and indicator sets proposed for use in a CHIP. Discussed first is the *community health profile*, with component indicators proposed by the committee, which can provide a broad overview of a community's characteristics and its health status and resources. The second part of the chapter focuses on the development of *indicator sets for performance monitoring*, which are intended for use with health improvement strategies for specific health issues. The committee presents some examples that illustrate how communities might approach selecting such performance indicators.

ROLE FOR A COMMUNITY HEALTH PROFILE

A community health profile is an integral component of the problem identification and prioritization cycle of the community health improvement process described in Chapter 4. The health profile is intended to be a set of indicators of basic demographic and socioeconomic characteristics, health status, health risk factors, and health resource use, which are relevant to most communities.

The committee's proposal is consistent with the efforts of others over the past several years to identify small sets of indicators for key issues. One source of interest has been health promotion and Healthy Cities/Healthy Communities activities by the World Health Organization (WHO, 1986) and others (e.g., Canadian Healthy Communities Project, 1988; National Civic League, 1993). In the United States in particular, the inclusion of 300 indicators in *Healthy People 2000* (USDHHS, 1991) led to interest in also selecting a smaller set of indicators that could be used to monitor health status (e.g., CDC, 1991; Stoto, 1992). In other work, a small set of indicators was proposed for monitoring access to health care (IOM, 1993).

The health profile can help a community maintain a broad strategic view of its population's health status and factors that influence health in the community. It is not expected to be a comprehensive survey of all aspects of community health and well-being, but it should be able to help a community identify and focus attention on specific high-priority health issues. The background information provided by a health profile can help a community interpret data on those issues.

A *community health profile* is made up of indicators of sociodemographic characteristics, health status and quality of life, health risk factors, and health resources that are relevant for most communities; these indicators provide basic descriptive information that can inform priority setting and interpretation of data on specific health issues.

Health profile data can help motivate communities to address health issues. For example, evidence of underimmunization among children or the elderly might encourage various sectors of the community to respond, through "official" actions (e.g., more systematic provider assessments of patients' immunization status) and through community action (e.g., volunteer groups offering transportation to immunization clinics). Even as raw numbers, these data may be an important signal to a community, especially when small numbers of cases make it difficult to construct meaningful rates. For example, *any* work-related deaths, births to teenagers, or cases of measles might be a source of concern. Working with small numbers of cases raises potential problems of privacy and confidentiality, which communities must consider. Further discussion of privacy and confidentiality considerations appears later in this chapter. Care should also be taken that evidence of health problems not be used as a basis for negative labels for particular population groups or neighborhoods in a community.

Comparisons based on health profile data may be another source of motivation and may help communities in assessing health priorities as well. These comparisons can be based on measurements over time within an individual community, comparisons with other communities or with state or national measurements, or comparisons with a benchmark or target value such as an objective from *Healthy People 2000* (USDHHS, 1991). A variety of specialized compilations of data may provide additional reference points (e.g., Andrulis et al., 1995; Annie E. Casey Foundation, 1996; Wennberg, 1996). The opportunity for such comparisons will be increased if there is widespread agreement across communities on a basic set of standard health profile indicators and their operational definitions.

In making comparisons, however, communities must consider underlying factors that might contribute to observed differences. Some factors, if recognized, can be captured in quantitative form. For example, there might be a greater number of hospitalizations in an older population than in a younger population even though the age-specific rates are the same in both groups. Less easily addressed is the effect on the validity of comparisons among communities of different physical, social, political, and cultural contexts and different local needs and priorities, all of which may influence community profile indicators and, for some, argue against standard indicator sets (Hayes and Willms, 1990). (See Appendix B for further discussion of methodological issues in selecting and using health profile and performance indicators.)

The committee emphasizes that communities should update their health profile data on a regular basis to maintain an accurate picture of community circumstances, including identifying positive or negative changes that might influence health improvement priorities. The health profile is not, however, intended to be a tool specifically to monitor changes in stakeholder performance or to establish responsibility and accountability for health outcomes. Some of the indicators that are included in a profile might, however, serve as performance indicators if they are applied to other CHIP activities. Immunization rates, for example, are a useful community health descriptor but could also be monitored as an outcome measure for targeted efforts to reduce the risk of vaccine-preventable disease.

PROPOSED INDICATORS FOR A COMMUNITY HEALTH PROFILE

To promote community use of health profiles, the committee is proposing a basic set of 25 indicators (see Table 5-1). They provide descriptive information on a community's demographic and socioeconomic characteristics and highlight important aspects of health status and various health determinants, including behavior, factors in the social and physical environments, and health care. Some the indicators include multiple measures within a broader category (e.g., causes of death and incidence of infectious diseases). Appendix 5A reviews each indicator individually.

TABLE 5-1 Proposed Indicators for a Community Health Profile

Sociodemographic Characteristics

1. Distribution of the population by age and race/ethnicity
2. Number and proportion of persons in groups such as migrants, homeless, or the non–English speaking, for whom access to community services and resources may be a concern
3. Number and proportion of persons aged 25 and older with less than a high school education
4. Ratio of the number of students graduating from high school to the number of students who entered 9th grade three years previously
5. Median household income
6. Proportion of children less than 15 years of age living in families at or below the poverty level
7. Unemployment rate
8. Number and proportion of single-parent families
9. Number and proportion of persons without health insurance

Health Status

10. Infant mortality rate by race/ethnicity
11. Numbers of deaths or age-adjusted death rates for motor vehicle crashes, work-related injuries, suicide, homicide, lung cancer, breast cancer, cardiovascular diseases, and all causes, by age, race, and gender as appropriate
12. Reported incidence of AIDS, measles, tuberculosis, and primary and secondary syphilis, by age, race, and gender as appropriate
13. Births to adolescents (ages 10–17) as a proportion of total live births
14. Number and rate of confirmed abuse and neglect cases among children

continued on next page

TABLE 5-1 *Continued*

Health Risk Factors

15. Proportion of 2-year-old children who have received all age-appropriate vaccines, as recommended by the Advisory Committee on Immunization Practices
16. Proportion of adults aged 65 and older who have ever been immunized for pneumococcal pneumonia; proportion who have been immunized in the past 12 months for influenza
17. Proportion of the population who smoke, by age, race, and gender as appropriate
18. Proportion of the population aged 18 and older who are obese
19. Number and type of U.S. Environmental Protection Agency air quality standards not met
20. Proportion of assessed rivers, lakes, and estuaries that support beneficial uses (e.g., fishing and swimming approved)

Health Care Resource Consumption

21. Per capita health care spending for Medicare beneficiaries (the Medicare adjusted average per capita cost [AAPCC])

Functional Status

22. Proportion of adults reporting that their general health is good to excellent
23. During the past 30 days, average number of days for which adults report that their physical or mental health was not good

Quality of Life

24. Proportion of adults satisfied with the health care system in the community
25. Proportion of persons satisfied with the quality of life in the community

NOTE: See Appendix 5A for additional information on each indicator.

Selection of Community Health Profile Indicators

The committee's selection of indicators reflects consideration of several factors. Measures were sought that would be relevant across a broad range of communities. Recognizing the diversity among communities in health needs, priorities, and resources, the committee selected a limited number of indicators that could be expected to be widely applicable. The list draws extensively from the "consensus set" of indicators for assessing community health status (CDC, 1991) that was developed in response to *Healthy People 2000* Objective 22.1. This objective calls for developing a set of health status indicators appropriate for use by federal, state, and local health agencies and implementing them in at least 40 states by the year 2000 (USDHHS, 1991). The committee gave these indicators a high priority because they and *Healthy People 2000* have had an important influence on community health assessment activities since 1991. The committee agreed, however, that the consensus indicators per se were not sufficient to constitute an adequate community health profile.

The committee considered four other factors in selecting indicators: consistency with the field model framework for the determinants of health; attention to the health needs of specific populations; existence of a measure with an operational definition; and availability of data. The mix of indicators was also examined to ensure relevance across the age spectrum (Stoto, 1992). Table 5-2 summarizes the field model domains and current or potential sources of data for each proposed health profile indicator.

The broad perspective on health embodied in the field model (Evans and Stoddart, 1994) is a fundamental component of the committee's approach to health improvement and performance monitoring. For the community health profile, proposed indicators were mapped to the domains of the field model (social and physical environment, genetic endowment, behavior, disease, health care, health and function, prosperity, and well-being) to identify potential gaps and to assess the distribution of indicators across domains. Only the domain of genetic endowment is not represented directly; its contribution can be seen, however, in indicators such as infant mortality, cardiovascular disease mortality, and obesity.

In its selections, the committee favored measures that are in use and have a recognized operational definition or lend themselves to the construction of such a definition. Being able to specify clearly how an indicator is measured will help communities determine what data they need and will help them identify points of comparison with other communities and at state and national levels. For some of the selected indicators, generally recognized measures have not been established. This applies in particular to the indicators on satisfaction with the quality of life in the community and with the health care system in the community. The committee felt, however, that these indicators were of sufficient importance for understanding health in the broadest sense that they should be proposed for inclusion in a community health profile to encourage the development of suitable measures. The Centers for Disease Control and Prevention (CDC) has developed survey questions on the influence of personal health on quality of life that are now in use in the Behavioral Risk Factor Surveillance System (BRFSS) and is attempting to identify community-level indicators of health-related quality of life (Hennessy

TABLE 5-2 Features of Proposed Community Profile Indicators

Indicator Topic	Field Model Domain	Data Sources
Sociodemographic Characteristics		
1. Age and race/ethnicity	Social environment (behavior, genetics)	Census; intercensal estimates
2. Groups whose access to community services or resources may be limited	Social environment (behavior, physical environment, prosperity)	Census; intercensal estimates
3. Educational attainment (high school graduation)	Social environment (behavior, physical environment, prosperity, well-being)	Census; intercensal estimates
4. High school dropouts	Social environment (disease, behavior, physical environment, prosperity)	Local school districts
5. Household income	Prosperity (behavior, social environment, physical environment, health care, health and function)	Census; intercensal estimates
6. Children in poverty	Social environment, prosperity (behavior, physical environment, health care, health and function)	Census; intercensal estimates
7. Unemployment rate	Social environment, prosperity (behavior, physical environment, health care, health and function, well-being)	State employment security office
8. Single-parent families	Social environment (behavior, physical environment, health care, prosperity, well-being)	Census; intercensal estimates
9. Persons without health insurance	Social environment, health care (disease, health and function, prosperity)	Behavioral Risk Factor Surveillance System (special sampling)

Health Status		
10. Infant mortality	Disease, genetics, social environment, behavior, physical environment, health care, prosperity	State vital records
11. Death rates, overall and for selected causes	Disease, genetics, behavior, social environment, physical environment, health care, prosperity	State vital records
12. Incidence of AIDS, measles, tuberculosis, syphilis	Disease, behavior, social environment, health care (prosperity, health and function, well-being)	State communicable disease records
13. Births to adolescents	Behavior, social environment (prosperity, well-being)	State vital records
14. Child abuse and neglect	Behavior, social environment (disease, physical environment, health care, well-being)	State or local child protection agency records
Health Risk Factors		
15. Preschool immunization	Behavior, health care (social environment, prosperity)	Community survey; retrospective estimates from school entry records; immunization registry
16. Older adult immunization	Behavior, health care (social environment, prosperity)	Medicare claims files; health plan records
17. Prevalence of smoking	Disease, behavior, social environment, physical environment, health and function (health care, prosperity)	Behavioral Risk Factor Surveillance System (special sampling)
18. Prevalence of obesity	Behavior, health and function (genetics, social environment, health care, well-being)	Behavioral Risk Factor Surveillance System (special sampling)
19. Air quality	Disease, physical environment (social environment, well-being)	State environmental quality agency; local air quality management agency
20. Water quality (for recreational uses)	Physical environment (behavior, social environment, well-being)	State environmental quality agency

continued on next page

TABLE 5-2 *Continued*

Indicator Topic	Field Model Domain	Data Sources
Health Care Resource Consumption		
21. Per capita Medicare spending	Health care, prosperity	Health Care Financing Administration
Functional Status		
22. Self-reported health status	Health and function, well-being	Behavioral Risk Factor Surveillance System (special sampling)
23. Recent poor health	Health and function, well-being	Behavioral Risk Factor Surveillance System (special sampling)
Quality of Life		
24. Satisfaction with health care system	Health care, well-being (social environment, prosperity, health and function)	Community survey
25. Satisfaction with quality of life	Well-being (behavior, social environment, physical environment, health care, prosperity, health and function)	Community survey

NOTE: Secondary field model domains are listed in parentheses; some indicators could be addressed by questions developed for the state-based surveys of the Behavioral Risk Factor Surveillance System (CDC, 1993), but special sampling methods would have to be adopted to obtain community-specific estimates.

et al., 1994; Moriarty, 1996). Once valid and reliable measures are available, issues of data collection can be addressed.

Availability of and Access to Data

The availability of data is a special concern at the community level. For most of the health profile indicators proposed by the committee, data are already being collected at the state or national level, but not necessarily by communities themselves or in a form that can produce community-level information or as frequently as might be desired. Few communities have the financial resources or expertise to collect such data on a routine basis or to perform the additional analysis that may be needed to make available data meaningful at the community level. In some cases, however, opportunities may exist to develop sources of data for communities. In selecting indicators for the community profile, the committee frequently chose to suggest such potential sources of data rather than limit its list of indicators to only those for which community-level data are typically available now.

As noted in Chapter 4, the committee believes that states have an obligation to ensure that communities have access to the data needed to construct health profiles. Some states have already assumed this responsibility, and an Assessment Initiative managed by the National Center for Health Statistics (NCHS, 1995a) is assisting other states in developing the capacity to provide such data. Information is often produced in printed reports, but some states such as Illinois and Massachusetts are also developing data systems that give local health departments online access to data. In Massachusetts, the MassCHIP (Massachusetts Community Health Information Profile) data system makes community-level health profile data available to the public as well as to the state's community health network areas (see Box 5-1 for additional information on MassCHIP). Minnesota is providing electronic access to county data from its Substance Abuse Monitoring System (Minnesota Department of Human Services, 1995). Evolving computer and communications technologies can be expected to facilitate access to information not only within states but across the country. Some states, federal agencies, and private companies are already making data available through the Internet.

One promising source of community-level data on adults may be the BRFSS, through which the states and CDC collaborate to produce state estimates for a variety of health status, health behavior, and health risk topics (CDC, 1993). Modifications to the

BOX 5-1
Massachusetts Community Health Information Profile

The Massachusetts Department of Public Health (MDPH) has established as a priority improving the availability of health status data for community-based health promotion and prevention. In 1996, MDPH implemented the Massachusetts Community Health Information Profile—MassCHIP—an information service to provide dial-up access to community-level data for assessing community health needs, monitoring health status indicators, and evaluating programs. In the initial phase, data on health status, health outcome, program utilization, and sociodemographic characteristics are available from 18 separate data sets. The system is designed to be used by anyone with modem access, which could include local governments, health plans, individual health care providers, researchers, community agencies and organizations, and the general public.

MassCHIP has the ability to create standard or customized reports for several different levels of geographic detail: 351 cities and towns; neighborhoods in Boston, Springfield, and Lowell; standard regional units (counties, MDPH regions, and Community Health Network Areas [CHNAs]); or user-defined combinations of cities, towns, and regions. Depending on the original data, variables such as age, sex, race or ethnicity, education, or income can be used to restrict reporting to groups of interest. All data elements are cross-linked to relevant *Healthy People 2000* objectives. Reports can be based on observed counts, crude or age-adjusted rates, age-specific rates, and standardized ratios. The system includes guidelines for suppressing small numbers as needed to ensure confidentiality. Among the standard reports are sets of health status indicators for CHNAs.

SOURCE: Massachusetts Department of Public Health (1995); D.K. Walker, personal communication (1996).

sampling methods and inclusion of additional questions could make it possible to generate county or other substate estimates. Illinois, for example, is adopting a program to produce periodic county-level estimates by oversampling different groups of counties for each BRFSS round. In Massachusetts, similar arrangements are being made for cities and regions of the state. The school-based Youth Risk Behavior Surveillance System (YRBSS)—a collaborative effort involving states, cities, and the CDC (1995)—may lend itself to similar approaches to generating community data for adolescents. Neither the BRFSS nor the YRBSS as they are currently designed will provide information on children. To obtain such data, modifications of those surveys or separate data collection methods will be needed. If local data remain unavailable or are not feasible to obtain, communities that are similar to the state as a whole may find some state-level data useful.

Adding location identifiers (e.g., zip codes, census tracts) to survey and other types of data could improve their usefulness at the community level. This approach may be especially valuable for some forms of environmental risk monitoring. The additional information may also make it possible to link data from state sources with local data systems such as an immunization registry. The committee strongly supports more extensive use of such "geocoding," particularly for data collected by states.

Community-level data collection may also be possible—perhaps essential—for obtaining some types of information. NCHS (1995b) is testing the feasibility of a telephone survey to obtain data related to the consensus indicators, particularly the supplemental indicators for which data sources were not available at the time the consensus indicators were issued. The committee has included some of these supplemental indicators in its health profile.

Because most of the proposed health profile indicators rely on population-based measures, health departments and other public agencies with responsibilities for an entire community will tend to be the principal sources of needed data. Nevertheless, health plans, insurers, employers, and others in the private sector could contribute to community data resources, particularly for numerator data needed to calculate rates. Rate calculations pose other challenges as well. For many indicators, small numbers of cases at the community level will mean that calculation of stable rates will require aggregating data over multiple years. If, however, data are collected only infrequently (e.g., every five years), aggregation may not be practical, either because of the delay created in producing a usable measurement or because circumstances in the community change sufficiently that combining data could be misleading. Communities may also need assistance in developing intercensal population estimates accurate enough to be used as rate denominators. These estimates are especially important if the population is changing rapidly in size or composition.

Further Development of the Community Health Profile

The community health profile proposed by the committee should be viewed as a starting point for further development, not a final product. The indicators chosen reflect the committee's judgment in balancing three considerations: (1) importance in shaping or contributing to understanding community health, (2) usefulness across a broad range of communities, and (3) feasibility of measurement. Communities may, through their health improvement activities, identify topics of local importance that should supplement the basic profile. Indicators that address issues beyond the traditional realm of "health" (e.g., education, literacy, employment, crime, housing, community participation) may be relevant. For example, the categories of measures for the National Civic League's (1993) Healthy Community Indicators include health, family income, housing and homelessness, food assistance, child care, education, youth employment, transportation, public safety, and environmental issues. The Sustainability Indicators developed by the Regional Municipality of Hamilton–Wentworth (1996) in Ontario, Canada, include measures such as air quality, water and electricity consumption, voter turnout, and applications for affordable housing.

Access to a wide array of data, perhaps through state sources, can also support an expanded health profile. In expanding the profile, however, communities should not be aiming to produce a comprehensive health assessment tool. Such assessments are valuable, but if resources are limited, comprehensive assessments should probably be prepared less frequently than updates to a health profile. For a profile, communities should focus on indicators that can contribute most to an understanding of the population's health status and the factors that affect it in a positive or negative way. As was the case with the basic profile, the field model will be a useful guide for examining a broader array factors that may be determinants of a community's health and for selecting indicators to add to a profile.

Part of the committee's intention in proposing a basic set of indicators for a community profile is to encourage the development of common indicator definitions and common practices in data collection, analysis, and reporting that will facilitate comparisons over time and among communities. State programs that provide data to communities can promote this kind of comparability. Activities at the national level related to *Healthy People 2000* and the consensus indicators, including reporting requirements for some block grants (e.g., CDC, 1994; MCHB, 1995), should also contribute to standardization of measures suitable for community health profiles. In addition, the work being done to develop indicators for state reporting for the proposed federal public health

Performance Partnership Grants (PPGs) can also be expected to promote standardization (USDHHS, no date; NRC, 1996).

The committee encourages reexamination and revision of its basic community profile. Individual indicators in the current set might be modified as new or better data and measures become available. The profile might also evolve toward a greater focus on positive measures of health and health promoting features of individual behavior and the community environment. For example, measures on diet and exercise, topics for which questions have been developed for the BRFSS, might be considered. In general, however, such measures are less well developed than those for health "problems." Work is also needed to further the development of community-level measures to supplement those for individuals (Patrick and Wickizer, 1995).

A formal process, which might be organized by federal agencies, national professional organizations, or foundations, could promote the development and improvement of measures suitable for community-level data and the adoption of standard measures. Participation by a broad array of public and private stakeholders representing national, state, and local perspectives should be encouraged.

The committee also sees a need for a variety of forms of technical assistance that can help communities understand how to use health profile indicators and obtain appropriate data. States may be able to provide some of the assistance that communities need, but states themselves may benefit from technical assistance in these areas. National efforts such as those suggested for the development of community-level measures would also be useful for improving analytic techniques and developing resources for technical assistance.

As presented here, the community health profile is based on a "community" defined by geographic or civic boundaries, frequently a county or city. This reflects the current form in which data are generally available and not a necessary or preferable basis on which to define a community. Discussions at the committee's workshops emphasized that data for much smaller units (e.g., neighborhoods) are often needed to generate support for health improvement activities. The committee encourages the development of data for a variety of "community" units. It believes that states should work toward developing interactive electronic data systems that will permit users to define the specific population, including demographic or socioeconomic groupings, for which they want data. The MassCHIP system (see Box 5-1), for example, is designed to provide data on cities and towns, neighborhoods in three large cities, predefined regions such as the state's Community Health Network Areas, and user-defined combinations of cities, towns, and regions (Massachusetts Department of Public Health, 1995).

INDICATOR SETS FOR PERFORMANCE MONITORING FOR SPECIFIC HEALTH ISSUES

Communities, through mechanisms such as the problem identification and prioritization cycle of a CHIP (see Chapter 4), need to identify the health issues that key stakeholders consider important. Data from a community's health profile can point to issues, but health priorities may also be identified by other means, such as community meetings or surveys. In working from the broad perspective of the field model, critical "health" issues may also be found not only among conditions that create a substantial burden in terms of illness or costs of care but also in areas such as education and housing. Some issues may be of great concern but will not yet be suitable choices for more targeted health improvement activities because effective interventions have not been developed.

Once a health issue has been selected, a CHIP moves on to the analysis and implementation cycle, and a community's information needs expand from the descriptive measures in a community profile to the more "actionable" indicators that are crucial to performance monitoring and health improvement activities. As noted

---

For the community health improvement process, a *performance indicator* provides a concrete measure of a specific capacity, process, or outcome related to an accountable entity that is part of a defined health improvement strategy for a specific health issue. Such indicators can be used to measure performance at varying levels of specificity: a community as a whole; particular categories of accountable entities (e.g., health departments, schools, or insurers); or specific entities in a community (e.g., a specific school or health plan). A *set* of performance indicators is used to assess the multiple dimensions of a health issue and monitor the contributions of various accountable entities to the health improvement strategy.

---

in Chapter 4, communities will have to assemble a set of performance indicators to address the multiple dimensions of a health issue. Discussed here are factors that should be considered in selecting sets of indicators for issue-specific performance monitoring. Prototype indicator sets in Appendix A to this report illustrate how communities might use the committee's approach.

Assessing the Scope of an Issue

Almost any health issue will have many dimensions and present many possible opportunities to respond. As an initial step in the analysis and implementation cycle of a CHIP, a community will need to think broadly about the nature of the problem, what can be done, who can take action, and what indicators can track progress most effectively. The field model provides a helpful framework for accomplishing the kind of systematic review that is needed. To gain a clear understanding of the features of a particular health issue so that an effective intervention strategy can be developed, it may be useful to gather additional information from key stakeholder groups. A community that wants to reduce adolescent tobacco use, for example, will need information on topics such as the age at which use begins, how adolescents obtain tobacco products, and the kinds of school-based prevention programs available.

As a community moves on to the process of identifying potential performance indicators, it should specifically include consideration of (1) the domains of the field model that could be addressed by those indicators and (2) the potential to engage the interest and action of a variety of community stakeholders. A narrow focus on any one stakeholder group or health factor may limit opportunities for effective action. For example, efforts to reduce the adverse impact of depression that look only at the quality of care provided by mental health specialists will neglect the contributions that might be made by primary care providers or by activities based in settings such as schools and workplaces.

Considering the Health Field Model

A narrow view of health interventions might be limited to the diagnosis and treatment of disease. Examining an issue in the framework of the field model, which presents health and well-being as the product of a more complex mix of forces, can point to a broader array of possible interventions and related performance indicators. Communities may find it beneficial to use the field model in conjunction with other assessment tools, such as the analysis of risk factors and direct and indirect contributing factors suggested by *APEXPH: Assessment Protocol for Excellence in Public Health* (NACHO, 1991). An assessment of a health issue may, however, point to important concerns for which satisfactory indicators and data have not yet been developed, often because of gaps in our understanding of the complex processes that produce "health."

Engaging Stakeholders

Successful health improvement efforts in a community will require the interest and support of a variety of stakeholder groups and, for some stakeholders, may require changing their responsibilities and activities. Therefore, health issues identified as community priorities and the performance indicators selected to assess progress should engage key stakeholders who must act or who can encourage action. The mix of stakeholders and their degree of involvement can be expected to vary depending on the health issue being addressed. Nursing homes, for instance, could be expected to be key participants in efforts targeting the health of the elderly but would probably have little role in improving prenatal care.

Selecting Performance Indicators

Many potential performance indicators, generally "process" and "outcome" measures,[1] will emerge in discussions about an issue, but some will be more appropriate than others. Selecting those that will be used is a critical stage in a CHIP. Sofaer (1995) points out that indicator selection is a normative process, reflecting community expectations as to which aspects of a health issue are

---

[1]The framework of structure, process, and outcome measures was originally developed for quality assurance in health care (Donabedian, 1980, 1982, 1985) but has proved useful in a variety of contexts. *Structure* applies to capacity to perform (e.g., whether smoking cessation counseling is available to pregnant women). *Process* applies to activities that are being performed (e.g., numbers of pregnant women receiving smoking cessation counseling). *Outcome* applies to results of those activities (e.g., proportion of counseled women who stop smoking or, more significantly, the rate of low-weight births among counseled women).

important and what stakeholder actions should achieve. A CHIP and the community coalition that is at its core should provide a framework within which a community can reach agreement on the values and expectations to be represented in performance indicators.

Indicator selection should also reflect a strategic consideration of the value of individual indicators and of the collection of indicators to be used in connection with a specific health issue (Sofaer, 1995). Individual indicators become more valuable to the extent that they are effective proxies for multiple dimensions of performance. A *set* of indicators will usually be needed to cover a range of relevant performance areas and must be assembled carefully to assure that, together, the indicators effectively serve the process of improving the community's health. The set should appeal to many stakeholders and reflect broad consideration of the domains of the field model, but it should be limited to a comprehensible number of indicators. Too many indicators become distracting and, in practical terms, could make collecting and analyzing data prohibitively burdensome (Sofaer, 1995).

Operational implications and costs of data collection and analysis also must be considered in selecting indicators and indicator sets. Even though indicators may be formulated with the intention of promoting actions that will have positive effects on community health, they must be based on an accurate understanding of their effect in the setting in which they will be applied. For example, reducing the number of cigarette vending machines as a way to limit youth access to tobacco will not have the anticipated impact if teenagers buy most of their cigarettes in convenience stores. It also is possible to frame indicators in a way that creates "perverse incentives" for action, which produce a "better" measured result but do not achieve intended health goals. For example, lower rates of sexually transmitted diseases might be "achieved" through less complete reporting rather than through true reductions in disease rates.

A reasonable balance must be struck between the information value of an indicator and the cost of collecting the necessary data. A conceptually appropriate indicator will not be helpful if a community cannot afford to obtain the data it requires. Costs of data generation may include designing data collection instruments, collecting or locating data, analyzing and summarizing the results, and reporting information to the community. In some communities and for some indicators, these activities may require new resources. In other cases, it may be possible to apply existing resources (e.g., funds, expertise, data systems) to producing CHIP data.

Another concern is how time factors are addressed in performance monitoring. Communities must approach performance monitoring with an understanding of when to expect measurable effects from health improvement. It is generally easier to examine factors that affect health in the short term (e.g., vaccination or care for acute illness), but some important influences on health operate over much longer time frames. For example, changes in lung cancer rates can lag changes in smoking patterns by 20–30 years, and the health benefits of interventions targeted at critical developmental periods in early childhood may not be seen until adolescence or adulthood. Interventions with important long-term benefits should not be neglected in favor of those that operate more quickly. Indicators based on intermediate goals such as changes in risk factors (e.g., decreased prevalence of smoking) can help bridge the period until changes in health outcomes can be measured.

In selecting indicators, communities will also have to consider factors such as how issues manifest themselves (e.g., social isolation among the elderly could be a function of lack of transportation but might also result from fear of street crime); what information resources are available; and what actions are organizationally, socially, politically, and economically feasible within the community (e.g., gun safety programs might be acceptable when gun control is not). These concerns should be addressed through the community processes described in Chapter 4.

Selection Criteria

The committee identified several specific criteria to consider in selecting individual performance indicators.[2] Ideally, every indi-

---

[2]The committee's indicator selection criteria are similar to those specified by other groups for related purposes. The Sustainable Development Indicators project in Hamilton-Wentworth, Ontario, Canada (Regional Municipality of Hamilton-Wentworth, 1996), listed the criteria of measurability, cost and ease of collection, credibility and validity, balance, and potential for effecting change.

The National Committee for Quality Assurance (NCQA, 1996) identified the following desired attributes of measures to be submitted for consideration for version 3.0 of the Health Plan Employer Data and Information Set (HEDIS): relevance (meaningful to users, health importance, financial importance, cost-effectiveness, strategically important, controllability, variance between plans, potential for improvement), scientific validity (reproducible, valid, accurate, risk adjustable, com-

cator should satisfy them, but compromises may be necessary until improvements such as better measures and data systems or stronger scientific evidence are available. Communities may need to act cautiously in the face of such limitations but should not neglect important health issues that cannot yet be addressed through quantitative approaches to performance monitoring.

The committee proposes the following criteria for selecting indicators:

- *Established validity and reliability.* To be of value, a performance indicator must be valid for its intended use; that is, it must measure what it purports to measure. It is also essential that performance indicators be reliable, that is, producing consistent responses when measured by different people or at different times. Indicators must also demonstrate validity and reliability in varying cultural contexts. These basic qualities of a good measure are particularly important in a monitoring system where progress, or lack thereof, is being followed closely and the results will affect important decisions.
- *Evidence-based link between performance and health improvement.* Performance indicators measure how well specific actions are being carried out by those who accept responsibility for them. There should be (under the best of circumstances) clear scientific evidence that the action being monitored will, indeed, lead to improvement in health. In some cases, available evidence may not be conclusive, but expert judgment represented in sources such as clinical practice guidelines (e.g., see IOM, 1992; U.S. Preventive Services Task Force, 1996) may suggest actions that could be expected to produce desired effects. Without such evidence or consensus in expert judgment, it is not reasonable to expect accountability for health improvement when, even under ideal circumstances, it may not be possible for the action taken to have the desired impact.

---

parability of data sources), and feasibility (precisely specified, reasonable cost, confidential, logistically feasible).

Criteria established by the Scientific Advisory Committee of the Medical Outcomes Trust (Perrin, 1995) for outcomes assessment instruments to be included in the Trust's collection are a conceptual and measurement model, reliability, validity, responsiveness (ability to detect change), interpretability, burden, alternative forms, and cultural and language adaptations.

• *Responsibility and accountability for performance.* A critical element of performance monitoring is identifying where responsibility and accountability lie for actions that can improve health. It should be possible to link performance indicators to specific community stakeholders who have accepted or been assigned responsibility for some aspect of health improvement. In some cases, a stakeholder may have responsibility for a defined portion of the total population (e.g., health plans and their enrolled members, schools and enrolled students). When similar health needs exist in the remainder of the population, communities will have to determine where responsibility for serving that portion of the population lies.

Under some circumstances, a stakeholder may have to assume responsibility for producing or assuring the existence of an enabling precondition for achieving health improvement, rather than assuming more direct responsibility for the health outcome itself. Determining whether an "intermediate" activity such as this will be monitored at the community level or by an individual stakeholder organization will depend on a community's approach to the health issue and the nature of the precondition to be achieved.

• *Robustness and responsiveness to change in health system performance, particularly in targeted populations.* A performance indicator must be able to detect the effect of reasonably small changes in the performance system so that progress can be measured, even in small increments. If the performance indicator is unable to detect small initial changes, failure may be declared prematurely. Consideration must also be given to whether the indicator can reflect the impact of system changes on small subgroups in the population. In addition, indicators should be sufficiently stable and well defined that they are not subject to substantial random variation.

• *Availability of data in a timely manner at a reasonable cost.* The need to collect performance indicator data on a recurring basis makes ease and cost of collection important considerations. Because financial constraints are a concern for most communities, it will be imperative that performance indicators be measurable at reasonable cost and in a timely manner. Communities should consider the roles that the public and private sectors should each have in supporting data collection, analysis, and reporting.

• *Inclusion in other indicator sets (monitoring sets).* Some health-related indicator systems are already being used to assess performance, although rarely community-wide. Using existing indicators makes it possible to benefit from the indicator development experience of the parent group and to avoid duplication of effort or variation in specification that may hinder comparisons. A few of these indicator sets include HEDIS, the Health Plan Employer Data and Information Set (NCQA, 1993, 1996), which is focused on managed care organizations and includes some measures framed specifically for Medicaid and Medicare enrollees; the accountability measurement sets being developed by the Foundation for Accountability (FAcct, 1995, 1996) for specific health issues; *Healthy People 2000* (USDHHS, 1991), which sets out roughly 300 health promotion and disease prevention objectives and is the starting point for objectives outlined in the Healthy People consensus indicators (CDC, 1991); *Healthy Communities 2000* (APHA et al., 1991); and the measures required for reporting on some federal grants (e.g., CDC, 1994; MCHB, 1995). The indicators established for the proposed PPGs may also prove helpful. Some of the additional indicator sets that communities might consult are noted in Chapter 4.

Using Indicator Sets

Once communities establish performance indicator sets for specific health issues, they are able to move further through the health improvement process outlined by the committee. The indicator data should reflect whether appropriate actions are being taken by accountable entities and whether those actions are having the intended health effect. To interpret performance monitoring results, communities will have to take their specific circumstances into consideration. The resources available to a community, the mix of risk factors, and the interventions chosen will all influence the results achieved through a given health improvement strategy. Information provided by the performance indicators should guide subsequent steps: moving on to a new health issue, continuing or modifying the current effort, or perhaps returning to an earlier stage in the process to reassess the intervention strategy and the appropriate indicators to use.

PROTOTYPE PERFORMANCE INDICATOR SETS

To illustrate the application of its proposed approach to performance monitoring and indicator selection, the committee has assembled, with advice from outside experts, examples of indicator sets for several health issues: breast and cervical cancer, depression, elder health, environmental and occupational lead poisoning, health care resource allocation, infant health, tobacco and health, vaccine-preventable diseases, and violence. Appendix A presents for each topic a discussion of the health issue, the application of the field model and stakeholder interests, and the selection of a limited number of specific performance indicators. Comments are offered on likely sources of data and special considerations in using specific indicators. Table 5-3 shows the relationship to the field model domains of the indicators suggested for health improvement activities for vaccine-preventable diseases.

These health issues were selected to be generally representative of the spectrum of health concerns facing many communities. Most are associated with significant morbidity or health care costs. The committee's selections were also made to illustrate varying perspectives from which health issues might be viewed, including factors affecting population groups (infant and elder health); acute and chronic illness (breast and cervical cancer, depression); prevention and health promotion (tobacco and vaccine-preventable diseases); environmental and occupational health risk (lead exposure); operation of the health care system; and broad societal issues that have health implications (violence). Similarly, the committee selected health issues that present an opportunity for a variety of stakeholders to respond, including public health and other government agencies, health care providers, schools, employers, community groups, and individuals.

The committee's aim has been to demonstrate how performance indicators can be selected and to present credible indicator sets as models for work on a variety of other health issues as well as the ones discussed here. The committee is not attempting to prescribe intervention strategies or specific indicator sets for these health issues because it cannot adequately address the unique combination of circumstances that each community will have to consider. Instead, the examples use *community-level* indicators to illustrate issues discussed by the committee. Individual communities will have to formulate performance indicators that are based on performance expectations for their particular accountable entities and that reflect specific needs and resources. Some of factors to be considered include who provides specific services, what data are available from what sources, and whether important stakeholders are willing to accept responsibility for particular tasks.

PRIVACY AND CONFIDENTIALITY

The performance monitoring component of the CHIP outlined by the committee will require increased access to potentially sensitive data such as an individual's income level, employment status, medical diagnoses (e.g., HIV status, other sexually transmitted diseases, genetic conditions, mental illness), and lifestyle information (e.g., sexual practices, drug and alcohol use). Ensuring that this information is not misused must be a priority.

Matters of both privacy and confidentiality must be considered. Privacy can be defined as the capacity of the individual to determine which personal information is communicated to whom (Westin, 1967). In the health care setting, privacy refers to the implicit right of an individual to have control over personal medical information. Confidentiality, however, refers to the duty of those who hold information about others to protect that information from inappropriate disclosure to third parties. Underlying this duty is the knowledge that uncontrolled access to some types of personal information can result in harm to individuals (IOM, 1994).

Data in the form of person-identified (or identifiable) records are the most vulnerable, but access to such data can be vital for the success of some activities, particularly linking information from separate sources. Immunization registries, for example, must be able to update a child's record each time a vaccine dose is administered, regardless of who the provider is. Techniques that create unique but anonymous identifiers can make it possible to omit personal information such as name, address, and social security number from stored records. Risks of misuse are lower for aggregated data and for individual records that do not include personal identifiers. Even in this form, however, distinctive combinations of characteristics such as age, race, occupation, and diagnosis could suggest the probable identity of an individual in a community. Thus, policies are needed regarding the level of detail provided even in supposedly anonymous data.

Developing appropriate procedures to safeguard data from misuse is important for two reasons—it will prevent harm to individuals and it will help maintain the integrity of the data system (Gostin, 1995). All states have privacy protection laws regarding health data held by government agencies (e.g., communicable disease reports); the specific protections and penalties for violations vary from state to state (Gostin et al., 1996). Various state provisions also protect privately held health data, but federal legisla-

TABLE 5-3 Field Model Mapping for Sample Indicator Set for Vaccine-Preventable Diseases

Field Model Domain	Construct	Sample Indicators	Data Sources	Stakeholders
Disease	Eliminate vaccine preventable diseases	Pneumonia and influenza death rates for persons age 65 and older	Death certificates	Health care providers Health care plans State health agencies Local health agencies Business, industry Community organizations Special health risk groups General public
Individual Response	Ensure that Medicare enrollees are immunized appropriately	Percentage of Medicare enrollees who received an influenza immunization during the previous year; percentage who have ever received a pneumococcal pneumonia immunization	Immunization registry or medical charts	Health care providers Health care plans State health agencies Local health agencies Community organizations Special health risk groups General public
	Ensure that children are immunized appropriately	Immunization rate for children at 24 months of age		
Social Environment	Ensure that populations with special health risks are immunized	Immunization rate at 24 months of age for children currently enrolled in Medicaid	Immunization registry or medical charts	Health care providers State health agencies Local health agencies Special health risk groups

	Reduce financial barriers to immunization	Among children with commercial health insurance, percentage with full coverage for immunization	Employers, insurance licensing authority	Health care plans Local government Business, industry General public
	Provide leadership for immunization efforts	Existence in the community of an active childhood immunization coalition		Health care providers Health care plans State health agencies Local health agencies Local government Business, industry Education agencies and institutions Community organizations Special health risk groups General public
Health Care	Ensure that the health care system is organized to provide high immunization rates	Immunization rate for children at 24 months of age	Immunization registry or medical charts	Health care providers Health care plans State health agencies Local health agencies Business and industry Community organizations Special health risk groups General public
		Immunization rate at 24 months of age for children currently enrolled in managed care organizations	Immunization registry or medical charts	Health care providers Health care plans Business and industry General public

continued on next page

TABLE 5-3 *Continued*

Field Model Domain	Construct	Sample Indicators	Data Sources	Stakeholders
Health Care *(continued)*		Existence in the community of a computerized immunization registry; if available, percentage of children in the community included	Immunization registry, birth records	Health care providers Health care plans State health agencies Local health agencies General public
	Ensure that Medicare enrollees are immunized appropriately	Percentage of Medicare enrollees who received an influenza immunization during the previous year; percentage who have ever received a pneumococcal pneumonia immunization		

NOTE: See Appendix A.8 for the full discussion of the prototype indicator set for vaccine-preventable diseases.

tion such as the Employee Retirement Income Security Act (ERISA) may take precedence without offering protection comparable to state laws (IOM, 1994). Federal legislation that would provide more comprehensive protection for health data has been proposed (e.g., U.S. Congress, 1995, 1996).

Recommendations from the Institute of Medicine (IOM, 1994) report *Health Data in the Information Age*, which outlines a role for community-based "health data organizations" (HDOs), aim for a balance between ensuring confidentiality of information and the security of automated databases and providing access to information for activities that will improve the health of communities. In particular, the report recommends that HDOs have explicit mechanisms for developing and implementing policies and procedures governing the acquisition and dissemination of information that will provide for protection of privacy and confidentiality. The report also recommends passage of preemptive federal legislation that is designed to ensure that data systems protect privacy and confidentiality and would impose penalties for inappropriate use or release of data (IOM, 1994).

Communities should ensure that a CHIP incorporates adequate protection for all data that are used. Access to technical assistance from state agencies and experts in academia and the private sector may help communities establish policies and implement technologies that provide needed protections.

CONCLUSIONS

The health improvement process outlined by the committee depends heavily on access to information provided by indicators such as those discussed in this chapter. Both the broad perspective of a community health profile and the narrower focus of issue-specific indicator sets are needed. To aid communities in assembling and using indicators and indicator sets, the committee has proposed specific indicators for a health profile and has illustrated how communities might develop indicator sets for specific health issues.

Communities will have to translate these proposals into the realities of their particular circumstances. An immediate aim should be to identify a manageable number of indicators to be included in a community profile and to begin collecting and publishing data for those indicators on a routine basis. Over time, a community will have an information resource that allows it to see whether strengths are being preserved, progress is being made, or problems are emerging. More challenging will be the development of appropriate measurement tools to support an issue-specific performance monitoring process.

The guidance offered in this chapter and, by example, in the prototype indicator sets in Appendix A should help communities begin. Further work should be undertaken at the national and state levels to develop ways to make expertise in measurement and analysis available to communities that desire it.

REFERENCES

Andrulis, D.P., Ginsberg, C., Shaw-Taylor, Y., and Martin, V. 1995. *Urban Social Health: A Chart Book Profiling the Nation's One Hundred Largest Cities.* Washington, D.C.: National Public Health and Hospital Institute.

Annie E. Casey Foundation. 1996. *KIDS COUNT Data Book: State Profiles of Child Well-Being.* Baltimore: Annie E. Casey Foundation.

APHA (American Public Health Association), Association of Schools of Public Health, Association of State and Territorial Health Officials, National Association of County Health Officials, United States Conference of Local Health Officers, Department of Health and Human Services, Public Health Service, Centers for Disease Control. 1991. *Healthy Communities 2000: Model Standards.* 3rd ed. Washington, D.C.: APHA.

Canadian Healthy Communities Project. 1988. *Canadian Healthy Communities Project Start-up Kit.* Ottawa: Canadian Healthy Communities Project.

CDC (Centers for Disease Control and Prevention). 1991. Consensus Set of Health Status Indicators for the General Assessment of Community Health Status—United States. *Morbidity and Mortality Weekly Report* 40:449–451.

CDC. 1993. Special Focus: Behavioral Risk Factor Surveillance—United States, 1991. *Morbidity and Mortality Weekly Report* 42(SS-4).

CDC. 1994. Organization and Implementation of the Uniform Data Sets (Preventive Health and Health Services Block Grant). Atlanta, Ga.: U.S. Department of Health and Human Services. November 1. (mimeo)

CDC. 1995. Youth Risk Behavior Surveillance—United States, 1993. *Morbidity and Mortality Weekly Report* 44(SS-1).

Donabedian, A. 1980. *Explorations in Quality Assessment and Monitoring.* Vol. 1. *The Definition of Quality and Approaches to Its Assessment.* Ann Arbor, Mich.: Health Administration Press.

Donabedian, A. 1982. *Explorations in Quality Assessment and Monitoring.* Vol. 2. *The Criteria and Standards of Quality.* Ann Arbor, Mich.: Health Administration Press.

Donabedian, A. 1985. *Explorations in Quality Assessment and Monitoring.* Vol. 3. *The Methods and Findings of Quality Assessment and Monitoring: An Illustrated Analysis.* Ann Arbor, Mich.: Health Administration Press.

Evans, R.G., and Stoddart, G.L. 1994. Producing Health, Consuming Health Care. In *Why Are Some People Healthy and Others Not? The Determinants of Health of Populations.* R.G. Evans, M.L. Barer, and T.R. Marmor, eds. New York: Aldine De Gruyter.

FAcct (Foundation for Accountability). 1995. Guidebook for Performance Measurement: Prototype. Portland, Ore.: FAcct. September 22.

FAcct. 1996. In Practice—Diabetes. *Accountability!* (Fall):1–29.

Gostin, L.O. 1995. Health Information Privacy. *Cornell Law Review* 80(3):451–528.

Gostin, L.O., Lazzarini, Z., Neslund, V.S., and Osterholm, M.T. 1996. The Public Health Information Infrastructure: A National Review of the Law on Health Information Privacy. *Journal of the American Medical Association* 275:1921–1927.

Hayes, M.V., and Willms, S.M. 1990. Healthy Community Indicators: The Perils of the Search and the Paucity of the Find. *Health Promotion International* 5(2):161–166.

Hennessy, C.H., Moriarty, D.G., Zack, M.M., Scherr, P.A., and Brackbill, R. 1994. Measuring Health-Related Quality of Life for Public Health Surveillance. *Public Health Reports* 109:665–672.

IOM (Institute of Medicine). 1992. *Guidelines for Clinical Practice: From Development to Use.* M.J. Field and K.N. Lohr, eds. Washington, D.C.: National Academy Press.

IOM. 1993. *Access to Health Care in America.* M. Millman, ed. Washington, D.C.: National Academy Press.

IOM. 1994. *Health Data in the Information Age: Use, Disclosure, and Privacy.* M.S. Donaldson and K.N. Lohr, eds. Washington, D.C.: National Academy Press.

Massachusetts Department of Public Health. 1995. Massachusetts Community Health Information Profile. Boston: Massachusetts Department of Public Health. (brochure)

MCHB (Maternal and Child Health Bureau). 1995. Annual Report Guidance for the Maternal and Child Health Services Block Grant Program. OMB No. 0915-0172. Rockville, Md.: U.S. Department of Health and Human Services.

Minnesota Department of Human Services. 1995. The Substance Abuse Monitoring System. *researchNEWS* (January). St. Paul: Minnesota Department of Human Services, Chemical Dependency Division.

Moriarty, D. 1996. CDC Studies Community Quality of Life. *NACCHO News* 12(3):10,13.

NACHO (National Association of County Health Officials). 1991. *APEXPH: Assessment Protocol for Excellence in Public Health.* Washington, D.C.: NACHO.

National Civic League. 1993. *The Healthy Communities Handbook.* Denver: National Civic League.

NCHS (National Center for Health Statistics). 1995a. The CDC Assessment Initiative: A Summary of State Activities. *Healthy People 2000: Statistics and Surveillance.* No. 7 (October). Hyattsville, Md.: U.S. Department of Health and Human Services.

NCHS. 1995b. Pilot Test of Community Survey. *Healthy People 2000: Activity Update.* (Brock, B.M. A Telephone Survey Methodology for Local Health Departments' Community Health Status and Risk Factor Assessments Related to *Healthy People 2000.* DHHS/PHS/CDC Contract #200-94-7064.) Hyattsville, Md.: U.S. Department of Health and Human Services.

NCQA (National Committee for Quality Assurance). 1993. *Health Plan Employer Data and Information Set and User's Manual, Version 2.0 (HEDIS 2.0).* Washington, D.C.: NCQA.

NCQA. 1996. HEDIS 3.0 Draft for Public Comment. Washington, D.C.: NCQA.

NRC (National Research Council). 1996. *Assessment of Performance Measures in Public Health.* Phase 1 Report. Draft for Comment. Washington, D.C.: National Academy Press.

Patrick, D.L., and Wickizer, T.M. 1995. Community and Health. In *Society and Health.* B.C. Amick, S. Levine, A.R. Tarlov, and D.C. Walsh, eds. New York: Oxford University Press.

Perrin, E.B. 1995. SAC Instrument Review Process. *Medical Outcomes Trust Bulletin* 3(4):1, I–IV.

Regional Municipality of Hamilton–Wentworth. 1996. *Signposts on the Trail to Vision 2020: Hamilton–Wentworth Sustainable Indicators, 1996.* Hamilton, Ont.: Regional Municipality of Hamilton–Wentworth Environment Department.

Sofaer, S. 1995. *Performance Indicators: A Commentary from the Perspective of an Expanded View of Health.* Washington, D.C.: Center for the Advancement of Health.

Stoto, M.A. 1992. Public Health Assessment in the 1990s. *Annual Review of Public Health* 13:59–78.

U.S. Congress, House of Representatives. 1996. H.R. 3482: Medical Privacy in the Age of New Technologies Act of 1996. 104th Congress, 2d Session, May 16.

U.S. Congress, Senate. 1995. S. 1360: Medical Records Confidentiality Act of 1995. 104th Congress, 1st Session, October 24.

USDHHS (U.S. Department of Health and Human Services). 1991. *Healthy People 2000: National Health Promotion and Disease Prevention Objectives.* DHHS Pub. No. (PHS) 91-50212. Washington, D.C.: Office of the Assistant Secretary for Health.

USDHHS. No date. *Performance Measurement in Selected Public Health Programs: 1995–1996 Regional Meetings.* Washington, D.C.: Office of the Assistant Secretary for Health.

U.S. Preventive Services Task Force. 1996. *Guide to Clinical Preventive Services.* 2nd ed. Baltimore: Williams and Wilkins.

Wennberg, J., ed. 1996. *The Dartmouth Atlas of Health Care.* Chicago: American Hospital Press.

Westin, A.F. 1967. *Privacy and Freedom.* New York: Atheneum.

WHO (World Health Organization). 1986. A Discussion Document on the Concept and Principles of Health Promotion. *Health Promotion* 1(1):73–76.

APPENDIX 5A
PROPOSED COMMUNITY HEALTH PROFILE INDICATORS

1. Distribution of the population by age and race or ethnicity. Data on the basic demographic characteristics of a community are important for understanding current or potential health concerns. For example, a community that has a significant percentage of young families may have a special interest in health issues related to children, pregnancy, teenagers, and injuries, whereas an older community may need to address health issues related to health care resources and utilization, and chronic disease associated with aging. The demographic composition of the population should be understood because significant disparities in health status between minority and nonminority populations may be due to factors including economic resources, health care access, discrimination, and genetic susceptibility to disease. **Field**

model domains: individual behavior, genetics, and social environment. **Data sources:** decennial census; states may also develop intercensal estimates for communities.

2. Number and proportion of persons in groups such as migrants, the homeless, or the non-English speaking, for whom access to community services and resources may be a concern.

Subpopulations such as migrants, the homeless, or those who do not speak English are at greater risk for more significant health problems than the general population, may have greater difficulty gaining access to community services and resources, and may benefit from a variety of specialized responses. If a community has a large population of this type, then an attempt should be made to collect health indicator data for that group. In most cases, however, special populations are small, which necessitates special care in the analysis of group-specific data. The size and composition of these populations may change more rapidly than the rest of the population, so care should also be exercised in using data that are not current. **Field model domains:** individual behavior, social environment, physical environment, and prosperity. **Data sources:** decennial census; local agencies that serve special populations. Caution may also be needed in using census data if there is reason to believe that a group may have been undercounted relative to others in the community.

3. Number and proportion of persons aged 25 and older with less than a high school education.

Adults with less than a high school education can be at increased risk of health problems because of illiteracy, low-paying jobs that do not provide health insurance, lack of health information, and poor living conditions. There is also evidence that children living with parents whose educational attainment is low have more health problems than other children, even after other socioeconomic factors have been taken into account (Zill, 1996). These problems can begin even before birth because low educational attainment is associated with poor maternal health. **Field model domains:** individual behavior, social environment, physical environment, prosperity, and well-being. **Data sources:** decennial census; intercensal data may be available from state or community data systems or estimates.

4. Ratio of the number of students graduating from high school to the number of students who entered 9th grade three years previously.

Teenagers who drop out of high school may be at increased risk of unwanted pregnancy, sexually transmitted diseases, substance abuse, low-paying jobs without health insurance, and violence. This indicator is a measure of cumulative dropouts from the beginning of the high school period. Adjustments will be needed to account for students who transfer to or from other schools. **Field model domains:** disease, individual behavior, social environment, physical environment, and prosperity. **Data sources:** local school districts; data should be collected by individual districts and for all districts combined.

5. Median household income.

Median household income in the community provides information on family economic resources and the distribution of income in the community. Household income can affect a family's ability to obtain suitable housing, nutrition, or health insurance and may be related to behaviors that affect health. Comparisons over time within a community, among population groups within a community, or with other communities may be helpful in gauging the possible relationship between income and health status or other factors. **Field model domains:** individual behavior, social environment, physical environment, prosperity, health care, and health and function. **Data sources:** decennial census; may be available from state surveys.

6. Proportion of children less than 15 years of age living in families at or below the poverty level.

This indicator is included in the consensus set recommended by the Centers for Disease Control and Prevention (CDC, 1991) for use by all states and communities. It is similar to median household income but focuses specifically on children in low-income households, whose risk for health problems is high and whose ability to address health risks is limited. Many of these children will be enrolled in Medicaid or qualify for other health-related programs such as WIC (Special Supplemental Food Program for Women, Infants, and Children). **Field model domains:** individual behavior, social environment, physical environment, prosperity, health care, and health and function. **Data sources:** decennial census; may be available from state or local surveys.

7. Unemployment rate.

For individuals, unemployment reduces household income, can limit access to health insurance, and can contribute to psychological stress. For a community, an increase in the unemployment rate can increase demands on social services and might signal broader economic problems. The unemployment rate can fluctuate considerably from month to month; therefore rates should be obtained by month or quarter for one to two years to determine the underlying trend. **Field model domains:** individual behavior, social environment, physical environment, prosperity, health care, and health and function. **Data sources:** state employment security office.

8. Number and proportion of single-parent families.

Single-parent families may experience many economic and social stresses that affect the health status of adults and children. **Field model domains:** individual behavior, social environment, physical environment, prosperity, health care, and well-being. **Data sources:** decennial census; data on divorce and births to unmarried mothers can be obtained from the state vital records office to monitor changes in family structure.

9. Number and proportion of persons without health insurance.

Having health insurance can be key for access to health care services. Without insurance, individuals often do not receive timely treatment or preventive care, which can compound adverse health conditions. **Field model domains:** disease, social environment, health care, health and function, and well-being. **Data sources:** no uniform community-level data collection tool is available; state assistance may be necessary to obtain data through community surveys. Oversampling in a state-level survey for the Behavioral Risk Factor Surveillance System (BRFSS) might be a source of information on adults; modifications would be required to obtain information on children.

10. Infant mortality rate by race or ethnicity.

This indicator is included in the consensus set recommended by the CDC (1991) for use by all states and communities. It is widely used as an indicator of child health. Because there are many reasons why infants die, infant mortality reflects the effectiveness of health departments, personal health care providers, outreach services, and preventive services for the mother before and during pregnancy and for the child during the first year of life. The number of deaths will be small in most communities so caution is required in analyzing these data. Usually, data will have to be aggregated for multiple years to produce a stable rate. **Field model domains:** disease, genetics, individual behavior, social environment, physical environment, health care, and prosperity. **Data sources:** state or local vital records.

11. Numbers of deaths or age-adjusted death rates for motor vehicle crashes (ICD-9 codes: E810–E825[1]), work-related injuries, suicide (E950–E959), homicide (E970–E978), lung cancer (162), breast cancer (174), cardiovascular diseases (390–448), and all causes, by age, race, and gender as appropriate.

This indicator is included in the consensus set recommended by CDC (1991) for use by all states and communities. These leading causes of death provide a basic understanding of the health status of the community. Data should be analyzed by age, race, and gender if possible to target preventive efforts. Although in some communities the numbers of deaths will always be too small to develop a stable rate, it is important to know the number of events. For example, although there may not be a large number of teenage suicides, any number is unacceptable. At the community level, the number of deaths for any specific cause will be small, and data will need to be aggregated for multiple years to produce stable rates. **Field model domains:** disease, genetics, individual behavior, social environment, physical environment, health care, and prosperity. **Data sources:** state or local vital records.

12. Reported incidence of AIDS, measles, tuberculosis, and primary and secondary syphilis, by age, race, and gender as appropriate.

This indicator is included in the consensus set recommended by CDC (1991) for use by all states and communities. Communicable diseases such as these affect the individuals who are infected and also place the entire community at risk. For some conditions, the numbers of cases may be too small to develop stable rates, but establishing the number of persons with the disease is important since nearly all cases are potentially prevent-

---

[1]Diagnostic codes assigned under the *International Classification of Diseases*, 9th Revision (USDHHS, 1995).

able. **Field model domains:** disease, genetics, individual behavior, social environment, health care, health and function, well-being, and prosperity. **Data sources:** state or local disease surveillance systems.

13. Births to adolescents (ages 10–17) as a proportion of total live births.

This indicator is included in the consensus set recommended by CDC (1991) for use by all states and communities. Births to young women of school age are usually unplanned and often unwanted. The pregnancy can have a negative impact on the health and well-being of the mother, father, grandparents, and child. Lack of economic and social support can manifest in various diseases and health conditions. **Field model domains:** individual behavior, social environment, well-being, and prosperity. **Data sources:** state or local vital records.

14. Number and rate of confirmed abuse and neglect cases among children.

This indicator is included among the priority data needs to augment the consensus indicators recommended by CDC (1991) for use by all states and communities. Children are the most vulnerable population in a community. Most abuse and neglect cases involve young children who cannot defend or choose for themselves; thus, a community response is required. Child abuse and neglect are thought to be underreported, and inconsistencies in reporting and confirmation practices make it difficult to assess changes in incidence (NRC, 1993). **Field model domains:** disease, individual behavior, social environment, physical environment, health care, and well-being. **Data sources:** state or local child protection agency.

15. Proportion of 2-year-old children who have received all age-appropriate vaccines, as recommended by the Advisory Committee on Immunization Practices.

This indicator is included among the priority data needs to augment the consensus indicators recommended by CDC (1991) for use by all states and communities. The immunization rate reflects the effectiveness of the public health system and personal health care providers in delivering immunization services. It also reflects the impact of family decisions, which can be influenced by personal circumstances, economic factors, and factors affecting access to services. The current series of immunizations recommended for completion by 2 years of age is four doses of diphtheria–tetanus–pertussis (DTP) vaccine; three doses of polio vaccine (oral or inactivated); three doses of Haemophilus influenzae type b (Hib) vaccine; three doses of hepatitis B vaccine; one dose of measles–mumps–rubella (MMR) vaccine; and one dose of varicella vaccine (CDC, 1996). **Field model domains:** individual behavior, social environment, prosperity, and health care. **Data sources:** retrospective school records surveys; community immunization register; community surveys; health plan records; reviews of patient records. Except where an immunization registry has been established, there is no routine reporting on immunizations.

16. Proportion of adults aged 65 and older who have ever been immunized for pneumococcal pneumonia; proportion who have been immunized in the past 12 months for influenza.

This indicator is included among the priority data needs to augment the consensus indicators recommended by CDC (1991) for use by all states and communities. The immunization rate reflects the effectiveness of the public health system and personal health care providers, as well as decisions of the elderly or their caretakers. **Field model domains:** individual behavior, social environment, prosperity, and health care. **Data sources:** Medicare claims files; health plan records; community surveys (questions have been developed for the BRFSS).

17. Proportion of the population who smoke by age, race, and gender as appropriate.

This indicator is included among the priority data needs to augment the consensus indicators recommended by CDC (1991) for use by all states and communities. Smoking is the greatest risk factor associated with the leading causes of death. It has been estimated that 19 percent of all deaths are related to smoking (McGinnis and Foege, 1993). It also contributes to morbidity from chronic lung disease and respiratory infections. Smoking adversely affects the health of smokers and also other persons who breathe secondhand smoke. The fetus of a pregnant woman can be adversely affected as well. Estimates of the prevalence of smoking among adolescents (ages 10–14 and 15–19) might serve as a proxy for more direct measures of smoking initiation. **Field model domains:** disease, individual behavior, social environment, physical environment, prosperity, health care, and health and function. **Data sources:** community surveys (e.g., oversampling for a state survey for the BRFSS) and school-based surveys (e.g., for the Youth Risk Behavior Surveillance System) for data on adolescents; maternal smoking status is recorded on birth certificates, but the quality of the data needs to be evaluated.

18. Proportion of the population age 18 and older who are obese.

This indicator is included among the priority data needs to augment the consensus indicators recommended by CDC (1991) for use by all states and communities. Obesity is associated with increased risk for cardiovascular diseases, diabetes, some cancers, and conditions such as arthritis. It also generally reflects a combination of dietary factors and limited physical activity that are themselves associated with increased health risks. It has been estimated that 14 percent of all deaths in the United States are related to diet and activity patterns (McGinnis and Foege, 1993). Obesity can be measured in terms of the body mass index, which can be constructed from weight and height data (kg/m^2). **Field model domains:** individual behavior, genetics, social environment, health care, health and function, and well-being. **Data sources:** community surveys (e.g., oversampling for a state survey for the BRFSS).

19. Number and type of U.S. Environmental Protection Agency air quality standards not met.

This indicator is included in the consensus set recommended by CDC (1991) for use by all states and communities. Air quality can have a significant impact on health, particularly for those who have chronic respiratory conditions. **Field model domains:** disease, social environment, physical environment, and well-being. **Data sources:** state environmental quality agency; local air quality management agency.

20. Proportion of assessed rivers, lakes and estuaries that support beneficial uses (e.g., fishing and swimming approved).

This indicator is included among the priority data needs to augment the consensus indicators recommended by CDC (1991) for use by all states and communities. Pollution in a community's rivers, lakes, and estuaries may directly cause disease and also affect the well-being of the community. **Field model domains:** disease, individual behavior, social environment, physical environment, and well-being. **Data sources:** state environmental quality agency.

21. Per capita health care spending for Medicare beneficiaries (the Medicare adjusted average per capita cost [AAPCC]).

Analysis shows considerable differences among communities in health care costs even after controlling for demographic factors (Wennberg, 1996). These analyses also indicate no discernible differences in mortality rates in communities that spend less money on health care. Communities should use this indicator in combination with other information (e.g., AAPCC and morbidity levels over time or across communities) in considering the appropriateness of resource use for health care. Because data do not exist on the total health care costs for most communities, the per capita health care spending for Medicare beneficiaries serves as a proxy for the community's total health care costs. **Field model domains:** health care and prosperity. **Data sources:** Health Care Financing Administration.

22. Proportion of adults reporting that their general health is good to excellent.

This indicator is a good overall indicator of the health status of persons in the community. **Field model domains:** health and function and well-being. **Data sources:** community surveys (e.g., oversampling for a state survey for the BRFSS).

23. During the past 30 days, average number of days for which adults report that their physical or mental health was not good.

This indicator is another approach to measuring the overall health of persons in the community. **Field model domains:** health and function and well-being. **Data sources:** community surveys (e.g., oversampling for a state survey for the BRFSS).

24. Proportion of persons satisfied with the health care system in the community.

Perceptions regarding the health care system can have an influence on perceived health status. This indicator is a broad measure of satisfaction, which could relate to many aspects of the health care system including access, cost, availability, quality, and options in health care. No standard measure of "satisfaction" has been established, but the committee endorses efforts to do so. **Field model domains:** social environment, health care, health and function, well-being, and prosperity. **Data sources:** community survey.

25. Proportion of persons satisfied with the quality of life in the community.

As proposed by the committee, health is more than just the biological events occurring or not occurring in a person. The ideal of health is a sense of well-being in a person's life. Although quality of life is a difficult concept to measure, this indicator represents an effort to address this state. Standard measures of satisfaction and quality of life would have to be developed to use this indicator. **Field model domains:** individual behavior, social environment, physical environment, prosperity, health care, health and function, and well-being. **Data sources:** community survey; questions related to quality of life have been developed for the BRFSS.

REFERENCES

CDC (Centers for Disease Control and Prevention). 1991. Consensus Set of Health Status Indicators for the General Assessment of Community Health Status—United States. *Morbidity and Mortality Weekly Report* 40:449–451.

CDC. 1996. Immunization Schedule—United States, January–June 1996. *Morbidity and Mortality Weekly Report* 44:940–943.

McGinnis, J.M., and Foege, W.H. 1993. Actual Causes of Death in the United States. *Journal of the American Medical Association* 270:2207–2211.

NRC (National Research Council). 1993. *Understanding Child Abuse and Neglect.* Washington, D.C.: National Academy Press.

USDHHS. 1995. *International Classification of Diseases, Ninth Revision, Clinical Modification.* 5th ed. DHHS Pub. No. (PHS) 95-1260. Washington, D.C.: National Center for Health Statistics and Health Care Financing Administration.

Wennberg, J., ed. 1996. *The Dartmouth Atlas of Health Care.* Chicago: American Hospital Press.

Zill, N. 1996. Parental Schooling and Children's Health. *Public Health Reports* 111:34–43.

6

Conclusions and Recommendations

As the analysis and examples in this report have demonstrated, a wide array of factors influences a community's health, and many entities in the community share responsibility for maintaining and improving its health. Responsibility shared among many entities, however, can easily become responsibility ignored or abandoned. The *community health improvement process* (CHIP) described in this report offers one approach for a community to address this collective responsibility and to marshal resources of specific, accountable entities to improve the health of its members.

Contributing to the interest in health improvement and performance monitoring is a wider recognition that health embraces well-being as well as the absence of illness. For both individuals and populations, health can be seen to depend not only on medical care but also on other factors including individual behavior and genetic makeup and social and economic conditions. The health field model, as described by Evans and Stoddart (1994) and discussed in Chapter 2, presents these multiple determinants of health in a dynamic relationship. It also suggests that a variety of public and private entities in the community, many of whose roles are not within the traditional domain of health activities, have a stake in and an influence on a community's health (Patrick and Wickizer, 1995).

Performance monitoring has gained increasing attention as a

tool for evaluating the delivery of personal health care services and for examining population-based activities addressing the health of the public (see Chapter 4). Although many performance monitoring activities are focused on specific health care organizations, there is a growing appreciation of their importance from a population-based perspective. Only at the population level is it possible to examine the effectiveness of health promotion and disease prevention activities and to determine whether the needs of all segments of the community are being addressed.

A FRAMEWORK FOR COMMUNITY HEALTH IMPROVEMENT

If a community's resources are to be mobilized for a continuing effort to improve its own health, potential participants must know what values they have in common and develop a clear and shared vision of what can be achieved. Based on its review of the determinants of health, of the forces in the community that can influence them, and of community experience with performance monitoring, the committee finds that a *community health improvement process* that includes performance monitoring, as outlined in this report, can be an effective tool for developing a shared vision and supporting a planned and integrated approach to improve community health. The committee's recommendations for operationalizing a CHIP are based on a variety of theoretical and practical models for community health improvement, continuous quality improvement, quality assurance, and performance monitoring in health care, public health, and other settings. However, the specifics of the committee's proposal have never been tested, in toto, in community settings. Thus, the final section in this chapter identifies a number of ways in which the process that the committee proposes can be evaluated and developed.

The committee suggests that a CHIP should include two principal interacting cycles based on analysis, action, and measurement. The *problem identification and prioritization cycle* focuses on identification and prioritization of health problems in the community, and the *analysis and implementation cycle* on a series of processes intended to devise, implement, and evaluate the impact of health improvement strategies to address the problems (see Figure 6-1).

OPERATIONALIZING THE CHIP CONCEPT

In developing a health improvement program, every commu-

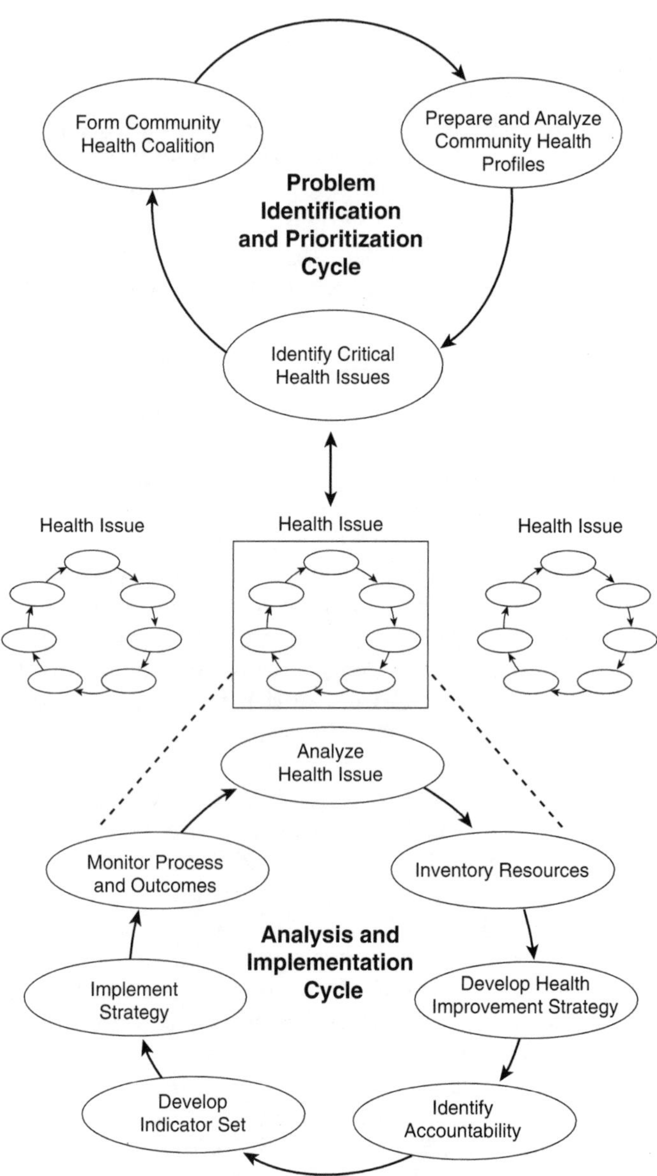

FIGURE 6-1 The community health improvement process (CHIP).

nity will have to consider its own particular circumstances, including factors such as health concerns, resources, social and political perspectives, and other competing concerns. The committee cannot prescribe what actions individual communities should take to address their health concerns or who should be responsible for what, but it does believe that communities need to address these issues and that an organized approach to health improvement that makes use of performance monitoring tools will help them achieve their goals.

Given the different perspectives and activities of personal health service, public health, and other organizations that can contribute to the health of communities and given differing views of the meaning of "health" in the community context, the committee recommends that

- **communities should base a health improvement process on a broad definition of health and a comprehensive conceptual model of how health is produced within the community.**

In the committee's view, the field model, as elaborated by Evans and Stoddart (1994), is a good starting point. They have drawn on evidence from social and behavioral as well as health sciences to construct a comprehensive model of the determinants of health, which provides a potential for engendering creative thinking about possible interventions to improve a community's health. The field model perspective makes it clear that most public and private organizational entities in a community, as well as individuals, share an interest in their community's health and are collectively responsible for it. Among these stakeholders in the community's health, those that can influence health outcomes can be thought of as "accountable entities." Although the field model's comprehensive approach to the determinants of health expands the list of stakeholders and the possibilities for interventions, the model's multifactorial nature also clarifies the need for careful analysis to specify (1) what *individual entities* can contribute and thus be held accountable for contributing, and (2) where *collaborative action* and shared responsibility are essential.

To operationalize the concept of shared responsibility and individual accountability for community health, stakeholders need to know, jointly and as clearly as possible, how the actions of each potentially accountable entity can contribute to the community's health. Thus, the committee recommends that

- **a CHIP should develop its own set of specific, quantitative performance measures, linking accountable entities to the performance of specific activities expected to lead to the production of desired health outcomes in the community.**

Developing community-level performance indicators through the lens of the field model leads to a multidimensional portrayal of the population's health—a highly desirable result, given the committee's working definition of health. To encourage full participation in the health improvement process, the selected performance measures should be balanced across the interests and contributions of the various accountable entities in the community, including those whose primary mission is not health specific. Selecting indicators also requires careful consideration of how to gain insight into progress achieved in the health improvement process. A set of indicators should balance population-based measures of risk factors and health outcomes and health systems-based measures of services performed. A balance is also needed among indicators that focus on short-term gains and those that target more fundamental changes in community health.

Knowing that stakeholder-level performance measures will, in many instances, be unique to a particular community and to the circumstances of stakeholders in that community, the committee devoted its energies to developing community-level performance indicators. Such performance measures would permit communities and their health coalitions to ask, "How are we, as a community, performing in assuring the health of our citizenry?" The prototype indicators also include measures specific to sectors in the community such as managed care organizations, schools, employers, and public health agencies. Depending on their circumstances, individual communities may want to go beyond this to include measures for specific managed care organizations, specific large employers, and so on.

Communities have to establish criteria that can guide the selection of indicators. In the committee's view, such criteria should include consistency with a conceptual framework, such as the field model, for understanding factors that contribute to the production of health, salience to community stakeholders, and support for the social change processes needed to achieve health improvements. Indicators should also be assessed against criteria of validity and reliability, evidence linking performance and health improvement, sensitivity to changes in community health status, and availability of timely data at a reasonable cost. It is also essential to develop an operational definition for each measure to determine what data are needed and how (or if) they can be obtained. A review of existing indicator sets may suggest measures that could be adapted for community use and may be a source of tested operational definitions.

Many of the important influences on health that the field model helps identify are often not amenable to change in the short run. For example, interventions aimed at critical developmental periods, such as educational programs in early childhood, may have long-term health benefits but produce little measurable effect in the near term. A desire to make observable progress can lead a CHIP to focus on other more immediately measurable problems or on problems that may be high on the political agenda but of uncertain importance to the community's overall health (e.g., a new renal dialysis unit). Participants in a CHIP must also ensure that the process does not become paralyzed by focusing on the undoable. To maintain momentum for coalitions set up to foster community health improvement, it may be reasonable to select some problems that are amenable to change and success in the short term. Thus, the committee recommends that

- **a CHIP should seek a balance between strategic opportunities for long-term health improvement and goals that are achievable in the short term.**

One way to achieve this balance is by including interim goals, such as risk reduction strategies, for major health problems. If a community were interested in reducing cancer mortality, for instance, reductions in smoking initiation among teenagers and the implementation of workplace smoking restrictions might be appropriate intermediate goals.

The proposed health improvement process and performance monitoring activities will require that communities have a sustainable organization or system that represents all major stakeholders and accountable entities. Thus, the committee recommends that

- **community coalitions guiding CHIPs should strive for strategic inclusiveness, incorporating individuals, groups, and organizations that have an interest in health outcomes, can take actions necessary to improve community health, or can contribute data and analytic capabilities needed for performance monitoring.**

Participants should assume responsibility for contributing to the health of the community, not just furthering the goals of the organizations they represent.

As described in Chapters 3 and 4, a CHIP focuses on horizontal peer relationships in a community rather than vertical hierarchical relationships. Experience suggests that performance monitoring used as a basis for inspection and discipline of those not producing as expected is less effective in achieving improvements than is monitoring used as a tool for learning and process change (Berwick, 1989; Osborne and Gaebler, 1992). Rather, a CHIP should use performance monitoring to encourage productive action and collaboration from many sectors. Because the proposed community health improvement process is new, the groups that carry it out should be "learning organizations" in the sense that the people, agencies, and community involved are organized to learn from their own experience and improve their operations.

All community initiatives require leadership, which may come from the public or the private sector. To institutionalize the health improvement process as a multiparty effort, the committee recommends that

- **a CHIP should be centered in a community health coalition or similar entity.**

Some communities will have appropriate coalitions in place, but others will need to expand existing groups or establish a workable forum for collective action for the first time. Strategies for improving the effectiveness of community coalitions for health improvement are discussed in Chapter 3.

ENABLING POLICY AND RESOURCES

Federal, state, and local public health agencies and boards of health are all stakeholders in a community's health and capable of taking action to improve it. Indeed, *The Future of Public Health* (IOM, 1988) implies that public health agencies have a responsibility to assure that something like a CHIP is in place.

In general, the roles of federal, state, and local public health agencies might be described as follows:

- At the federal level, the Public Health Service can provide leadership and resources (e.g., research funding, technical assistance, data and data collection) that promote the implementation of community-level activities and especially the development of measures and measurement tools.

• At the state level, health departments should promote community-based activities and, in the committee's view, have a particular responsibility to facilitate community access to data such as that needed for the proposed community health profile. The experience in states such as Illinois, Massachusetts, and Washington (see Appendixes C and D) suggests that leadership from the state health department can promote activities at the local level.

• At the local level, the health department must be a part of the community coalition that is addressing health issues and must be prepared, as one of the community's accountable entities, to perform functions consistent with the needs of the community; these will vary widely.

In particular, the committee recommends that

• **state and local public health agencies should assure that an effective community health improvement process is in place in all communities. These agencies should at a minimum participate in CHIP activities and, in some communities, should provide its leadership and/or organizational home.**

For the CHIP to be effective, communities need certain resources, especially data for community health profiles and performance measures. Since all parties share in the goal of improving community health, it is reasonable that public and private resources be combined to support the data collection and analysis needed for communities to obtain health profile information, to conduct health status assessments and communicate results, and to sustain performance monitoring programs. Such resources could include funding, personnel, data, and data processing and analysis.

Both public and private sectors can contribute critical data for performance monitoring. Public health agencies, as part of the public health assessment function called for in *The Future of Public Health*, should promote, facilitate—and where necessary and appropriate—perform community health assessments and monitor changes in key performance measures. Much of the necessary data and expertise exist at the state health department. Thus, the committee recommends that

- **in support of community-level health improvement processes, state health agencies, in cooperation and collaboration with local health departments, should assure the availability of community-level data needed for health profiles.**

Currently, most of the data for these profiles are aggregated by standard geopolitical units such as counties, municipalities, and so on. To the extent possible, community health data should be made available in a form that allows communities to prepare health profiles and performance measures according to their own definitions (e.g., geographic, socioeconomic, cultural) of the community. Geocoding of health data gathered for other purposes would be an important step toward improving the data for performance monitoring. For data available only at the community level, state health departments should provide models and technical assistance that communities can use in their own data collection activities.

Because data on and from all accountable entities are essential for effective performance monitoring, states and the federal government (in their policy development and regulatory roles) can assist communities by facilitating access to relevant data held by the private sector. In particular, the committee recommends that

- **states and the federal government, through health departments or other appropriate channels, should require that health plans, indemnity insurers, and other private entities report standard data on the characteristics and health status of their enrolled populations, on services provided, and on outcomes of those services, as necessary for performance monitoring in the community health improvement process.**

Providing these data should be seen as part of the responsibility that these private-sector organizations have to the community (IOM, 1996; Showstack et al., 1996). Adequate safeguards for privacy and confidentiality will be necessary for all CHIP data (IOM, 1994).

The relationship between the CHIP and public or private community organizations should be reciprocal. In addition to data that these organizations can provide to a CHIP, the organizations can use other community data that are gathered, and this in turn should reinforce CHIP goals. For instance, health policymakers at the federal and state levels could consider community-level performance indicators when planning and evaluating publicly funded health services programs such as managed care for Medicaid populations. State agencies designing these programs can specify what performance measures will be used in evaluating the contractors and what data the contractors must report. Similarly, state-level licensure and accreditation of health systems could be tied to performance monitoring systems that stipulate measurable targets for performance and hold systems accountable for achieving targets during the term of licensure. Private health service organizations could use CHIP data in assessing their own contributions to the community's health under "community benefit" guidelines and regulations or in their own service planning and resource allocation decisions. Community performance measures could also contribute to the management of federal block grants and the proposed federal Performance Partnership Grants (USDHHS, no date).

DEVELOPING THE COMMUNITY HEALTH IMPROVEMENT PROCESS

The community health improvement process and its use of performance monitoring, as laid out in this report, are a work in progress. In preparing this report, the committee reviewed existing efforts at the national, state, and community levels and found much of value. The committee also found, however, that a conceptual framework for using performance monitoring concepts to improve community health as a whole (as opposed to monitoring the performance of specific entities such as managed care organizations or public health agencies) was lacking. The development of such a conceptual framework, and the illustration of its application through sets of prototype indicators, is the major contribution of this report, but this framework remains largely untested. The overall community health improvement process, its performance monitoring component, and the indicator sets should be tested and improved over time. Thus, the committee recommends that

- **the CHIP concept developed in this report should be implemented in a variety of communities across the country, and these efforts should be carefully documented and independently assessed.**

The assessment process should strive to include sites that vary both in the nature of the community (size and political jurisdiction, socioeconomic and racial composition, region of the country, specific health issues addressed) and in the structures and processes used for performance monitoring (composition of the group responsible for identifying and monitoring performance measures, leadership role of state and local health departments, and so on). The assessment should also include estimates of the full range of public and private costs of carrying out the CHIP and should explore ways to achieve efficiencies in these efforts. The goals of these "natural experiments" would be to learn how local circumstances, including opportunities and barriers experienced, affect the way the CHIP is adapted by different communities; to identify the "necessary and desirable conditions" for implementation of the CHIP; and to assess whether or not the CHIP indeed results in a refocusing of attention on root causes of health problems and, ultimately, in important improvements in community health.

The current evaluations of community health interventions ought to inform this field through their findings on specific interventions to address health problems, on the community intervention process itself, and on the analytic techniques to apply to community studies. Among the programs being evaluated are interventions to reduce coronary heart disease sponsored by the National Heart Lung and Blood Institute in California (Fortmann et al., 1995), Minnesota (Murray, 1995), and Rhode Island (Elder et al., 1993); the Community Intervention Trial for Smoking Cessation (COMMIT, 1995a,b) sponsored by the National Cancer Institute; and the Kaiser Family Foundation's Community Health Promotion Grant Program (Wagner et al., 1991; Wickizer et al., 1993). The work of the recently established Task Force on Community Preventive Services, organized by the Centers for Disease Control and Prevention, will be compiling evidence on the effectiveness of a variety of community-level activities. The CHIP in its entirety can also be thought of as a "comprehensive community initiative," and many of the ideas regarding the evaluation of such initiatives can be applied (see Connell et al., 1995).

For the proposed community health improvement process to be effective, performance measurement tools for community health must be developed further. Thus, the committee recommends that

- **the Public Health Service, in conjunction with state and**

local health agencies, national professional organizations, and foundations, should develop standard measures for community health profiles and topic-specific model indicator sets that perform well in individual communities and are suitable for cross-community comparison.

These standard measures would be a resource available to communities, not a set of prescribed measures. The prototype indicator sets described in Appendix A of this report should be viewed as a starting point. Particular attention should be given to issues for which valid measures are not currently available, but the refinement of existing measures should also be addressed. The development of measures of "quality of life" and consumer satisfaction for use in community surveys is particularly important. Research to develop and improve techniques of measurement and analysis (e.g., small area analysis) that can be applied to community-level performance monitoring should also be supported. Noack and McQueen (1988) have observed that the development of health promotion indicators has often been approached as a technical matter, ignoring the need to clarify basic concepts of health and the purpose of such indicators. To further indicator development, they encourage a dialogue between health researchers and policymakers.

More generally, technical expertise based on experience with the CHIP must be developed and shared. Although a wide variety of excellent resources on community health assessment and CQI currently exist, those materials generally do not link assessment and CQI concepts and techniques in the way that is envisioned for a CHIP. Thus, the committee recommends that

- **the Public Health Service, in conjunction with state and local health agencies, national professional organizations, and foundations, should develop workbooks, seminars, and other forms of technical assistance to catalog and convey to communities information on best CHIP practices, specific model performance measures for a variety of health issues and ways to interpret changes in these measures, and available data resources.**

Universities can, in a variety of activities and through a variety of disciplines, play an important role in helping communities implement a CHIP and in developing and sharing technical expertise. Schools of public health, which have been urged to turn their attention to public health practice issues (IOM, 1988; Sorensen and Bialek, 1991), could begin by working with their local communities as part of a CHIP. CDC's university-based health promotion and disease prevention research centers (CDC, 1996) are another vehicle through which universities might contribute.

In the long run, effective dissemination of the CHIP concept will depend on the development of a workforce whose attitudes, values, and skills support its implementation. Thus, the committee recommends that

- **educational programs for professionals in public health, medicine, nursing, health administration, public management, and related fields should include CHIP concepts and practices in their curriculum for preservice and midcareer students.**

These programs should introduce the concept of CHIP as a way of thinking about the application of a group of academic disciplines (epidemiology, biostatistics, environmental health, health behavior, and so on) to the practice of community health improvement. Among the other fields in which CHIP might be addressed are maternal and child health, behavioral sciences, and mental health and substance abuse counseling and program administration.

REFERENCES

Berwick, D.M. 1989. Continuous Improvement as an Ideal in Health Care. *New England Journal of Medicine* 320:53–56.

CDC (Centers for Disease Control and Prevention). 1996. *Health Promotion and Disease Prevention Research Center Program: Annual Report 1996.* Atlanta, Ga.: CDC, National Center for Chronic Disease Prevention and Health Promotion.

COMMIT (Community Intervention Trial for Smoking Cessation). 1995a. I. Cohort Results from a Four-Year Community Intervention. *American Journal of Public Health* 85:183–192.

COMMIT. 1995b. II. Changes in Adult Cigarette Smoking Prevalence. *American Journal of Public Health* 85:193–200.

Connell, J.P., Kubisch, A.C., Schorr, L.B., and Weiss, C.H., eds. 1995. *New Approaches to Evaluating Community Initiatives: Concepts, Methods, and Contexts.* Washington, D.C.: Aspen Institute.

Elder, J.P., Schmid, T.L., Dower, P., and Hedlund, S. 1993. Community Heart Health Programs: Components, Rationale, and Strategies for Effective Interventions. *Journal of Public Health Policy* 14:463–479.

Evans, R.G., and Stoddart, G.L. 1994. Producing Health, Consuming Health Care. In *Why Are Some People Healthy and Others Not? The Determinants of Health of Populations.* R.G. Evans, M.L. Barer, and T.R. Marmor, eds. New York: Aldine De Gruyter.

Fortmann, S.P., Flora, J.A., Winkleby, M.A., Schooler, C., Taylor, C.B., and Farquhar, J.W. 1995. Community Intervention Trials: Reflections on the Stanford Five-City Project Experience. *American Journal of Epidemiology* 142:576–586.

IOM (Institute of Medicine). 1988. *The Future of Public Health.* Washington, D.C.: National Academy Press.

IOM. 1994. *Health Data in the Information Age: Use, Disclosure, and Privacy.* M.S. Donaldson and K.N. Lohr, eds. Washington, D.C.: National Academy Press.

IOM. 1996. *Healthy Communities: New Partnerships for the Future of Public Health.* M.A. Stoto, C. Abel, and A. Dievler, eds. Washington, D.C.: National Academy Press.

Murray, D. 1995. Design and Analysis of Community Trials: Lessons from the Minnesota Heart Health Program. *American Journal of Epidemiology* 142:569–575.

Noack, H., and McQueen, D. 1988. Toward Health Promotion Indicators. *Health Promotion* 3(1):73–78.

Osborne, D., and Gaebler, T. 1992. *Reinventing Government: How the Entrepreneurial Spirit is Transforming the Public Sector.* Reading, Mass.: Addison-Wesley.

Patrick, D.L., and Wickizer, T.M. Community and Health. 1995. In *Society and Health.* B.C. Amick, S. Levine, A.R. Tarlov, and D.C. Walsh, eds. New York: Oxford University Press.

Showstack, J., Lurie, N., Leatherman, S., Fisher, E., and Inui, T. 1996. Health of the Public: The Private Sector Challenge. *Journal of the American Medical Association* 276:1071–1074.

Sorensen, A.A., and Bialek, R.G., eds. 1991. *The Public Health Faculty/Agency Forum: Linking Graduate Education and Practice.* Final Report. Gainesville: University Press of Florida.

USDHHS (U.S. Department of Health and Human Services). No date. *Performance Measurement in Selected Public Health Programs: 1995–1996 Regional Meetings.* Washington, D.C.: Office of the Assistant Secretary for Health.

Wagner, E.H., Koepsell, T.D., Anderman, C., et al. 1991. The Evaluation of the Henry J. Kaiser Family Foundation's Community Health Promotion Program: Design. *Journal of Clinical Epidemiology* 44:685–699.

Wickizer, T.M., Von Korff, M., Cheadle, A., et al. 1993. Activating Communities for Health Promotion: A Process Evaluation Method. *American Journal of Public Health* 83:561–567.

Appendixes

A

Prototype Performance Indicator Sets

This report proposes an organized activity—a community health improvement process—that uses performance monitoring to assess the impact of health improvement activities on health outcomes and to promote accountability among a diverse array of community stakeholders for participation in those activities (see Chapter 4). The process operates through two interacting cycles: (1) a broader *problem identification and prioritization cycle*, through which a community maintains an overview of its health and health-related activities and determines which health issues are of special concern; and (2) more narrowly focused *analysis and implementation cycles*, through which these specific health concerns are addressed.

An essential component of the analysis and implementation cycle is the development of sets of indicators that a community can use to monitor the performance of its accountable entities (see Chapter 5). As proposed by the committee, these indicator sets should reflect the broad definition of health and its determinants that is embodied in the field model as presented by Evans and Stoddart (1994; also see Chapter 2 of this report) and should address the roles that multiple community stakeholders can play in shaping a community's health.

The committee has developed prototypes for such indicator sets to illustrate how communities might apply these proposals.

Presented in this appendix are the committee's indicator sets for nine specific health issues:

1. breast and cervical cancer,
2. depression,
3. elder health,
4. environmental and occupational lead exposure,
5. health care resource allocation,
6. infant health,
7. tobacco use,
8. vaccine-preventable diseases, and
9. violence.

These issues were selected with several considerations in mind. The committee wanted to use as examples topics that are of concern at the community level and that can be addressed by community-level action. The committee also wanted to give examples that relate to the interests and roles of a diverse group of community stakeholders. A further consideration was illustrating different ways in which health issues might be framed (e.g., on the basis of population groups, risk factors, forms of morbidity, economic factors, societal concerns). The committee's examples also illustrate the interrelated nature of many health concerns. For example, reducing vaccine-preventable diseases carries benefits for both infant and elder health. Thus, interventions initiated in one context can have implications for other issues that may be of concern to a community.

Once specific health issues had been selected, the committee developed its indicator sets using an approach like the community-based process described in Chapters 4 and 5. The domains of the field model provided a guide for examining each issue to formulate a broad list of potential performance indicators. From this list, about 10 indicators were selected as a proposed indicator set. The committee notes that for most of the health issues, the domain of genetic endowment includes few indicators because opportunities for intervention are currently limited. With growing knowledge in this field, however, additional interventions may emerge, making it possible to consider developing performance indicators.

The selection criteria considered were those presented in Chapter 5: established validity and reliability of a measure to be used; an evidenced-based link between performance to be measured and health improvement; robustness and responsiveness of a measure to meaningful change in performance or health status; availability of data in a timely manner at a reasonable cost; opportunities to assign responsibility and accountability for performance; and inclusion in other monitoring systems (monitoring sets). Indicators must also be measurable; that is, it must be possible to formulate an operational definition that identifies units to be counted, a rate's numerator and denominator, or other appropriate components of a measurement.

Ideally, an indicator should meet all of these criteria, with the exception of inclusion in another monitoring system; in practice, limitations in knowledge and available data may make it appropriate to begin with usable measures while efforts are under way to develop better ones. Resources that communities might draw on to identify potential indicators include documents that cover many health issues, such as *Healthy People 2000* (USDHHS, 1991) and its "midcourse" review (USDHHS, 1995); *Healthy Communities 2000: Model Standards* (APHA et al., 1991); and the *Health Plan Employer Data and Information Set and Users Manual* (HEDIS; NCQA, 1993, 1996). More specialized resources are also available (e.g., Walker and Richmond, 1984; National Committee for Injury Prevention and Control, 1989; AMBHA, 1995; Fawcett et al., 1995). In using these sources, communities need to look beyond measures of health status to indicators that link performance and outcomes, and beyond measures for a small set of stakeholder groups to indicators that encompass the entire community.

In a community setting, a variety of stakeholders should have the opportunity to participate in the selection of indicators through a mechanism such as a health coalition. For the examples presented here, a member of the committee or the study staff assumed primary responsibility for developing the materials on a given issue but was not necessarily an expert in that field. Comments were provided by other committee members, and for each health issue, advice was received from a small number of outside experts. As a result, the proposed indicators represent an informed but not definitive selection.

The committee focused its attention on performance measures applicable at the community level or to a broad category of community stakeholders (e.g., health plans, Medicaid participants, schools, employers, the elderly), not on measures applicable to a specific accountable entity in any stakeholder group. Recognizing that communities will differ in how a health issue presents itself, what resources and policy options are available, and who the accountable entities are, the committee concluded that it could not, and should not try to, propose indicators that link specific stakeholders to specific types of performance. Some likely points of accountability are noted, however. Each community will have to tailor indicators to its particular circumstances.

To improve the resources available to communities seeking to implement a performance monitoring program, the committee has recommended a national effort to develop model indicator sets with standard measures. The work of scientific panels convened to review evidence linking performance and health outcomes and to address technical issues in measurement and data analysis of particular relevance at the community level will have to be integrated with guidance from community representatives on matters of acceptance and implementation. The extensive consultation on and analysis of performance measures undertaken by the U.S. Department of Health and Human Services for the proposed Public Health Performance Partnership Grants (see NRC, 1996; USDHHS, no date) and by the National Committee for Quality Assurance (NCQA, 1996) for HEDIS 3.0 illustrate the level of effort that could be needed.

In this appendix, each of the committee's prototype indicator sets is presented with a brief review of the health issue that touches on points such as the population health burden, social costs, and opportunities for change. That section is followed by a discussion of potential indicators suggested by the domains of the field model and of the likely roles of various stakeholders. The next part of each presentation focuses on the 10 or so community-level measures that were selected from among the potential indicators. Comments are provided on why individual indicators were selected and their relationship as an indicator "set." Also noted are special considerations in obtaining data or interpreting the measures used.

A summary table maps each of the proposed indicators to a domain of the field model and, in some cases, suggests stakeholders that are likely to have an interest. Each indicator has been assigned to a specific domain but may be relevant to other domains as well. Additional or alternative stakeholders may also be appropriate. The field model domains and an illustrative set of stakeholder groups that the committee used as reference points are listed in Table A-1.

All of the health issues were addressed in the same general manner, but each topic poses unique problems and committee authors each brought a particular perspective to the task of formulating a prototype indicator set. As a result, the character of

TABLE A-1 Field Model Domains and Examples of Stakeholder Groups Used in Developing Prototype Performance Indicator Sets

Field Model Domains	Stakeholder Groups
Disease	Health care providers
Individual behavior and response	Health care plans
Genetic endowment	Local government
Social environment	State public health agencies
Physical environment	Local public health agencies
Health care	Environmental health agencies and organizations
Health and function	Education agencies and institutions
Well-being	Business and industry
Prosperity	Community-based organizations
	Populations with special health risks
	Disease or patient organizations
	General public

the presentations and indicators varies across issues, offering illustrations of different approaches that might prove useful in a community.

REFERENCES

AMBHA (American Managed Behavioral Healthcare Association). 1995. Performance Measures for Managed Behavioral Healthcare Programs. Washington, D.C.: AMBHA.

APHA (American Public Health Association), Association of Schools of Public Health, Association of State and Territorial Health Officials, National Association of County Health Officials, United States Conference of Local Health Officers, Department of Health and Human Services, Public Health Service, Centers for Disease Control. 1991. *Healthy Communities 2000: Model Standards.* 3rd ed. Washington, D.C.: APHA.

Evans, R.G., and Stoddart, G.L. 1994. Producing Health, Consuming Health Care. In *Why Are Some People Healthy and Others Not? The Determinants of Health of Populations.* R.G. Evans, M.L. Barer, and T.R. Marmor, eds. New York: Aldine De Gruyter.

Fawcett, S.B., Sterling, T.D., Paine-Andrews, A., et al. 1995. *Evaluating Community Efforts to Prevent Cardiovascular Diseases.* Atlanta, Ga.: Centers for Disease Control and Prevention, National Center for Chronic Disease Prevention and Health Promotion.

National Committee for Injury Prevention and Control. 1989. *Injury Prevention: Meeting the Challenge.* New York: Oxford University Press.

NCQA (National Committee for Quality Assurance). 1993. *Health Plan Employer Data and Information Set and Users Manual, Version 2.0 (HEDIS 2.0)*. Washington, D.C.: NCQA.

NCQA. 1996. HEDIS 3.0 Draft for Public Comment. Washington, D.C.: NCQA.

NRC (National Research Council). 1996. *Assessment of Performance Measures in Public Health*. Phase 1 Report. Draft for Comment. Washington, D.C.: National Academy Press.

USDHHS (U.S. Department of Health and Human Services). 1991. *Healthy People 2000: National Health Promotion and Disease Prevention Objectives*. DHHS Pub. No. (PHS) 91-50212. Washington, D.C.: Office of the Assistant Secretary for Health.

USDHHS. 1995. *Healthy People 2000: Midcourse Review and 1995 Revisions*. Washington, D.C.: USDHHS, Public Health Service.

USDHHS. No date. *Performance Measurement in Selected Public Health Programs: 1995–1996 Regional Meetings*. Washington, D.C.: Office of the Assistant Secretary for Health.

Walker, D.K., and Richmond, J.B., eds. 1984. *Monitoring Child Health in the United States: Selected Issues and Policies*. Cambridge, Mass.: Harvard University Press.

A.1

Prototype Indicator Set: Breast and Cervical Cancers

BACKGROUND

Breast and cervical cancers are major causes of death and suffering among women in the United States. Although each disease has a distinct etiology, screening currently is the principal preventive intervention for both. Communities may want to develop an integrated approach to diseases such as these that are of concern to a specific segment of the population.

Breast Cancer

Breast cancer is the second leading cause of cancer death among women. It accounts for 31 percent of all newly diagnosed cancers in women and 17 percent of women's cancer deaths (American Cancer Society, 1996). It is estimated that over a lifetime one out of nine women is affected by breast cancer (American Cancer Society, 1995). Screening procedures such as clinical breast examination and mammography can help detect breast cancer at an early stage, which significantly increases chances for successful treatment and cure. Use of mammography screening and clinical breast examination have been associated with reductions of 20–30 percent in breast cancer mortality in women over age 50 (Kerlikowske et al., 1995). In general, cancers are detected at more advanced stages among minority and poor women, and these women also have higher mortality rates.

Major risk factors for breast cancer include older age, Caucasian race, higher socioeconomic status, and never marrying. Early onset of menstruation, late menopause, no full-term pregnancies before age 30, and never having given birth are additional risk factors. A family history of breast cancer in a woman's mother or sister is an important risk factor for about 5–10 percent of total cases (Colditz et al., 1993; Slattery and Kerber, 1993). In general, these risk factors are not easily modifiable, but two behavioral factors, alcohol consumption and breast feeding, may offer opportunities to reduce risk. Consuming more than two alcoholic beverages a day appears to increase the risk of developing breast cancer (Longnecker et al., 1995), and breast feeding appears to have a protective effect (Newcomb et al., 1994). Identifying risk factors for breast cancer can provide some guidance for prioritizing screening and early intervention programs, but current screening guidelines rely primarily on age.

Cervical Cancer

Cervical cancer is one of the most curable cancers in women, if caught in time through early screening and intervention. Cervical cancer carries a five-year survival rate of about 90 percent if localized, but only 40 percent of women with invasive disease survive five years (Ries et al., 1994). Of concern is evidence that since 1986 the previous downturn in the incidence of cervical cancer in women over age 50 has reversed and that it is now increasing about 3 percent each year (Washington State Department of Health, 1994). Early intervention through effective screening is critical for influencing health and survival.

Attention should also be given to the opportunities for prevention of cervical cancer. Risk factors include early age of sexual intercourse, multiple sex partners, human papilloma virus (HPV) infection (i.e., genital warts), lower socioeconomic status, and nonwhite race (Kjaer et al., 1992). Use of barrier methods of contraception appears to have a protective effect, perhaps due to decreasing exposure to HPV and other viruses (Slattery et al., 1989a). In addition, there may be an association between cigarette smoking and cervical cancer (Slattery et al., 1989b). An understanding of the risk factors for cervical cancer can point to interventions that can promote prevention. It can also help prioritize screening and early intervention programs, but efforts might also focus on increasing the proportion of women screened regardless of specific risk factors.

"FIELD" SET OF PERFORMANCE INDICATORS

The field model encourages a shift from a focus on individuals to the community as a whole. The potential stakeholders for such an effort include all segments of the community. By using the domains of the field model, it is possible to identify a variety of measures that might serve as performance indicators for a community's efforts to improve the health of women by reducing the toll of breast and cervical cancers.

Disease and Health Care

Falling under the disease and health care domains of the field model are essential tasks for addressing breast and cervical cancer prevention. Currently, principal focus is on secondary prevention through screening programs. These programs require patient–provider interactions, support from the social environment, and cooperation of individuals. Possible indicators include the following:

1. Number of cases and rates (incidence and mortality) for breast and cervical cancers, including stage at diagnosis.

Data on incidence are an important indicator of overall system-wide performance, however, this indicator is not likely to be sensitive to small changes or to small-area improvements. Nevertheless, incidence remains an essential indicator because it allows comparisons over time and over large populations. The collection and analysis of these data tend to be the responsibility of the public health system. Examples of more specific performance indicators that could be used in communities include the following:

- For each managed care organization (MCO) and the community as a whole, the number of cases and the incidence of breast and cervical cancers, by stage at diagnosis.
- For the community as a whole, the number of deaths and the death rate from breast and cervical cancers, by stage at diagnosis.

2. Access to affordable and quality-controlled mammography

screening, clinical breast examination, cervical cancer screening (Pap test), and pelvic examination.

Access to these four primary screening services is essential for utilization and follow-up to occur. Access is the first step in an effective early intervention breast and cervical cancer program. The qualifiers "affordable" and "quality controlled" were included to indicate that access is defined by certain expectations. Major stakeholders include health care providers, health plans, state health agencies, environmental health agencies, and community-based organizations.

Health care providers and health plans are responsible for developing and offering screening programs. There is consensus that mammography should be performed every one to two years for women between the ages of 50 and 69 (U.S. Preventive Services Task Force, 1996), but consensus has not emerged regarding guidelines for women under age 50 or over age 69. A Pap test is suggested at least every three years for sexually active women (U.S. Preventive Services Task Force, 1996).

Health care providers are also responsible for following quality standards established for breast and cervical cancer screening. The state public health system usually participates in setting regulatory standards such as mammography screening and laboratory standards. The state health department may also be involved in programs to reduce barriers to accessing services and to identify women who do not use services and the reasons why. Environmental health agencies may be involved in inspections regarding the safety of facilities and equipment. Community-based organizations such as community clinics and voluntary organizations such as the American Cancer Society may also be involved in identifying women in need of screening and in the standard-setting process.

Although this indicator is primarily related to disease and health care, it also involves the social environment and prosperity. Barriers related to access, geography, and safety can be overcome by working with stakeholders from the social environment. Prosperity may dictate whether communities offer services at sufficient sites and whether women can afford to take advantage of the services.

More specific performance indicators that could be used by communities include the following:

- Proportion and number of facilities offering mammography and Pap tests that meet federal and state regulatory standards.

• Proportion of health plans or insurers that cover 80 percent or more of the cost of breast and cervical cancer screening.

3. Referral and follow-up rates on results from positive mammography and Pap test screening.

For women who have been screened, follow-up by health care providers and health plans of the results and recommendations from screening programs is essential to early intervention in the event of disease or evidence of high risk of disease. Local public health agencies are another important stakeholder; they may coordinate tracking programs that remind women about screening or may follow up women who are in need of care and lost to the system.

An example of a performance indicator that could be used in communities is the following:

• For each health plan or insurer, the proportion of enrolled women with positive results for mammography or Pap testing who receive appropriate and timely follow-up care.

4. Rates at which physicians refer women for screening mammograms.

Physicians are in a good position to educate, counsel, and refer women for mammography screening. This indicator engages individual providers as well as health plans, which must encourage physicians to make this a routine part of counseling for women in targeted populations. The advice of a primary care physician can be a strong incentive for women to seek preventive screening (American Cancer Society, 1993). The data for this indicator would be contained in medical records.

Examples of performance indicators that could be used in communities are the following:

• For each MCO, family practitioner, internist, and obstetrician–gynecologist, the proportion of women served who should have mammography who were referred for mammography in the past 12 months.

• For each MCO, family practitioner, internist, and obstetrician–gynecologist, the proportion of referred women who received mammography within 30 days of referral.

Behavior and Genetic Endowment

A number of risk factors for cervical cancer are behavioral in nature and potentially modifiable. For example, age at first sexual intercourse, number of sex partners, cigarette smoking and contraceptive methods are modifiable if communities can effectively translate health promotion messages into behavior changes. Benefits conferred by changing these behaviors will extend well beyond a decreased risk of cervical cancer; risks of sexually transmitted diseases, lung disease, and unwanted pregnancy will also be reduced.

Fewer of the risk factors for breast cancer are modifiable. Alcohol consumption and breast feeding are factors that can be modified; to an extent, age at first pregnancy may be modified. The influence of family history on the occurrence of breast cancer represents a potential focus for community activities. Women with a family history of breast cancer should be encouraged to modify their risk of disease, to the extent possible, through behavior changes. Another aspect of behavior that can change is seeking and using preventive and screening services.

Potential indicators include the following:

1. Rates of tobacco use and alcohol consumption among women.

Cigarette smoking and alcohol consumption (of two or more drinks per day) are especially important lifestyle factors. To date, evidence of their relationship to cervical and breast cancers remains only suggestive of an association (Slattery et al., 1989b; Longnecker et al., 1995), but cigarette smoking and alcohol consumption are known to be linked to numerous other causes of morbidity and mortality.

2. Proportion of sexually active women who use barrier methods of contraception.

Epidemiologic data indicating that barrier methods of contraception (i.e., condoms or diaphragms) reduce a woman's risk of cervical cancer are consistent with researchers' understanding of the viral etiology of the disease. Studies reviewed by the U.S. Preventive Services Task Force (1996) showed substantial reductions in risk for both condom users (20–60 percent) and diaphragm users (30–80 percent). It has also been suggested that spermicides have antiviral properties that can contribute a protective effect.

3. Utilization of screening programs by women at risk for breast and cervical cancer.

Access is only the first step in an effective program. Women must use the services once access is established; therefore, their individual behavior and response are important.

The following are examples of performance indicators that could be used in communities:

- For each health plan or insurer, the proportion of enrolled women who should have breast and cervical cancer screening who received appropriate screening services in the past 12 months.
- For women who are not enrolled in a health plan or insurance group, the proportion who should have breast and cervical cancer screening who received appropriate screening services in the past 12 months.

Social Environment

The social environment is an important domain of the field model and has a role to play in reducing the burden of breast and cervical cancers in a community. Stakeholders in the social environment may provide (1) information to make women aware of the need for and availability of screening activities and (2) supportive services that enable women to use screening services.

1. Availability of breast and cervical cancer public education programs for target populations that include information on breast self-exam, the importance and availability of screening programs, and the value of screening as a tool to protect health and well-being.

Public education programs involve all stakeholders. Health care providers and health plans often are a source of education for patients. State and local public health agencies, including environmental health agencies, are involved in public education campaigns at the population level. Local government may provide financial support for public education programs. Educational programs can be offered at the work site, in providers' offices, and at sites used by education organizations and institutions. Populations at risk for the diseases are responsible for receiving the information and subsequently putting it to use. Patient or disease organizations often contribute data and information for inclusion in educational programs. Thus, many segments of the community share responsibility for this aspect of efforts to improve the health status of women at risk for breast and cervical cancers.

Some of these data are tracked by state health departments and health plans. Overall, however, the ability to collect and analyze data for this indicator is somewhat troublesome, and therefore, it may be weak when standing alone. This indicator also may have limited sensitivity to changes in the performance of the system and may be difficult to track given the array of individuals, organizations, and institutions involved in educational programs.

Examples of performance indicators that could be used in communities are the following:

- Proportion of employers, community-based organizations, school parent–teacher associations (PTAs), or faith organizations that provided in the past 12 months health promotion programs in the community about the value of screening, breast self-exam, and the availability of screening programs to prevent breast and cervical cancer among women.
- For each health plan or insurer and the community as a whole, the proportion of women who have a risk factor for breast or cervical cancer that can be modified through lifestyle changes.

2. Availability of effective patient and family support programs.

In response to the American Cancer Society (1989) report *Cancer and the Poor*, hospitals that serve poor patients began to respond to their special needs (e.g., diagnosis at a later stage of disease, lack of insurance, unfamiliarity with negotiating the health care system) by developing expanded inner-city screening programs and innovative "patient navigator" programs. The patient navigator programs have proven effective as a mechanism for helping patients who receive an abnormal screening result complete a confirming biopsy and treatment in a timely manner (Freeman et al., 1995). Communities may want to duplicate such programs as a way of responding to the special needs of their medically underserved populations. Communities also may want to monitor the number of support programs for women and the utilization rate of such programs.

SAMPLE INDICATOR SET

A proposed set of performance indicators is listed below. The set was derived by combining similar indicators and selecting those that are relevant at the community level and for which data are available. Some data may be available through the National Breast and Cervical Cancer Early Detection Program, which is now established in at least 35 states and for nine American Indian Tribes (CDC, 1996). The program was created to improve access to screening services for underserved women.

1. Number of cases and rates (incidence and mortality) for breast and cervical cancers, including stage at diagnosis.

This information is available, often for the county level, from cancer registries and statistics offices at the state health agency. Examples of performance indicators that could be used in communities are the following:

- For each MCO and the community as a whole, the number of cases and the incidence of breast and cervical cancer, by stage at diagnosis.
- For the community as a whole, the number of deaths and the death rate from breast and cervical cancer, by stage at diagnosis.

2. Access to affordable and quality-controlled mammography screening, clinical breast examination, cervical cancer screening (Pap test), and pelvic examination.

This indicator requires a new source of data. Measuring access, quality, and barriers will require cooperation among health care providers including health plans, hospitals, and individual clinicians, public health agencies, and the insurance industry. Questions about access are available in the Behavioral Risk Factor Surveillance System (BRFSS), for which surveys are conducted in 50 states, the District of Columbia, and three territories.

Examples of performance indicators that could be used by communities include:

- Proportion and number of facilities offering mammography and Pap tests that meet federal and state regulatory standards.
- Proportion of health plans or insurers that cover 80 percent or more of the cost of breast and cervical cancer screening.

3. Referral and follow-up rates on results from positive mammography and Pap test screening.

This measure requires a survey or a review of medical records.

The following is an example of a performance indicator that could be used in communities:

- For each health plan or insurer, the proportion of enrolled women with positive test results for mammography or Pap testing who received appropriate and timely follow-up care.

4. Rates at which physicians refer women for screening mammograms.

This measure requires a survey or a review of medical records. Examples of performance indicators that could be used in communities are the following:

- For each MCO, family practitioner, internist, and obstetrician–gynecologist, the proportion of women who should have mammography who were actually referred for mammograms in the past 12 months.
- For each MCO, family practitioner, internist, and obstetrician–gynecologist, the proportion of referred women who received mammography within 30 days of referral.

5. Rates of tobacco use and alcohol consumption among women.

This information might be obtained by modifying state BRFSS surveys to produce community-level data.

6. Proportion of sexually active women who use barrier methods of contraception.

This measure requires a survey or a review of medical records.

7. Utilization of screening programs by women at risk for breast and cervical cancer.

Health plans may be able to rely on HEDIS (Health Plan Employer Data and Information Set) measures for these data (NCQA, 1993, 1996). Data on women without health plan or insurance coverage might be available from the BRFSS. Examples of performance indicators that could be used in communities include the following:

- For each health plan or insurer, the proportion of enrolled women who should have breast and cervical cancer screening who received appropriate screening services in the past 12 months.
- For women who are not enrolled in a health plan or insur-

ance group, the proportion who should have breast and cervical cancer screening who received appropriate screening services in the past 12 months.

8. Availability of breast and cervical cancer public education programs for target populations that include information on breast self-exam, the importance and availability of screening programs, and the value of screening as a tool for health and well-being.

The ability to collect and analyze data for this indicator is somewhat troublesome; therefore, it may be weak when standing alone. This indicator is less sensitive to changes in the performance of the system and somewhat more difficult to track given the array of individuals, organizations, and institutions involved in educational programs. Some of these data are tracked by state health departments and health plans.

The following are examples of performance indicators that could be used in communities:

- Proportion of employers, community-based organizations, school PTAs, or faith organizations that provided in the past 12 months health promotion programs in the community about the value of screening, breast self-exam, and the availability of screening programs to prevent breast and cervical cancer among women.
- For each health plan or insurer and the community as a whole, the proportion of women who have a risk factor for breast or cervical cancer that can be modified through lifestyle changes.

9. Availability of effective patient and family support programs.

Communities may want to monitor the number of support programs for women and the utilization rate of such programs. These data may not be available to communities unless they conduct a survey of provider sites (e.g., managed care organizations, public and private hospitals and clinics).

The proposed indicators on breast and cervical cancers address the potentially modifiable risk factors of tobacco use and barrier contraception methods, as well as behaviors that promote early detection (utilization of screening programs). The proposed set also includes measures related to the development and implementation of screening programs (indicators 2–4), utilization of screening programs, and social supports for screening programs. In addition, the direct effects of disease are included.

REFERENCES

American Cancer Society. 1989. *Cancer and the Poor: A Report to the Nation.* Atlanta, Ga.: American Cancer Society.

American Cancer Society. 1993. *Breast and Cervical Cancer Screening: Barriers and Use Among Specific Populations.* AMC Cancer Research Center, Literature Review Supplement (Oct. 1991–May 1992) Supplement 2 (June 1992–May 1993).

American Cancer Society. 1995. *Cancer Facts and Figures 1995.* Atlanta, Ga.: American Cancer Society.

American Cancer Society. 1996. *Cancer Facts and Figures 1996.* Atlanta, Ga.: American Cancer Society.

CDC (Centers for Disease Control and Prevention). 1996. Update: National Breast and Cervical Cancer Early Detection Program—July 1991–September 1995. *Morbidity and Mortality Weekly Report* 45:484–487.

Colditz, G.A., Willett, W.C., Hunter, D.J., et al. 1993. Family History, Age, and Risk of Breast Cancer: Prospective Data from the Nurses' Health Study. *Journal of the American Medical Association* 270:338–343. (published correction in *Journal of the American Medical Association* 1993;270:1548)

Freeman, H.P., Muth, B.J., and Kerner, J.F. 1995. Expanding Access to Cancer Screening and Clinical Follow-up Among the Medically Underserved. *Cancer Practice* 3(1):19–30.

Kerlikowske, K., Grady, D., Rubin, S.M., Sandrock, C., and Ernster, V.L. 1995. Efficacy of Screening Mammography: A Meta-Analysis. *Journal of the American Medical Association* 273:149–154.

Kjaer, S.K., Dahl, C., Engholm, G., Bock, J.E., Lynge, E., and Jensen, O.M. 1992. Case-Control Study of Risk Factors for Cervical Neoplasia in Denmark. II. Role of Sexual Activity, Reproductive Factors, and Venereal Infections. *Cancer Causes and Control* 3:339–348.

Longnecker, M.P., Newcomb, P.A., Mittendorf, R., et al. 1995. Risk of Breast Cancer in Relation to Lifetime Alcohol Consumption. *Journal of the National Cancer Institute* 87:923–929.

NCQA (National Committee for Quality Assurance). 1993. *Health Plan Employer Data and Information Set and Users Manual, Version 2.0 (HEDIS 2.0).* Washington, D.C.: NCQA.

NCQA. 1996. HEDIS 3.0 Draft for Public Comment. Washington, D.C.: NCQA.

Newcomb, P.A., Storer, B.E., Longnecker, M.P., et al. 1994. Lactation and a Reduced Risk of Premenopausal Breast Cancer. *New England Journal of Medicine* 330:81–87.

Ries, L.A.G., Miller, B.A., Hankey, B.F., Kosary, C.L., Harras, A., and Edwards, B.K., eds. 1994. *SEER Cancer Statistics Review, 1973–1991: Tables and Graphs.* NIH Pub. No. 94-2789. Bethesda, Md.: National Cancer Institute.

Slattery, M.L., and Kerber, R.A. 1993. A Comprehensive Evaluation of Family History and Breast Cancer Risk: The Utah Population Database. *Journal of the American Medical Association* 270:1563–1568.

Slattery, M.L., Overall, J.C., Jr., Abbott, T.M., French, T.K., Robinson, L.M., and Gardner, J. 1989a. Sexual Activity, Contraception, Genital Infections, and Cervical Cancer: Support for a Sexually Transmitted Disease Hypothesis. *American Journal of Epidemiology* 130:248–258.

Slattery, M.L., Robinson, L.M., Schuman, K.L., et al. 1989b. Cigarette Smoking and Exposure to Passive Smoke Are Risk Factors for Cervical Cancer. *Journal of the American Medical Association* 261:1593–1598.

U.S. Preventive Services Task Force. 1996. *Guide to Clinical Preventive Services.* 2nd ed. Baltimore: Williams and Wilkens.

Washington State Department of Health. 1994. *The Washington State Public Health Improvement Plan.* Olympia: Washington State Department of Health.

TABLE A.1-1 Field Model Mapping for Sample Indicator Set: Breast and Cervical Cancers

Field Model Domain	Construct	Sample Indicators	Data Sources
Disease, Health Care	Impact of disease on the community	Number of cases and rates (incidence and mortality) for breast and cervical cancers, including stage at diagnosis: *For each MCO and the community as a whole, number of cases and incidence of breast and cervical cancers, by stage at diagnosis.* *For the community as a whole, number of deaths and death rate from breast and cervical cancers, by stage at diagnosis.*	Cancer registries, state health department
	Screening programs for early detection of disease	Access to affordable and quality controlled mammography screening, clinical breast examination, cervical cancer screening (Pap test), and pelvic examination: *Proportion and number of facilities offering mammography and Pap tests that meet federal and state regulatory standards.* *Proportion of health plans or insurers that cover 80 percent or more of the cost of breast and cervical cancer screening.*	BRFSS, surveys, medical records review
	Follow-up services for screening tests	Referral and follow-up rates on results from positive mammography and Pap test screening: *For each health plan or insurer, proportion of enrolled women with positive test results for mammography or Pap testing who received appropriate and timely follow-up care.*	Community or provider survey, review of medical records

		Rates at which physicians refer women for screening mammograms: *For each MCO, family practitioner, internist, and obstetrician–gynecologist, proportion of women who should have mammography who were referred for mammograms in past 12 months.* *For each MCO, family practitioner, internist, and obstetrician–gynecologist, proportion of referred women who received mammography within 30 days of referral.*	Community or provider survey, review of medical records
Behavior, Genetic Endowment	Behaviors that reduce risk and promote health	Rates of tobacco use and alcohol consumption among women	BRFSS
		Proportion of sexually active women who use barrier methods of contraception	Community survey, review of medical records
		Utilization of screening programs by women at risk for breast and cervical cancer: *For each health plan or insurer, proportion of enrolled women who should have breast and cervical cancer screening who received appropriate services in the past 12 months.* *For women who are not enrolled in a health plan or insurance group, proportion who should have breast and cervical cancer screening who received appropriate screening services in the past 12 months.*	HEDIS or BRFSS

continued on next page

TABLE A.1-1 *Continued*

Field Model Domain	Construct	Sample Indicators	Data Sources
Social Environment	Social support that enables activities that reduce risk, detect disease early, and promote health	Availability of breast and cervical cancer public education programs for target populations that include information on breast-self exam, importance and availability of screening programs, and value of screening as tool for health and well-being: *Proportion of employers, community-based organizations, school PTAs, faith organizations that provided in the past 12 months health promotion programs in the community about the value of screening, breast self-exam and availability of screening programs to prevent breast and cervical cancer among women.* *For each health plan or insurer and the community as a whole, proportion of women who have a risk factor for breast or cervical cancer that can be modified through lifestyle changes.*	Community survey, state health departments, health plans
		Availability of effective patient and family support programs: *Number of support programs.* *Utilization rate for such programs.*	Survey needed

NOTE: BRFSS, Behavioral Risk Factor Surveillance System; HEDIS, Health Plan Employer Data and Information Set; MCO, managed care organization; PTA, parent–teacher association.

A.2

Prototype Indicator Set: Depression

BACKGROUND

Depression is a serious, frequently recurring mental health problem. Estimates are that about 11 percent of adults aged 15 to 54 experience depression within a 12-month period (Kessler et al., 1994). It occurs among all age groups, races, ethnic groups, and levels of education and income, and its impact is felt by individuals and their families, health care providers, employers, and others in the community. In the form of either depressive symptoms or actual depressive disorder, it impairs physical, cognitive, social, and occupational functioning to an extent comparable to chronic illnesses such as diabetes and coronary heart disease (Wells et al., 1989). It is also associated with suicide and higher mortality rates for other causes of death. The economic impact of depression includes direct costs of treatment and indirect costs of reduced productivity, absence from work or school, and premature death (Johnson et al., 1992; Conti and Burton, 1994). Depression and depressive symptoms are also associated with physical complaints that contribute to increased use of health care services (Johnson et al., 1992; Simon et al., 1995a).

A diverse mix of biological, psychosocial, and environmental factors are associated with increased risk for depression (IOM, 1994). It is more common in women and in people with a family history of depressive disorder. It tends to appear first in early adulthood, but a first episode may occur in childhood, adolescence, or later years of adulthood. The postpartum period is a time of increased risk for new mothers, and some people experience recurrent depression associated with seasonal changes (seasonal affective disorder). Stressful life events or circumstances are also recognized as risk factors: death of a spouse or child, divorce or other marital disruptions, assault or abuse, social isolation, job loss or stress, and poverty (IOM, 1994). Community conditions, such as a poor economy or violence, can reinforce individual experience.

Depression may occur with or result from some medical conditions and other mental disorders, and some medications can produce depression. Use of tobacco and alcohol is more common among persons reporting depressed moods (Schoenborn and Horm, 1993), and substance abuse may produce symptoms of depression (Depression Guideline Panel, 1993a). Recurrence of depression, incomplete recovery between episodes, and previous suicide attempts are associated with increased risk for future depressive disorder (Depression Guideline Panel, 1993a).

Because 50 percent of those who experience one episode of depression have a second episode (Depression Guideline Panel, 1993a), primary prevention is an important goal. Particular personality traits or good social support may limit the impact of some risk factors. Overall, evidence for the effectiveness of primary prevention is not conclusive (IOM, 1994), but targeted prevention may have promise (e.g., Beardslee et al., 1993; Clarke et al., 1995). In addition, interventions in a variety of settings (e.g., schools, workplaces, homes, neighborhoods) have been shown to reduce depressive symptoms (Muñoz, 1993; IOM, 1994).

Once depression occurs, appropriate treatment can improve outcomes among people of all ages and can reduce the risk of relapse or recurrence (IOM, 1990; Depression Guideline Panel, 1993a; Sturm and Wells, 1995). Treatment with medication or psychotherapy is generally effective for depressive disorder, and other interventions (e.g., enhancing social support) can reduce depressive symptoms (Muñoz, 1993; IOM, 1994). Several factors may, however, hinder access to optimal treatment. Some people do not seek care or do not continue treatment to avoid the stigma still attached to mental health care. Lack of health insurance or limited coverage for mental health services may create financial constraints. Language and cultural barriers may also contribute (e.g., Padgett et al., 1994). In addition, many cases are not diagnosed or are not treated appropriately (Depression Guideline

Panel, 1993a; Sturm and Wells, 1995). The underdiagnosis and undertreatment of depression in primary care settings has led to the development of a set of clinical practice guidelines (Depression Guideline Panel, 1993a,b). Insufficient awareness among providers that the elderly will benefit from treatment is also a concern (e.g., Callahan et al., 1996).

The committee has chosen to consider performance indicators for depression because it and other mental disorders impose a substantial burden on the health and well-being of individuals and the community. Opportunities to reduce that burden are available and should receive attention from many parts of the community, including health care providers, employers, insurers, public-sector agencies that provide health and social services, schools, community groups, and the public at large.

"FIELD" SET OF PERFORMANCE INDICATORS

By reviewing the domains of the field model, it is possible to suggest a varied set of indicators that might be used to examine a community's efforts to address the prevention and treatment of depression and the reduction of high levels of depressive symptoms. Currently, there is better evidence supporting the efficacy and effectiveness of treatment and symptom reduction than of preventive interventions. Additional research may identify effective preventive interventions, especially for groups at increased risk for depression.

Disease

The disease burden of depression is reflected in both individuals whose symptoms meet diagnostic criteria for depressive disorder and those with high symptom levels without a diagnosable disorder. In the United States as a whole, about 11 percent of the adult population is estimated to have a depressive disorder over a 12-month period (Kessler et al., 1994). Lifetime prevalence is about 19 percent overall and reaches 24 percent among women (Kessler et al., 1994). Depressive symptoms also contribute to morbidity in the population (Wells et al., 1989; Johnson et al., 1992; Sherbourne et al., 1994). Johnson and colleagues (1992) estimated that about 23 percent of the population (not including those with a depressive disorder) had ever experienced periods with two or more depressive symptoms. Rates may rise over time; there is evidence that in younger birth cohorts, depression is occurring at higher rates and with an earlier age of onset (Cross-National Collaborative Group, 1992). Data for 1993 from the Youth Risk Behavior Surveillance System (YRBSS) indicate that 24 percent of high school students thought seriously about attempting suicide in the year preceding the survey (CDC, 1995).

The prevalence in the community of depressive symptoms and depressive disorders could be valuable health status measures with which to monitor the need for and impact of therapeutic and preventive interventions. Obtaining detailed prevalence data on a community-wide basis would require a community survey with valid and reliable screening questions. It might be possible to assess depression in subgroups of the population through periodic screening in settings such as health plans, work sites, human services agencies, and faith groups. Screening in schools, which might be appropriate for adolescent populations, would require instruments that have been validated for use with that age group.

Prevalence estimates will vary depending on the diagnostic tools and criteria used. *The Diagnostic and Statistical Manual of Mental Disorders,* Fourth Edition (DSM-IV; APA, 1994) is the current standard for diagnostic criteria, but various instruments have been used in surveys to screen for symptoms (Zung, 1965; Beck et al., 1974; Radloff, 1977) and to establish a diagnosis of depression (Robins et al., 1981; WHO, 1990). A less formal assessment of the prevalence of depressive symptoms in the community might be based on a question available for the Behavioral Risk Factor Surveillance System (BRFSS) on the number of days in the past month with depressed mood. Special sampling in individual state BRFSS surveys or adding residence information (e.g., zip codes) might be a way to obtain county-level data.

Indicators might include the following:

1. Proportion of the adult population (18 years of age and older) with current depressive symptoms meeting diagnostic criteria (DSM-IV) for depressive disorder.

2. Proportion of the adult population currently experiencing two or more depressive symptoms, but not meeting diagnostic criteria for a depressive disorder.

These two indicators would be based on the results of surveys using the more formal types of screening and diagnostic tools noted above. Using a minimum of three or four symptoms would give a more conservative estimate of the prevalence of depression.

3. Proportion of high school students who report having thought seriously during the previous 12 months about attempting suicide.

Thinking seriously about suicide is a symptom of depression. Although not all students who think about suicide will have a depressive disorder, this group is likely to be at higher risk for depression than other students. The question is based on one used by the YRBSS.

4. Proportion of the adult population reporting 14 or more days, during the past 30 days, of feeling sad, blue, or depressed.

This measure is based on a BRFSS question. The 14-day duration of depressed feelings reflects the DSM-IV criterion that symptoms persist for at least two weeks for diagnosis of major depression. This indicator could help identify groups in the population that might be at increased risk for depression. It would not provide a strict measure of symptom levels or diagnosable depression comparable to those based on more detailed screening and diagnostic assessments, but it would be easier to obtain at the community level.

Health and Function, Well-Being

The impact of depression on health and function and on well-being is felt by depressed individuals themselves and by others such as family members or other care givers, employers, and health care providers. A community prevalence survey might be used to obtain information on functional impairments related to depression. The Medical Outcomes Study, which found that impairment from depression was at least as severe as several common chronic illnesses, examined functioning in terms of physical limitations, ability to fill usual role (work, school, etc.), social limitations, and bed days (Wells et al., 1989). Well-being was assessed based on perceptions of current health and pain.

Other measures might also be used as indicators of the impact of depression on function and well-being. Questions have been developed for the BRFSS on impairment due to depression or other emotional problems. Numbers or rates of hospitalizations for depressive disorders, which could be obtained in some states from a hospital discharge data system, might suggest levels of severe depression. Declining use of inpatient treatment for depression may, however, limit the future usefulness of such a measure.

Length of disability claims related to depressive disorders could be another indicator of the impact on function and well-being.

Communities might also try to determine what proportion of the population with depressive symptoms or a depressive disorder is not receiving treatment and, therefore, is at increased risk for impairment of function and well-being. Examining the demographic and socioeconomic characteristics of those not being treated could help communities assess where additional services are needed, whether specific provider groups should give greater attention to depression among their patients, and whether steps might be required to improve access to or acceptance of appropriate services. Managed care organizations (MCOs), schools, and others serving defined populations might assess the extent of untreated depression in those populations.

One manifestation of the impact of depression on function and well-being is its association with higher mortality rates from a variety of causes, with the link to suicide being particularly strong. About half of all suicides are estimated to be associated with depression (U.S. Preventive Services Task Force, 1996). Numbers of recorded suicides would be available from state vital record systems. Numbers of calls to suicide hot lines might be another indicator to consider, but it would be necessary to determine whether changes in call volume could be correlated with changes in the incidence of suicide or attempted suicide. Some portion of other intentional and unintentional injuries may also be linked to depression.

Indicators might include the following:

1. Proportion of the adult population experiencing two or more depressive symptoms who also report limitations in physical activity, role function (work, school, or home), or social activities.

An instrument such as the SF–36 (Ware and Sherbourne, 1992), used in conjunction with the screening and diagnostic tools described above, might provide information on functional limitations.

2. Annual number of hospital discharges with a depressive disorder as the principal diagnosis.

Hospital diagnostic codes, which are based on the *International Classification of Diseases, 9th Revision, Clinical Modification* (ICD-9-CM; USDHHS, 1995) would have to be matched to equivalent DSM-IV codes. To use state-based hospital discharge data at the community level, information on residence (e.g., zip code) will be needed. A state-level data system such as this has the advantage of being able to identify hospital care provided outside a specific community. Numbers of hospital discharges are likely to be influenced by a variety of factors unrelated to the prevalence of depressive disorders, such as availability of hospital beds and insurance coverage for hospital care. Currently, no information system comparable to hospital discharge data is available to provide easy access to community-wide data on diagnosis and outpatient care. Such data might be available for specific populations, including members of MCOs or users of community mental health services.

3. For all employers in the community, proportion of total days of short-term disability attributable to depressive disorders.

This indicator measures the impact of depression on the ability to work relative to other causes of short-term disability. It reflects the effect on both employees and employers but may understate the impact of depression if employees are reluctant to make a claim for a mental health condition. A decrease can reflect either growth in claims for other conditions or a reduction in claims related to depression. Care should be taken not to create incentives to reduce claims by discouraging appropriate care. Employers would probably have to provide these data.

4. Proportion of the population meeting criteria for a current depressive disorder who are not receiving treatment.

A community prevalence survey of the type that has been described above might also be able to collect information on treatment. Determining which of several factors (e.g., economic constraints, reluctance to seek care, no diagnosis made) account for lack of treatment would require further assessment.

5. Number (or rate) of suicides in the community, by age and race or ethnicity.

Data will be available from state vital statistics systems but may understate true levels of suicide because some of those deaths are likely to be attributed to other causes. In most communities, the annual number of suicides will be too low to produce stable rates unless data are aggregated over multiple years. If rates are to be compared over time or across communities, they should be age-adjusted using a standard population.

Risk Factors: Disease, Genetic Endowment, Individual Behavior, Social Environment, and Physical Environment

Factors associated with several of the field model domains have been found to increase the risk of developing depression. Among these factors are specific medical disorders and medications, a family history of depression, previous episodes of depression, prior suicide attempts, social isolation, death of a spouse or child, marital disruption, job stress, unemployment, and poverty. Communities cannot expect to eliminate many of these risk factors, but they can respond through various channels in ways that reduce their impact.

Health departments, health plans, social service agencies, schools, nursing homes, and employers, among others, might be expected to facilitate access to services intended to resolve problems or moderate their impact. Health care providers, for example, may be able to withdraw medications that produce symptoms of depression. Employee assistance programs may be able to provide stress reduction services for on-the-job problems or assistance for personal concerns such as marital problems. Schools and school-based clinics might, for example, give special attention to children and adolescents with family disruptions (e.g., divorce or death) or with a personal or family history of depression.

Some potential performance indicators related to risk factors are presented in the sections on the field model domains listed above.

Individual Response

Individual behavior contributes both to increased risk for depression and to successful treatment or symptom reduction. Communities concerned about depression might, for example, try to assess rates of alcohol or substance abuse, both of which appear to induce depression in some people (but do not appear to be caused by depression) (Depression Guideline Panel, 1993a). Physical activity, on the other hand, appears to have therapeutic benefits and may be able to reduce the risk of depression (USDHHS, 1996). Participation in activities that reduce social isolation also moderates the risk of a depressive episode.

Healthy People 2000 (USDHHS, 1991) proposed objectives for an increase in (1) the proportion of people who seek help for emotional problems, (2) the proportion of people with mental health problems who use community support programs, and (3) the proportion of people with depression who obtain treatment. (Obtaining treatment is also a function of access to care and the quality of care available.) Individuals' willingness to seek care and follow recommended treatment is another necessary element in the success of any community response to depression. Evidence suggests that many patients treated in primary care settings discontinue prescribed medications before positive effects can be expected (e.g., Simon et al., 1995b).

Indicators that might be considered include the following:

1. Proportion of the adult population (18 years of age and older) who report feeling sad, blue, or depressed and also report not engaging in regular exercise.

This indicator might monitor the need for, or impact of, public education or counseling about the mental health benefits of exercise. Data might be obtained through questions that have been developed for the BRFSS. As noted elsewhere, special sampling in the state survey may be able to produce community-level data. Alternatively, communities might be able to include BRFSS questions in a local survey.

2. Proportion of the adult population meeting diagnostic criteria for depressive disorder who have sought treatment.

Seeking treatment reflects factors such as awareness of symptoms of depression, willingness to seek care, and availability of affordable care. Specific types of treatment covered by this indicator would have to be defined. Among those that might be included are medication, psychotherapy with a mental health professional, counseling from a primary care provider, or counseling through other community sources (e.g., school, work site, faith organization).

3. Of adults with a diagnosis of depressive disorder for whom antidepressant medication has been prescribed, the proportion who take prescribed doses for at least 30 days.

Antidepressant medications are not always used in the treatment of depressive disorders but are effective for many people if taken in adequate doses for at least four to six weeks. Minimum dosage guidelines for adults have been established for most antidepressant medications. Information on diagnosis and prescriptions filled may be available from some MCOs (see Simon et al.,

1995b) but might be difficult to monitor for a community as a whole.

Social Environment

Many aspects of the social environment have implications for the impact of depression in a community and for steps that might be taken if depression is considered a high priority. Monitoring the extent of risk factors may be a useful step. Community-wide indicators might include the divorce rate; rates of violent crime, particularly domestic violence; number of guns in the community; unemployment rates or number of layoffs; proportion of the population near or below the poverty line; and proportion of the population that has lived in the community less than one year. Some of these indicators might be included in a community profile. The profile indicators proposed by the committee include the unemployment rate and the proportion of children living at or below the poverty level.

Also part of the social environment are resources available to people who are at increased risk for depression. As noted above, health care providers, schools, employers, social service agencies, and others may be able to identify high-risk individuals and facilitate access to supportive services that can mitigate a risk or respond to depression that has developed. Children and adolescents may benefit from access to mental health services through school-based clinics or other school health services. For the elderly, the need may be for programs that address social isolation or that monitor symptom levels in nursing home residents. Programs for children of depressed parents offered by social service agencies, or perhaps by health plans, respond to current cases of depression and are an effort to reduce the risk of future depression. In communities with diverse subpopulations, the availability of culturally appropriate social and health services can improve social support and may reduce the risk of depression or facilitate access to acceptable forms of care.

Employers are affected by depression through lost productivity and through health care and disability claims. Employers also influence access to treatment through coverage for mental health services included in their health insurance plans. Communities may wish to assess what proportion of the population has mental health benefits through employment-based insurance and determine whether those benefits are comparable to coverage for other forms of medical care. The availability of work site resources such as employee assistance programs or counseling services for workers who have been laid off may also be a concern.

Indicators might include the following:

1. Proportion of adults, aged 21–65, who are unemployed (looking for but not able to find work).

As noted, an unemployment measure appears in the committee's proposed community profile. In communities experiencing major changes in employment patterns, it may be appropriate to monitor the number of people who were laid off during the previous year. Job loss and unemployment increase the risk of depression through loss of income and through less tangible losses of social support and self-esteem.

2. Proportion of the population living at or below poverty levels.

A community-based study has suggested that 10 percent of new cases of depression may be attributable to poverty (Bruce et al., 1991). Low income not only increases the risk of developing depression but can also hinder access to treatment.

3. Proportion of the ever-married adult population becoming separated, divorced, or widowed in the previous year.

Marital disruption increases the risk of depression and can affect children as well as spouses. Data should be available from the state vital statistics system. Communities in which informal unions are common might want to supplement official vital statistics data with periodic surveys that include questions on changes in such relationships.

4. Proportion of school-age children (6–18 years of age) with access to school-based mental health services.

5. Proportion of employed persons with access to employee assistance programs.

These two indicators are measures of the capacity to provide assistance but not of assistance actually sought or received. They should be used in conjunction with other measures that reflect services provided and health status outcomes. Data might be obtained from schools and employers in the community. A community survey might also provide data; results would reflect awareness of services as well as their availability.

6. Proportion of employees in the community whose health

insurance includes coverage for mental health services for themselves; for their families.

Lack of insurance coverage for mental health services can limit access to care. Use of this indicator would require a clear definition of "coverage." For example, differences may exist in number of visits or hospital days allowed and in copayments and deductibles. BRFSS questions on access to care might be expanded or adapted to address coverage for mental health services.

Physical Environment

Physical activity appears to have therapeutic benefits and may be able to reduce the risk of depression (USDHHS, 1996). Therefore, community recreation resources, including both built facilities and natural spaces, could be of interest in efforts to reduce the impact of depression.

Features of the physical environment can also be risk factors for depression. Seasonal affective disorder, for example, typically recurs with the shorter periods of daylight in fall and winter and is seen more often among persons living further north (Depression Guideline Panel, 1993a). Depression may also occur in response to individual trauma, such as assault (which might also be considered a social environment factor), or to events on a larger scale, such as natural disasters (IOM, 1994).

Indicators that might be used include the following:

1. Availability of public recreational facilities in the community.

This is an indirect measure of community resources that could support efforts to encourage increased physical activity for people with depression. This measure focuses on public facilities because they should be accessible to most of the community without the financial barriers that may exist for private facilities. If a standard definition of "recreational facility" can be established, the indicator might be restated as "the number of public recreational facilities available in the community." Because availability does not ensure use, studies may be needed to determine whether the availability of recreational resources contributes to increased physical activity by depressed persons.

2. Annual number of visits to public or private recreational facilities.

Numbers of visits might be determined from a community survey or from estimates by the agencies and organizations managing the facilities.

Health Care

Because *treatment* of depression currently is better understood than prevention, the health care system (in both the public and the private sectors) plays a significant role in how a community addresses depression. Several measures of performance might be proposed. Comprehensive community-level data are not likely to be readily available, but several separate sources can be tapped. Some of these include hospital discharge data, health plan data systems, and the state mental health agency client data system. Comparability across sources may be a concern, however.

Communities may want to consider several aspects of mental health care and the organizations that provide it. Access to care is essential. The potential financial barriers posed by limited insurance coverage have been noted, and other barriers may exist. Location of services may pose problems for individuals who lack transportation, and language or other cultural barriers can exist. People also can be reluctant to seek care for mental health problems. Some people who might benefit from care for depression may need better information about the value and availability of services. Health departments and community mental health programs may need information programs and mental health services designed specifically for hard-to-reach populations such as the homeless or recent immigrants.

People with depression receive care from a variety of providers, including primary care clinicians, community mental health clinics, and physician and nonphysician mental health specialists. Many people are seen only in a primary care setting. These providers need adequate training in recognizing and treating depression, but no recommendation has been made for or against routine screening of asymptomatic patients (U.S. Preventive Services Task Force, 1996). As noted earlier, treatment guidelines have been developed for primary care providers in response to evidence of underdiagnosis and undertreatment of depression (Depression Guideline Panel, 1993a,b). Some patients can be treated adequately in a primary care setting, but others will benefit from access to mental health specialty care. In all settings, adequate duration of care contributes to better outcomes.

HEDIS (Health Plan Employer Data and Information Set) indicators (NCQA, 1993) have included a measure for short-term ambulatory follow-up after hospitalization for depression. Assessment of longer-term follow-up may also be useful. With decreased use of hospitalization, other indicators based on outpatient services may be needed. Appropriateness of prescribed medications is another possible indicator. Indicators for outcomes of care should be considered as well. Changes in symptom levels or diagnostic status at specific intervals following initiation of treatment might be measured. Recurrence of symptoms or disorder can, however, reflect not only potential shortcomings in care but also the onset of a new episode in response to new stressors.

Health departments or state mental health agencies might be expected to monitor services provided by hospitals and other facilities. Accreditation standards are also being proposed for behavioral health care provided by MCOs and by managed behavioral health organizations (NCQA, 1996; IOM, 1997). In the future, compliance with those standards should promote the delivery of appropriate care. A means of assessing the quality of outpatient services provided by individual therapists could be valuable to a community but will be difficult to develop.

In the public sector, the implementation of Medicaid managed care is dividing responsibility for mental health services between Medicaid and state mental health agencies (SMHAs), but their activities and funding are not always being coordinated (AMBHA and NASMHPD, 1995). SMHA practices emphasizing provider continuity, for example, are not consistent with the competitive contracting often used in Medicaid managed care, which could lead to more frequent changes in service providers. Communities (and states) may want to monitor the impact of these new arrangements on the use of and satisfaction with services and on outcomes of care.

Indicators that might be used include the following:

1. Proportion of persons who have completed treatment for a diagnosed depressive disorder who have not experienced a relapse (return of symptoms within six months of completion of treatment).

This indicator of the outcome of care could point to inadequate treatment, including its premature termination. Medical record review could identify those cases in which relapse treatment was sought from the same provider. Cases in which people seek care from a different source or decline to seek new care would be harder to identify.

2. Proportion of patients receiving ambulatory follow-up within 30 days of discharge for hospitalization for depression.

Patients who require hospitalization tend to be those with more severe depression. Good follow-up care can reduce the risk of relapse and improve outcomes. Inclusion of this indicator in the HEDIS set means that most MCOs should be able to provide such information. It is not routinely collected for patients of fee-for-service providers, however. Increasing reliance on outpatient management of depression means that this indicator will apply to a small and decreasing portion of people treated for depression.

3. Of patients diagnosed with a depressive disorder and prescribed antidepressant medication, the proportion who receive prescriptions for therapeutically effective doses.

Appropriate doses of antidepressant medications are effective for many patients, but some prescriptions are written for inadequate dosages or are not continued for a sufficient length of time. This may delay the alleviation of a depressive episode while increasing the cost of care. A related concern not addressed by this indicator is the prescription of inappropriate medication (e.g., minor tranquilizers). This indicator is intended to distinguish provider practices from patient decisions not to follow prescribed dosages. Allowance must be made, however, for initial adjustments in dosage levels and for changes in medication that may be required to reduce side effects. Health plan and prescription service records could provide this information for some patients. For fee-for-service providers, record reviews, or possibly patient surveys, would be needed to obtain data.

4. Proportion of managed care organizations or managed behavioral health organizations serving the community that are accredited by a nationally recognized organization (e.g., the National Committee for Quality Assurance [NCQA] under its proposed Behavioral Health Accreditation program).

In both the public and private sectors, an increasing share of mental health services is being provided by MCOs and managed behavioral health organizations. Meeting nationally recognized accreditation standards should increase the likelihood that patients will receive good care. NCQA has proposed but not yet implemented its accreditation program (NCQA, 1996). Once it or other programs are in place, communities should be able to request accreditation information from a provider organization or the accrediting body.

SAMPLE INDICATOR SET

Nine of the indicators listed above are proposed as a set that a community might use to monitor efforts to reduce the impact of depression among its population. Each indicator is listed with comments on data and measurement considerations and on its implications for accountability. The indicators are a mix of health status, capacity, and process measures that address roles that several segments of the community might be expected to play.

Treatment indicators are emphasized over indicators on primary prevention because of the more extensive evidence for the effectiveness of treatment. Over time, however, the mix of indicators should change to reflect new information on opportunities for effective action. In operationalizing a performance monitoring program based on the proposed indicators, a community would have to consider the generally limited availability of standard measures and necessary data. Resource constraints could preclude frequent community surveys, which might otherwise be the most direct source of information. Another consideration should be whether other measures would address depression risks or services that are of more pressing concern in a specific community.

1. Proportion of the adult population (18 years of age and older) reporting 14 or more days, during the past 30 days, of feeling sad, blue, or depressed.

This indicator is an assessment of the extent of at least minimal depressive symptoms in the community; it does not, however, apply formal diagnostic criteria. In conjunction with data on age, ethnicity, socioeconomic status, and so on, it could help identify groups in the population that might be at increased risk for depression. The use of a cumulative 14-day experience ensures that very brief periods of depressed mood do not obscure more persistent problems. As noted earlier, this measure is based on a question developed for the BRFSS. It might, therefore, be incorporated into an existing state survey program that could be adapted to provide substate estimates. As a community-wide measure, it would reflect the combined effect of both adverse and positive influences from many sectors.

2. Proportion of high school students who report having thought seriously during the previous 12 months about attempting suicide.

This indicator would provide some indication of the risk of

depression in adolescents. The measure would not, however, reflect the proportion of students with depressive symptoms that do not include thoughts of suicide. Schools might be expected to facilitate access to mental health services for these students. The school-based survey for the YRBSS includes a question on this topic, and oversampling in conjunction with the state survey or a community-specific survey might be used to collect data. A shorter reference period (e.g., previous month, previous 3 months) would provide more current information, but its impact on the reliability of the data collected should be considered.

3. Proportion of the adult population (18 years of age and older) meeting criteria for a depressive disorder who are not receiving treatment.

Untreated episodes of depression generally last several months and are often accompanied by marked functional impairment. They may also increase the risk for subsequent depressive episodes. Not every case of depression requires formal treatment, but in many instances, treatment can shorten the length of an episode and improve long-term outcomes. This indicator will not identify why treatment is not being received (e.g., economic constraints, reluctance to seek care, no diagnosis made), but it could help communities assess the extent of unmet need. Data would probably have to be collected through periodic surveys. In terms of accountability, this indicator would address the role that many sectors of the community (e.g., health care providers, employers, schools, nursing homes, social service agencies, criminal justice agencies) have in facilitating access to care.

4. Number (or rate) of suicides in the community, by age and race or ethnicity.

Suicides are an extreme adverse outcome for depression and other mental health problems, and youth suicide is often a special concern. As noted above, about half of all suicides are associated with depression. Many suicide attempts are unsuccessful, but access to firearms increases the likelihood of death. This measure is included in the committee's proposed community profile indicators and is part of the *Healthy People 2000* consensus indicator set (CDC, 1991). Data are available from state vital records systems. In most communities, suicide will be a rare event, but it might be treated as a signal to give greater attention to sources of risk for depression and to identification of persons with current depressive disorders. The greatest accountability for addressing risks for suicide might be considered to lie with health care providers, criminal justice facilities, and others who serve groups with known risk factors.

5. Proportion of employed persons with access to employee assistance programs.

Employee assistance programs (EAPs) are a resource for work site interventions that might address risks for depression (e.g., stress reduction) and can facilitate access to risk reduction or treatment services outside the workplace. To have an impact, however, employees must be willing and able to use these services. If a community has many small businesses, which are less likely to have an EAP, the proportion of workers with access to such programs will tend to be lower. Estimates might be developed from reports from employers in the community. This indicator targets a specific contribution that employers might be expected to make to community efforts to reduce the adverse impact of depression.

6. Proportion of employees in the community whose health insurance includes coverage for mental health services for themselves; for their families.

This indicator is of interest because lack of insurance coverage for mental health services can create a financial barrier to care. In assessing the extent of coverage, communities would have to take into account differences in the kinds of services covered, number of visits allowed, amount of copayment required, and limits on total payments for services. To obtain data, it might be possible to expand or adapt BRFSS questions on access to care. Data might also be obtained from employer reports. State insurance authorities might be able to provide some information but are less likely to be able to provide information on self-insured companies. This indicator addresses the role that employers and insurers have in reducing the financial barriers to mental health services.

7. Proportion of patients receiving ambulatory follow-up within 30 days of discharge for hospitalization for depression.

Good follow-up care can reduce the risk of relapse and improve outcomes. This indicator was selected because it has already been operationalized as a HEDIS measure, which should make it easier for communities to implement. Its current use by health plans should also reduce the burden of collecting data.

Communities should, however, be considering alternative measures. Hospitalized patients are some of the most severely ill, but with the decreasing use of hospitalization, they are a small and declining proportion of all people receiving treatment for depression. As an indicator on follow-up care, this measure addresses accountability among health care organizations and providers.

8. Of patients diagnosed with a depressive disorder and prescribed antidepressant medication, the proportion who receive prescriptions for therapeutically effective doses.

This indicator addresses an issue of particular concern in the treatment of depression. Appropriate doses of antidepressant medications are effective for many patients, but some providers do not prescribe adequate dosages and do not continue medications for adequate periods of time. Use of medications in a manner that is not likely to be effective is a poor use of health care dollars. Guidelines on minimum dosage levels (e.g., see Depression Guideline Panel, 1993b) can provide criteria for evaluating prescriptions. Length of time a medication is used, which is also important in achieving a good response, has not been included in the indicator to simplify the measurement process. Health plan and prescription service records could be a source of data. Because only physicians can prescribe medications, this indicator specifically addresses physician accountability for appropriate treatment practices.

9. Proportion of managed care organizations or managed behavioral health organizations serving the community that are accredited by a nationally recognized organization (e.g., NCQA under its proposed Behavioral Health Accreditation program).

This indicator addresses concerns about quality of care. Accreditation should assure the community that past performance has met accepted standards and that specific capacities are in place to provide service in the future. Reference to nationally recognized accreditation standards would permit comparisons across communities. Once an accreditation program is in place, information on specific provider organizations in a community should be readily available from the accrediting group. Provider accountability is addressed by this indicator.

As a set, these proposed indicators on depression can give a community a sense of the extent of the current health problem (depressed mood, thoughts of suicide, number of suicides), of risk factors affecting health outcomes (lack of treatment, follow-up care, use of medication), and of resources available to apply to the problem (employee assistance programs, insurance coverage, accreditation of services). The proposed indicators focus on concerns that are specific to depression, but they should be used with other, more general measures of community status that are also depression risk factors (e.g., unemployment and poverty). Some of these general measures are included as indicators in the community profile proposed by the committee.

In terms of performance, the set of indicators reflects the community-wide impact of activities and opportunities for action by many stakeholders. For example, the indicators on depressed mood (indicator 1), thoughts of suicide (indicator 2), and lack of treatment for diagnosable depressive disorder (indicator 3) measure the result of actions that might be taken not only by health care providers but also by community groups (e.g., employers, schools, social service agencies, faith groups) to facilitate access to treatment or, perhaps, to offer supportive services that might reduce the need for treatment.

Because treatment practices will be relevant to most communities, it is useful to suggest some specific indicators (follow-up care, use of medication) without reference to a community's risk factors. Similarly, the indicator on EAPs (indicator 5) reflects a widely applicable opportunity offered by the workplace to address risks for depression, whether they arise at the workplace or elsewhere. In contrast, many activities that respond to risk factors need to be tailored to the specific form of risk (e.g., social isolation, unemployment, death of a spouse). Communities should supplement (or modify) the proposed set of indicators with others that are appropriate for local circumstances.

REFERENCES

AMBHA and NASMHPD (American Managed Behavioral Healthcare Association and National Association of State Mental Health Program Directors). 1995. Public Mental Health Systems, Medicaid Re-structuring and Managed Behavioral Healthcare. *Behavioral Health Care Tomorrow* (Sept/Oct):63–69.

APA (American Psychiatric Association). 1994. *Diagnostic and Statistical Manual of Mental Disorders: DSM-IV*. 4th ed. Washington, D.C.: APA.

Beardslee, W.R., Salt, P., Porterfield, K., et al. 1993. Comparison of Preventive Interventions for Families with Parental Affective Disorders. *Journal of the American Academy of Child and Adolescent Psychiatry* 32:254–263.

Beck, A.T., Rial, W.Y., and Rickels, K. 1974. Short Form of Depression Inventory: Cross Validation. *Psychological Reports* 34:1184–1186.

Bruce, M.L., Takeuchi, D.T., and Leaf, P.J. 1991. Poverty and Psychiatric Status: Longitudinal Evidence from the New Haven Epidemiologic Catchment Area Study. *Archives of General Psychiatry* 48:470–474.

Callahan, C.M., Dittus, R.S., and Tierney, W.M. 1996. Primary Care Physicians' Medical Decision Making for Late-Life Depression. *Journal of General Internal Medicine* 11:218–225.

CDC (Centers for Disease Control and Prevention). 1991. Consensus Set of Health Status Indicators for the General Assessment of Community Health Status—United States. *Morbidity and Mortality Weekly Report* 40:449–451.

CDC. 1995. Youth Risk Behavior Surveillance—United States, 1993. *Morbidity and Mortality Weekly Report* 44 (No. SS-1).

Clarke, G.N., Hawkins, W., Murphy, M., Sheeber, L.B., Lewinsohn, P.M., and Seeley, J.R. 1995. Targeted Prevention of Unipolar Depressive Disorder in an At-Risk Sample of High School Adolescents: A Randomized Trial of a Group Cognitive Intervention. *Journal of the American Academy of Child and Adolescent Psychiatry* 34:312–321.

Conti, D.J., and Burton, W.N. 1994. The Economic Impact of Depression in a Workplace. *Journal of Occupational Medicine* 36:983–988.

Cross-National Collaborative Group. 1992. The Changing Rate of Major Depression: Cross-National Comparisons. *Journal of the American Medical Association* 268:3098–3105.

Depression Guideline Panel. 1993a. *Depression in Primary Care: Volume 1. Detection and Diagnosis.* Clinical Practice Guideline, No. 5. AHCPR Pub. No. 93-0550. Rockville, Md.: U.S. Department of Health and Human Services.

Depression Guideline Panel. 1993b. *Depression in Primary Care: Volume 2. Treatment of Major Depression.* Clinical Practice Guideline, No. 5. AHCPR Pub. No. 93-0551. Rockville, Md.: U.S. Department of Health and Human Services.

IOM (Institute of Medicine). 1990. *The Second Fifty Years: Promoting Health and Preventing Disability.* R.L. Berg and J.S. Cassells, eds. Washington, D.C.: National Academy Press.

IOM. 1994. *Reducing Risks for Mental Disorders: Frontiers for Prevention Intervention Research.* P.J. Mrazek and R.J. Haggerty, eds. Washington, D.C.: National Academy Press.

IOM. 1997. *Managing Managed Care: Quality Improvement in Behavioral Health.* Washington, D.C.: National Academy Press.

Johnson, J., Weissman, M.M., and Klerman, G.L. 1992. Service Utilization and Social Morbidity Associated with Depressive Symptoms in the Community. *Journal of the American Medical Association* 267:1478–1483.

Kessler, R.C., McGonagle, K.A., Zhao, S., et al. 1994. Lifetime and 12-Month Prevalence of DSM-III-R Psychiatric Disorders in the United States: Results from the National Comorbidity Survey. *Archives of General Psychiatry* 51:8–19.

Muñoz, R.F. 1993. The Prevention of Depression: Current Research and Practice. *Applied and Preventive Psychology* 2:21–33.

NCQA (National Committee for Quality Assurance). 1993. *Health Plan Employer Data and Information Set and User's Manual, Version 2.0 (HEDIS 2.0).* Washington, D.C.: NCQA.

NCQA. 1996. NCQA Issues First National Accreditation Standards for Managed Behavioral Health Organizations. Washington, D.C. April 10. (press release)

Padgett, D.K., Patrick, C., Burns, B.J., and Schlesinger, H.J. 1994. Ethnicity and the Use of Outpatient Mental Health Services in a National Insured Population. *American Journal of Public Health* 84:222–226.

Radloff, L.S. 1977. The CES-D Scale: A Self-Report Depression Scale for Research in the General Population. *Applied Psychology Measures* 1:385–401.

Robins, L.N., Helzer, J.E., Croughan, J., and Ratcliff, K.S. 1981. National Institute of Mental Health Diagnostic Interview Schedule: Its History, Characteristics, and Validity. *Archives of General Psychiatry* 38:381–389.

Schoenborn, C.A., and Horm, J. 1993. Negative Moods as Correlates of Smoking and Heavier Drinking: Implications for Health Promotion. *Advance Data from Vital and Health Statistics*, No. 236. Hyattsville, Md.: National Center for Health Statistics.

Sherbourne, C.D., Wells, K.B., Hays, R.D., Rogers, W., Burnam, M.A., and Judd, L.L. 1994. Subthreshold Depression and Depressive Disorder: Clinical Characteristics of General Medical and Mental Health Specialty Outpatients. *American Journal of Psychiatry* 151:1777–1784.

Simon, G., Ormel, J., VonKorff, M., and Barlow, W. 1995a. Health Care Costs Associated with Depressive and Anxiety Disorders in Primary Care. *American Journal of Psychiatry* 152:352–357.

Simon, G.E., Lin, E.H.B., Katon, W., et al. 1995b. Outcomes of "Inadequate" Antidepressant Treatment. *Journal of General Internal Medicine* 10:663–670.

Sturm, R., and Wells, K.B. 1995. How Can Care for Depression Become More Cost-Effective? *Journal of the American Medical Association* 273:51–58.

USDHHS (U.S. Department of Health and Human Services). 1991. *Healthy People 2000: National Health Promotion and Disease Prevention Objectives.* DHHS Pub. No. (PHS) 91-50212. Washington, D.C.: Office of the Assistant Secretary for Health.

USDHHS. 1995. *International Classification of Diseases, Ninth Revision, Clinical Modification.* 5th ed. DHHS Pub. No. (PHS) 95-1260. Washington, D.C.: National Center for Health Statistics and Health Care Financing Administration.

USDHHS. 1996. *Physical Activity and Health: A Report of the Surgeon General.* Executive Summary. Atlanta, Ga.: Centers for Disease Control and Prevention and President's Council on Physical Fitness.

U.S. Preventive Services Task Force. 1996. *Guide to Clinical Preventive Services.* 2nd ed. Baltimore: Williams and Wilkins.

Ware, J.E., and Sherbourne, C.D. 1992. The MOS 36 Item Short-Form Health Survey (SF-36). *Medical Care* 30:473–483.

Wells, K.B., Stewart, A., Hays, R.D., et al. 1989. The Functioning and Well-being of Depressed Patients: Results from the Medical Outcomes Study. *Journal of the American Medical Association* 262:914–919.

WHO (World Health Organization). 1990. *Composite International Diagnostic Interview (CIDI, Version 1.0).* Geneva: WHO.

Zung, W.W.K. 1965. A Self-Rating Depression Scale. *Archives of General Psychiatry* 12:63–70.

TABLE A.2-1 Field Model Mapping for Sample Indicator Set: Depression

Field Model Domain	Construct	Sample Indicators	Data Sources	Stakeholders
Disease	Reduce prevalence of depression	Proportion of adult population reporting 14 or more days of depressed mood in past month	Community survey (BRFSS)	Health care providers Health care plans State health agencies Local health agencies Business and industry Education agencies and institutions Community organizations Special health risk groups General public
		Proportion of high school students reporting thoughts of suicide during past 12 months	School survey (YRBSS)	
Health and Function, Well-Being	Reduce functional impairment from depression	Proportion of adults meeting criteria for depressive disorder who are not receiving treatment	Community survey	Health care providers Health care plans Local health agencies Business and industry Education agencies and institutions Community organizations Special health risk groups Disease, patient organizations General public
	Reduce adverse outcomes of depression	Number (or rate) of suicides	Death certificates	
Social Environment	Improve access to services	Proportion of employed persons with access to employee assistance programs	Employers	Local health agencies Business and industry Community organizations Special health risk groups

continued on next page

TABLE A.2-1 *Continued*

Field Model Domain	Construct	Sample Indicators	Data Sources	Stakeholders
	Reduce financial barriers to treatment	Proportion of employees with insurance coverage for mental health services for themselves; for their families	Employers, insurance licensing authority	Health care plans Local government Business and industry General public
Health Care	Ensure that the health care system is following appropriate treatment practices	Proportion of patients receiving ambulatory follow-up within 30 days after discharge for hospitalization for depression	Patient records; claims files	Health care providers Health care plans Special health risk groups General public
		Proportion of depressed patients prescribed anti-depressant medications who receive prescriptions for therapeutically effective doses	Patient records; prescription services; claims files	Health care providers Health care plans Special health risk groups General public
		Proportion of MCOs or managed behavioral health organizations that are accredited by a nationally recognized organization	Behavioral health care providers; accrediting organizations	Health care plans Business and industry Special health risk groups General public

NOTE: BRFSS, Behavioral Risk Factor Surveillance System; MCO, managed care organization; YRBSS, Youth Risk Behavior Surveillance System.

A.3

Prototype Indicator Set: Elder Health

BACKGROUND

The age structure of the United States, indeed that of North America, is "graying." The most rapidly growing segment of the general population is the group age 85 and over. If present trends continue, approximately 20 percent of the population will be 65 years of age or older by the time this dynamic change has peaked in the year 2050 (Bureau of the Census, 1995). Providing appropriate health supports for this growing population, especially the frail elderly, will challenge many sectors within society.

The demographic shift has several important implications for health and health care. First, health care expenditures will be driven upward by the demographic shift since the elderly are provided health care resources out of proportion to their numbers. Next, the need for a full continuum of care for the frail elderly will become fully apparent in the next several decades, greatly expanding the demand for nursing home capacity, congregate care facilities, adult day care programs, and respite as well as other care giver support programs. The growth of capacity across this full continuum will be accelerated by the further penetration of managed care, since integrated systems of managed care will continue to drive down hospital use. Third, the health care workforce is not adequately prepared to meet the need for geriatric care, including assessment and care management services. Considerable investment will have to be made in undergraduate and graduate programs if appropriate services and care are to be available. Finally, the scope of "health care services" for the elderly is broad. Curative services remain important, but as the burden of chronic diseases increases with age, maintenance of function and satisfaction with care loom large as the primary outcomes in assessing the appropriateness and effectiveness of health care services. Critical services will be diverse, including clinical and personal care, functional assessment, education and social services, transportation, housing, social support, income supplementation, and others. Further, it is possible that social investments outside clinical geriatrics (e.g., in lay care giver training or in housing or social environments) will, in the end, be more effective in improving elder health than those in the medical care sector. Even within the domain of clinical activities, some critical services for sustaining elder health (e.g., annual influenza vaccination) may be the "product" of multiple providers such as the public health department or senior citizen centers, as well as the responsibility of clinical organizations.

"FIELD" SET OF PERFORMANCE INDICATORS

Given the size of the elder population, its political salience, and importance to medical care expenditures, many stakeholders would see the health status and effectiveness of services provided to this population as important, including providers, insurers, and state and local public health authorities. The frail elderly are an at-risk population in head-to-head competition with education of youth in state budget plans. Even employers and local industry, to the extent that they are committed to medical care for their retired employees and are concerned about current employees' obligations to care for elderly relatives, have a stake in the health of the elderly.

By using the domains of the field model, it is possible to identify a variety of measures that might serve as performance indicators for a community's efforts to improve the health of the elderly. Because of the nature of aging, both the medical and the social needs of elders must be addressed.

Health Care and Disease

An extraordinarily diverse set of performance indicators could be considered for use as part of a monitoring system that addresses health care and disease among the elderly. At a state level, both U.S. Medicare and Medicaid data sets have been used to characterize small-area variations in care, utilization of specific health care services by the elderly, mortality rates for specific procedures, hospital mortality rates, and even individual provider performance. Medicare data are specifically applicable to elders. Medicaid data are a source of information on the use of long-term care resources. Other potential sources of information on available resources at a community level would include health department information and "community resource" directories available in Area Agency on Aging offices in the United States.

In these data sets or others, potential indicators include a large universe of utilization and outcomes measures expressed as annual rates per thousand Medicare- or Medicaid-eligible persons living in a geographically defined residence community, ideally divided into two age strata, 65–84 years of age and 85 and over. These might include annual rates for mortality, hospitalization, nursing home days, physician visits, myocardial infarction, stroke, hip fracture, transurethral resection of the prostate, cholecystectomy, and coronary artery bypass surgery.

Kaiser Permanente's Northern California Region performance area "bundles" (see Table A.3-1), including those for cardiovascular disease, cancer, and common surgical procedures, suggest indicators that could be appropriate for elderly age groups (Center for the Advancement of Health and Western Consortium for Public Health, 1995). HEDIS-like indicators such as cholesterol screening, mammography, colorectal cancer screening, and provision of influenza vaccination annually would be highly appropriate. If cancer registry information is available, the incidence per thousand of late-stage breast cancer and advanced-stage colorectal cancer would be appropriate indicators. Health care providers and health care plans alike would be interested in community-level measures of self-rated health status and disability days, should these be available. With the exception of functional status measures at a community level, virtually all the potential indicators cited above make use of available data of reasonably good quality.

Social Environment and Prosperity

Indicator sets in general use have emphasized medical care utilization measures, relatively underrepresenting key social and economic determinants of the functional health of the elderly.

TABLE A.3-1 Kaiser Permanente Northern California Region Areas of Performance Measurement

Member Satisfaction
- Confidence in medical care
- Access to care
- Service
- Overall satisfaction

Childhood Health
- Rates of preventable diseases
- Immunization rates
- Disease outbreaks per 100,000 members
- Pediatric asthma
- Accidental poisoning
- Perceptions of experience of pediatric care

Maternal Care
- Rates of prenatal care
- Prenatal screening rates
- Birth outcomes (LBW, VLBW, neural tube defects, complex newborn rates, percentage of births to ICU, in-hospital mortality rate, perinatal mortality rate)
- Cesarian section rates
- Vaginal birth after cesarian section rate
- Perceptions of experience of obstetric inpatient care

Cardiovascular Disease
- Cholesterol screening rate
- AMI inpatient discharge rate
- AMI in-hospital mortality rate
- AMI mortality rate within 30 days of admission
- CABG inpatient discharge rate
- CABG mortality rate within 30 days of admission
- Heart disease mortality rate
- Hypertension screening rate
- Hypertension screening follow-up rate
- Hypertension treatment effectiveness (normal blood pressure after one year)
- Cerebrovascular accident inpatient discharge rate
- TIA inpatient discharge rate
- Cerebrovascular disease mortality rate

Cancer
- Mammography screening rate
- Breast cancer stage at diagnosis (local, regional, distant stages)
- Breast cancer five-year survival rate (by local, regional, distant stages at diagnosis)
- Breast cancer mortality rate

TABLE A.3-1 *Continued*

Cancer (continued)
Pap smear screening rate
Cervical cancer stage at diagnosis (local, regional, distant stages)
Cervical cancer mortality rate
Sigmoidoscopy screening rate
Colorectal cancer stage at diagnosis (local, regional, distant stages)
Colorectal cancer mortality rate
Lung cancer rate
Lung cancer mortality rate
Common Surgical Procedures
Laminectomy rate
Laminectomy average length of stay
Appendix rupture rate
Appendectomy average length of stay
Negative appendectomy rate
Cholecystectomy rate
Percentage of cholecystectomies performed laparoscopically
Cholecystectomy average length of stay
Laparoscopic cholecystectomy average length of stay
Hysterectomy rate
Percentage of hysterectomies performed vaginally
Percentage of vaginal hysterectomies laparoscopically assisted
Hysterectomy average length of stay
Other Adult Health
Diabetes inpatient discharge rate
Percentage of diabetics receiving annual retinal exam
Rate of flu shots in adults > 65
Pneumonia/pleurisy inpatient discharge rate
Adult asthma/bronchitis inpatient discharge rate
Average length of survival for AIDS patients
Mental Health and Substance Abuse
Rate of outpatient follow-up after inpatient discharge
Suicide rate

NOTE: AMI, acute myocardial infarction; CABG, coronary artery bypass graft; ICU, intensive care unit; LBW, low birth weight; TIA, transient ischemic attack; VLBW, very low birth weight.

SOURCE: Adapted from Center for the Advancement of Health and Western Consortium for Public Health (1995). Used with permission.

Acute general hospital event-based measures, moreover, have been used more frequently than measures that relate to health maintenance, rehabilitation, and long-term care.

As people enter elderly age groups, it is likely that they will face chronic diseases and conditions such as arthritis, diabetes, osteoporosis, and senile dementia (Bureau of the Census, 1995). Elderly persons with such conditions are likely to need assistance in performing the activities of daily living. Among noninstitutionalized elderly, 9 percent of those aged 65 to 69 and 50 percent of those 85 years or older needed assistance with daily activities such as bathing, preparing meals, and doing chores around the house (Bureau of the Census, 1995). This information raises concerns about the availability, accessibility, and quality of services for the elderly who need assistance with daily activities but are able to live in noninstitutional settings. Although only 1 percent of people aged 65 to 74 lived in nursing homes in 1990, nearly 25 percent who were age 85 or older did. These data point to the growing need for a range of social and health services for people between the ages of 65 and 84, as well as the growing need for institutional services for the "oldest old."

As the elderly grow in number, it will also be necessary and appropriate to monitor the development of an expanded capacity in the full continuum of care—that is, nonmedical services to assist with daily activities (e.g., bathing, meals, chores, transportation), low-intensity periodic nursing or medical services (e.g., checking vital signs, blood sugar, or medication compliance; changing dressings), and institutional services (e.g., adult day care, congregate care, senior housing with modified physical and social environments, nursing home care, respite care). In addition, coordination with the long-term care community is needed to ensure that adequate, appropriate-level, high-quality care for the elderly is available in the community.

Cooperation among federal, state, and local health agencies; social and housing agencies; community residents; and the medical care community is essential for achieving improved elder health. Communities could compile information from special studies that link health and other sectors; indicator measures might include various rates (expressed as an annual incidence per thousand persons aged 65 and older), including crimes against persons, residential burglaries, senior citizens bus ridership, participation in library services, access to sporting and cultural events (counting "senior citizen discount" tickets issued), voting in public elections, and property ownership.

Physical Environment

People negotiate the challenges of the physical environment every day as they drive automobiles and heavy equipment, walk on busy streets, do chores around the house or farm, and work in high-crime metropolitan areas. As individuals age, the challenges presented by the physical environment can become overwhelming due to changes in vision, hearing, bone density, muscle tone, and response time. Modifications in the physical environment and in individual behavior may be necessary to ensure that the elderly are able to maintain their independence and quality of life (IOM, 1990; Nuffield Institute for Health, 1996).

SAMPLE INDICATOR SET

1. Self-rated health status.

This indicator was chosen for its direct salience to the aims of health and social services for the elder population. Under current circumstances, measuring self-rated health status would require a special community-wide survey, although attempts could be made to "model" the community-based result from data routinely available at health departments (from the Behavioral Risk Factor Surveillance System), Area Agencies on Aging, senior citizen centers, or medical care plans operating in the community. Establishing accountability for maintaining health status would certainly be difficult, but it could be achieved if health status information were available for all *and* if individual organizational performance could be characterized on the basis of health status maintained in served populations (adjusted for age and gender). In a less precise approach, the distribution of poor health status in the community could be compared with catchment areas for clinical organizations, to determine whether community health organizations were serving vulnerable populations.

2. Physician visits per annum.

These data should be available from Medicare. This indicator is a utilization-based measure of access to health services.

3. Area-adjusted average per capita medical care expenditures for the elderly

This is a direct measure of medical care expenditure intensity available from Medicare. It can be interpreted as a measure of population need, the resource intensity of conventional medical practice, or both.

4. Influenza vaccination.

This is an efficacious service with major implications for morbidity and mortality from respiratory disease (influenza or pneumonia). Medicare claims data should be able to provide an approximation of the influenza vaccination rate in the community, but these data will not reflect vaccinations provided by hospitals, health departments, or managed care organizations. Accountability for achieving high vaccination rates among the elderly is shared. More specific measurements could be made within health care delivery systems in order to attach accountability more directly to organizational performance, but this approach would not provide community-wide information about coverage achieved.

5. Advanced-stage cancers of the breast.

A cancer registry (state health department) should be a reliable source of information about breast cancer in a community; other sources might include Medicare. This is a "sentinel event" measure of relevance to older women's health care. Accountability within systems of care for improving the performance of mammography and clinical examination screening could be established if individual-level data can be linked to a source of care.

6. Percentage of elderly residing in a nursing home on a given date.

For at least a subset of the population, these data should be available from Medicaid. State health department surveys of nursing homes and the decennial census are alternate sources of data. The indicator is a measure of population frailty, the lack of available alternative services for the frail elderly, or both.

7. Presence of the full continuum of care.

As the elderly increase in number, it will also be necessary and appropriate to monitor the development of an expanded capacity in the full continuum of care—that is, nonmedical services to assist with daily activities (e.g., bathing, meals, chores, transportation), low-intensity periodic nursing or medical services (e.g., checking vital signs, blood sugar, or medication compliance; changing dressings), and community long-term care services (e.g., adult day care, congregate care, senior housing with modified physical and social environments, nursing home care, respite care). In addition, coordination with the long-term care community is needed to ensure that adequate, appropriate-level, high-quality care for the elderly is available in the community.

This is a measure of "care capacity," one that could presumably be based on information from the Area Agency on Aging. Accountability for developing and maintaining the full continuum of care can best be described as a shared responsibility, since government, voluntary organizations, and the health care industry may all be needed to create the capacity.

8. Library readership, voting.

Social participation is a health-enhancing feature of an elder's lived experience and a manifestation of expanded function. This indicator cluster is a direct attempt to characterize the participation of elders in the social life of the community. Other possible measures might include senior theater, cinema, or other special event tickets per population base; bus ridership; church membership; and membership in the American Association of Retired Persons. Final selection of the measures included in this indicator should be appropriate to the community's social structure (e.g., bus ridership may not be appropriate in rural areas with no regular bus routes).

9. Senior citizen income and property ownership.

It is very difficult to measure the "prosperity" of the elderly. Income data are available but may underrepresent the wealth and savings of the elderly. Property ownership is an indirect measure of economic well-being but is a major component of the personal estate of older people in our society. Other possible approaches to assessing economic well-being might be to use Internal Revenue Service data to characterize income or bank data to measure savings, but both of these approaches seem less feasible. Accountability for economic well-being at a community level is difficult to establish, but the identification of populations in special need or at special risk would seem to be feasible if economic well-being can be measured.

10. Crimes against elderly persons or residential burglaries.

This measure of well-being is focused on personal safety, a major quality-of-life issue among the elderly, who may be viewed as "easy targets" by criminals. This information should be available from the public safety databases within a community. Accountability, at the first level of analysis, may reside with the police. At deeper levels of "ecological analysis," features of housing, transportation, and economic development within neighborhoods or urban subareas may also be relevant.

11. Falls among the elderly that result in hospitalization.

Falls among the elderly are a major cause of morbidity, disability, and mortality (IOM, 1990). Although hip fracture is the most devastating consequence of nonfatal falls, other consequences such as soft tissue injury, loss of mobility, and fear of falling can have a serious impact on quality of life. The prevention of falls provides an opportunity for multisectorial collaboration and cooperative efforts (Nuffield Institute for Health, 1996). Falls may have causes that are health related, pharmacologic, environmental, behavioral, or activity related (IOM, 1990).

This set of indicators has been composed to represent several underlying constructs, including health status (self-rated health, nursing home days), access to medical care (physician visits), resource use (per capita medical care expenditures), health care system capacity (continuum of care availability), states of well-being (economic, personal safety, social participation), critical health care services (influenza vaccination), and sentinel events (advanced-stage breast cancer). The indicator set substantially underrepresents the universe of potential indicators drawn directly from a medical care sector. This latter choice was a conscious one and could be controversial.

Taken together, the complex of indicators creates a profile of elder health production in a community, at least as one can characterize this process as cross-sectional. In the aggregate, it is an attempt to characterize the performance of health-relevant systems from a determinants-of-health perspective. In the aggregate, these indicators provide a relatively rich characterization of the health, health care utilization, social participation, and social welfare of the elderly population residing in a community. Health improvement initiatives might easily focus on any of these indicator sectors—from long-term care capacity to improving the quality of life for frail elderly residing in nursing homes. Any of these measures take on additional meaning if they can be compared (from one community to another or to a statewide average measure).

Specific organizational accountability for elder health is hard to assign on the basis of these indicators. Very few of the measures are likely to be precise enough to characterize the performance of single-provider organizations or even health care plans of modest size. Establishing accountability for performance by such a disparate set of "providers" as nursing homes, hospitals, physicians, metropolitan transportation systems, libraries, and the police will require forging an accountable community *coalition* within which collaborative action can arise and joint accountability be felt.

REFERENCES

Bureau of the Census. 1995. *Sixty-Five Plus in the United States.* Statistical Brief. SB/95-8. Washington, D.C.: U.S. Department of Commerce.

Center for the Advancement of Health and Western Consortium for Public Health. 1995. *Performance Indicators: An Overview of Private Sector, State and Federal Efforts to Assess and Document the Characteristics, Performance and Value of Health Care Delivery: Report on Field Research.* Washington, D.C.: Center for the Advancement of Health.

IOM (Institute of Medicine). 1990. *The Second Fifty Years: Promoting Health and Preventing Disability.* R.L. Berg and J.S. Cassells, eds. Washington, D.C.: National Academy Press.

Nuffield Institute for Health and NHS Centre for Reviews and Dissemination. 1996. Preventing Falls and Subsequent Injury in Older People. *Effective Health Care* 2(4):1–16.

TABLE A.3-2 Field Model Mapping for Sample Indicator Set: Elder Health

Field Model Domain	Construct	Sample Indicators	Data Sources	Stakeholders
Health Care, Disease	Reduce impact of disease among the elderly	Self-rated health status	Community survey (BRFSS data from health department), Area Agencies on Aging, senior citizen centers, medical care plans	Health care providers Health care plans State health agencies Local health agencies Medicare Agency on Aging Community organizations Special health risk groups General public
		Physician visits per annum	Medicare	
		Area-adjusted average per capita medical care expenditures for the elderly	Medicare	
		Influenza vaccination	Medicare	
		Advanced-stage cancers of the breast	State cancer registry, Medicare	
		Percentage of elderly residing in a nursing home on a given date	State health department surveys, census, Medicare	

Social Environment, Prosperity	Improve the quality of life of elderly by providing supportive social services	Presence of the full continuum of care	Area Agency on Aging	Health care providers Health care plans Medicare Local health agencies Social service agencies Area Agency on Aging Business and industry Nursing homes and caretaking organizations Community organizations Disease or patient organizations General public
		Library readership, voting	Community survey, voting rolls	
		Senior citizen income and property ownership	Community surveys, census, local property tax office, possibly IRS	
Physical Environment	Decrease hazards to elderly in the physical environment	Crimes against elderly persons or residential burglaries	Uniform crime reports, other police data	Health care providers Health care plans Medicare Local health agencies Social service agencies Police departments Area Agency on Aging Business and industry Community organizations General public
		Falls among the elderly that result in hospitalization	Hospital discharge data using ICD-9-CM E-codes, if available (otherwise N-codes for hip fractures)	

NOTE: BRFSS, Behavioral Risk Factor Surveillance System; ICD-9-CM, International Classification of Diseases, Ninth Revision, Clinical Modification; IRS, Internal Revenue Service.

A.4

Prototype Indicator Set: Environmental and Occupational Lead Poisoning

BACKGROUND

Decreased levels of lead in gasoline, air, food, and industrial releases have been linked to an overall lowering of mean blood lead levels in the United States from more than 15 μg/dL in the 1970s to less than 5 μg/dL in the 1990s. However, elevated blood lead level continues to be a prevalent childhood health problem (CDC, 1988). In addition, elevated blood lead levels pose an occupational risk to employees in a variety of industries. The problems of childhood and occupational lead poisoning and strategies to address these problems are discussed below.

Child Lead Intoxication

Elevated blood lead level is one of the most prevalent environmental threats to the health of children in the United States (CDC, 1988). Extremely elevated lead levels in children can result in serious medical conditions such as coma, convulsions, potentially irreversible mental retardation, seizures, and death (CDC, 1988). Lower levels of exposure may result in delayed cognitive development; reduced IQ scores; impaired hearing; adverse effects on hematocyte, vitamin D, and calcium production; and growth deficits (CDC, 1988).

Lead in and around the home environment remains a major

source of childhood exposure in the United States (USDHHS, 1995). An important route of exposure in young children is the ingestion of lead-based paint chips, lead-impregnated plaster, and contaminated dirt or dust found in homes built before 1950 (NCHS, 1984). Although all economic and racial subgroups of children are at risk of exposure, the prevalence of elevated lead levels remains highest for poor children living in the inner city. It is unlikely that childhood lead intoxication can be eliminated without further reductions in the lead content of paint, dust, and soil in inner-city areas (IOM, 1995).

The problem of childhood lead intoxication is reflected in Objective 11.4 of *Healthy People 2000: National Health Promotion and Disease Prevention Objectives* (USDHHS, 1991):

> Reduce the prevalence of blood lead levels exceeding 15 μg/dL among children aged 6 months through 5 years to no more than 500,000 by the year 2000. In addition, reduce blood lead levels exceeding 25 μg/dL among children (6 months through 5 years) to zero by year 2000.

At the time this objective was established, data for 1984 showed that 3 million young children had blood lead levels exceeding 15 μg/dL, and 234,000 had levels exceeding 25 μg/dL.

Current strategies to reduce the exposure of children to lead include abatement of lead hazards in homes and further reduction of lead levels in soil and drinking water. Abatement of lead in homes requires substantial resources, since the cost of abatement of a single residential structure can range from $3,000 to $15,000 (CDC, 1991). Title X of the Housing and Community Development Act of 1992 makes some provisions for funding residential lead abatement in communities. In addition, the act creates a process for involving federal agencies (e.g., the Department of Housing and Urban Development [HUD] and the Environmental Protection Agency [EPA]), local governments, and private owners in the abatement process.

Population-based strategies to reduce the availability of lead in soil and drinking water are under way in communities across the United States. Implementing these strategies is expensive and may raise controversies that position residents against government officials (or the business community). For example, soil remediation at Smuggler Mountain, a Superfund site near Aspen, Colorado, caused public outcry when residents learned that current blood lead levels of children were relatively low and that the process of soil remediation might result in a temporary increase in the level of exposure (IOM, 1995). This concern encouraged community members to become active participants in the remediation process and to work with officials to design strategies that minimize the risk of exposure during remediation.

Adult Lead Intoxication

Lead intoxication is a less prevalent problem among adults than among children. Among adults, lead exposure is associated most commonly with work at battery manufacturing plants, smelting operations, construction sites, radiator repair shops, ceramics production shops, firing ranges, and foundries (Pirkle et al., 1985; CDC, 1988). The exposure of adults to lead can affect a variety of organ systems, including cardiovascular, reproductive, renal, neurological, hematological, and musculoskeletal (CDC, 1988). In addition to personal health risks, adults who are exposed to lead in the workplace may "take home" lead dust on work clothes and shoes, thereby contributing to the exposure of family members.

According to the lead standard enforced by the Occupational Safety and Health Administration (OSHA, 1995), any worker with an average blood lead level greater than 50 μg/dL must be removed from exposure to lead. However, the medical literature suggests that serious health hazards such as neurological abnormalities, hypertension, and adverse reproductive effects for both genders are associated with blood lead levels as low as 30 μg/dL (CDC, 1988). Concern about the health hazards that occur at blood lead levels less than 50 μg/dL is reflected in Objective 10.8 of *Healthy People 2000* (USDHHS, 1991):

> Eliminate exposures resulting in workers having blood lead concentrations greater than 25 μg/dL by the year 2000.

As a comparison, there were 4,804 workers with elevated blood lead levels in seven states in 1988.

"FIELD" SET OF PERFORMANCE INDICATORS

By using the domains of the field model, it is possible to identify a variety of measures that might serve as performance indicators for a community's efforts to reduce the magnitude and sources of lead exposure for children and adults, thereby reducing the burden of lead intoxication in the United States. Because of the nature of lead intoxication, both the health outcomes and the exposure sources must be addressed. Educational efforts and strategies that modify the risk of exposure play an important role in community-based prevention efforts.

Achieving the childhood lead poisoning prevention objective requires coordination among federal, state, and local health agencies; environmental agencies; housing agencies; community residents (including parents); and the medical care community. In addition, coordination with occupational health groups is necessary to ensure safe removal of lead-containing paint from homes and other buildings. The prevention of adult lead exposure requires surveillance, evaluation, and control activities to identify high-risk industries and occupational groups. Control measures for high-risk occupations may include the substitution of less hazardous materials (e.g., using water-based instead of lead-based paint) or the use of personal protective measures (e.g., air filters and uniforms for hazardous work sites). Through collaborative efforts of public agencies, private organizations, and community members, the dual goals of preventing childhood and workplace lead intoxications can be achieved.

The following material reviews various types of health and exposure indicators that may be monitored in the community.

Disease and Health Care

Reducing the deleterious effects of lead intoxication for children and adults is the health outcome of primary interest. As mentioned earlier, lead intoxication in children can lead to serious conditions with lifelong impacts such as coma, potentially irreversible mental retardation, delayed cognitive development, reduced IQ scores, impaired hearing, and growth deficits. In adults, lead intoxication can lead to cardiovascular, reproductive, renal, neurological, hematological, and musculoskeletal system problems. The serious nature of lead-related medical conditions emphasizes the importance and need for primary prevention efforts. Through prevention, a community can avert potentially devastating and long-term health problems for its residents and can conserve health care, social service, and educational resources.

As part of an effort to reduce adverse health effects of lead, a community will need to compile accurate surveillance information about the extent of lead intoxication among its residents. The following indicators might be used:

1. Proportion and number of children (under 6 years of age)

who have blood lead testing as recommended by the Centers for Disease Control and Prevention (CDC).

CDC (1991) recommends universal screening of children at 12 months of age using a blood lead test, except in communities where no childhood lead poisoning problem exists. Children at high risk should receive earlier and more frequent testing. This recommendation is consistent with those of many organizations. For example, the American Academy of Pediatrics (1993) guidelines recommend that (a) all children should be screened for lead exposure at 12 months and again at 24 months of age; (b) providers should take a history of lead exposure for children between the ages of 6 months and 6 years to identify children living in high-risk situations; and (c) parents should receive educational materials on safe environmental, occupational, nutritional, and hygiene practices to protect their children from lead exposure. In addition, Medicaid's Early Periodic Screening, Diagnostic, and Treatment Program, which provides services to many poor inner-city children in high-risk environments, requires periodic screening of children with a blood lead measurement.

The American Medical Association, the American Academy of Family Physicians, and the Canadian Task Force on the Periodic Health Examination are consistent and recommend less in the way of testing than CDC and the groups mentioned above. The three organizations recommend blood lead testing for children who are at high risk of exposure (as found through history taking) as opposed to all children. The U.S. Preventive Services Task Force (1996) considered this option and decided against it, concluding that there is insufficient evidence to recommend a specific community prevalence level below which targeted screening can be substituted for universal screening.

2. Proportion and number of employees who have blood lead testing as recommended by the Occupational Safety and Health Administration (OSHA).

Occupational lead exposures are associated most commonly with work at battery manufacturing plants, smelting operations, construction sites, radiator repair shops, ceramics production shops, firing ranges, and foundries (Pirkle et al., 1985; CDC, 1988). OSHA has developed standards (29 CFR 1910.1025 and 29 CFR 1926.62) that provide medical surveillance guidelines for groups that are exposed to lead in the workplace (e.g., California Department of Health Services, 1995). In any workplace where air concentrations of lead exceed the OSHA standard, employees should have a blood lead monitoring program.

3. Proportion and number of tested children and adults with an elevated blood lead level.

Medical laboratories and health care providers have information about the proportion and number of elevated blood lead level tests. CDC has suggested that all blood lead tests for children be reported to state and local health agencies, and there is a growing national movement to make such reporting mandatory. Currently, about 35 states require that blood lead levels be reported to a state authority by medical laboratories. However, the reporting requirements vary from state to state. Most states require reporting to the health department, although in Maryland, for example, the Department of the Environment is the designated agency. It is noteworthy that in some states, *all* blood lead tests of children, including those that show no evidence of lead, are reportable to state authorities. Generally, this is not true for adults. In some states, reporting is required at specific levels (e.g., all blood lead test results above 20 µg/dL must be reported).

Communities may be interested in monitoring a variety of blood lead levels. For instance, a community may want to compile information about blood lead levels that correspond to national health objectives so that its progress can be compared to that of the nation, and it may want to compile information about the type of environmental or medical intervention required so that the performance of clinical, public health, and social service organizations can be measured. Some of the blood lead levels for children that should be considered follow:

- *Less than 10 µg/dL:* 10 µg/dL is the current level of concern at CDC. CDC considers children's blood lead levels less than 10 µg/dL to be "normal."
- *Greater than 15 µg/dL and greater than 25 µg/dL:* These levels correspond to health objectives for the nation's children.
- *10–19 µg/dL, 20–39 µg/dL, and 40 µg/dL or greater:* These correspond to levels at which CDC recommends environmental or medical interventions (discussed under item 4, below). At levels of 10–19 µg/dL, CDC suggests that health agencies provide educational information to parents about lead poisoning prevention. At levels of 20–39 µg/dL, CDC recommends environmental and medical management. At levels of 40 µg/dL or greater, CDC sug-

gests chelation therapy in addition to appropriate environmental and medical management.

For adults, communities may want to monitor blood lead levels greater than 25 μg/dL (the maximum level targeted by national health objectives) and greater than 50 μg/dL (the level at which workers are removed from workplace lead exposures under the OSHA Lead Standard).

If health care providers in the community adhere to CDC's recommendation for universal testing of children for blood lead levels, then the indicator provides an accurate measure of disease burden in the community for children at 12 months of age (recommended age of testing). If clinicians do not adhere to the CDC recommendation, the data may underrepresent the magnitude of lead poisoning in the community (for children 1 year of age). However, the indicator will contain additional testing results as well. Clinicians are likely to test blood lead levels of children living in high-risk environments, adults working in high-risk environments, and patients with symptoms of lead poisoning. The additional tests are important for disease surveillance. Since lead poisoning is a reportable condition in most states, state and local health agencies should have additional epidemiologic data for all children and adults who test positive for lead poisoning. With these data, communities can examine issues that are relevant to better identifying the geographic areas and populations at high-risk and designing intervention strategies. The availability of this information will vary from state to state.

Communities that conduct surveillance and follow-up activities may encounter many complex problems, such as public misunderstanding of the problem and prevention strategies; inadequate health care provider knowledge of prevention, diagnosis, and treatment; inadequate blood lead testing of high-risk groups (including children and workers); inadequate medical or public health case management; and incomplete surveillance information. To address problems such as these, a community may choose to use the indicators below.

4. Proportion of children and adults with elevated blood lead levels who receive follow-up services (monitoring, treatment, and reduction of exposure) in accordance with CDC guidelines.

Appropriate medical and public health case management is essential for minimizing the impact of lead exposure on the health of children and adults. In most states, case management is provided by the local health agency or managed care organization (MCO), although it may be coordinated through the state health or environmental agency. Follow-up procedures will vary from state to state. However, CDC recommends the following:

- At levels of 10–19 μg/dL, CDC suggests that health agencies provide educational information to parents and caretakers about lead poisoning prevention.
- At levels of 20–39 μg/dL, CDC recommends environmental and medical management. The local health agency should make a home visit to examine the environment for hazards and to work with the child's parents and caretakers to remove such hazards. Environmental management may also involve working with other state agencies, landlords, HUD, and EPA to coordinate the abatement of lead paint from houses, if that is the source of a child's lead poisoning. Health department staff should provide parents and caretakers with information about lead poisoning, hygienic practices that can reduce risk, and nutritional or dietary factors that modify risk.

Medical management includes an extensive history for the child, a careful physical exam for possible sequelae of lead poisoning, a nutritional assessment, and possible intervention. The nutritional status of the child can modify his risk of lead poisoning, thereby presenting an opportunity to intervene. The absorption of lead into a child's body is less likely if the child has frequent meals because an empty stomach facilitates lead absorption. Adequate calcium, which competes with lead for absorption, and sufficient iron also reduce the risk of lead poisoning.

At levels of 20–39 μg/dL, decisions about chelation therapy should be made by an informed health care provider. Although most providers would agree that chelation therapy is not beneficial at blood lead levels of 20–25 μg/dL, there is no consensus about its benefits at levels of 26–39 μg/dL. Medical management should include follow-up blood tests within three to four months to monitor lead levels.

- At levels of 40 μg/dL or greater, CDC suggests chelation therapy in addition to appropriate environmental and medical management. In chelation therapy, drugs are administered that bind and remove lead from the body (through the liver or kidneys). Chelation is generally performed in the hospital. Untreated children with levels greater than 40 μg/dL are at risk for coma, convulsions, and death.

For adults, workers are removed from the workplace at blood lead levels greater than 50 μg/dL, and they cannot return until their levels drop to 40 μg/dL or less. Chelation therapy protocols are more variable in adults. Eliminating lead exposures at the work site and using personal protective measures (e.g., respirator, goggles, protective work clothes, boots) may decrease the occurrence of occupational lead poisoning.

5. Existence of standard professional training opportunities for health care staff, public health staff, and environmental staff in areas related to child and adult lead poisoning.

Communities should ensure that professional staff who are responsible for issues related to lead poisoning receive adequate training in state-of-the-art approaches to the problem. Communities may want to consider the following:

- Are clear guidelines disseminated to area clinicians by medical associations and public health departments to ensure appropriate diagnosis, treatment, and reporting of lead poisoning in the community?
- What proportion and number of medical and related training programs provided by hospitals, MCOs, or other organizations incorporate state-of-the-art education into the curriculum?
- What proportion and number of courses that provide continuing medical education (CME) credit or other relevant and mandatory professional education credit incorporate state-of-the-art education into the curriculum?
- What proportion and number of state licensing examinations for physicians, nurses, and related providers include lead poisoning questions?

The answers to these questions may provide some direction for potential interventions.

6. Per capita public funding (state and local governments) for lead poisoning prevention that is dedicated to case management: identification of source, medical monitoring, treatment, and reduction of exposure.

One approach to monitoring performance is to review and compare the number and complexity of tasks (e.g., case management), the resources allocated to those tasks, and their outcomes. Information about public-sector funding for case management of lead poisoning prevention provides a starting point for such inquiries.

However, it is difficult to track the allocation and use of funds from state coffers in local programs. Communities should approach this measure with some caution.

Additional issues that are relevant to the disease and health care discussion include the level at which pregnant women are considered to have elevated blood lead, whether blood lead results should be based on confirmed (venous) or screening (capillary) blood tests, and whether ICD-9 diagnostic codes are adequate to identify health care provider visits for lead-associated health conditions. Although these issues are of vital interest and relevant, they were not included in the indicator set because they have not been resolved by the scientific community and reliable data are not available.

Physical Environment

Lead poisoning can be prevented by reducing exposure to lead in the environment (IOM and National Institute of Public Health, 1996). Recent efforts to reduce the number of lead exposure sources, focused on the physical and social environments, have been relatively successful. According to the midcourse review of the national objectives described in *Healthy People 2000*, the number of children who have blood lead levels greater than 15 μg/dL has been reduced from 3 million to 503,000, and the number of children who have blood lead levels greater than 25 μg/dL has been reduced from 234,000 to 93,000 (USDHHS, 1995). Communities can further reduce the risk of lead exposure among children by reducing the remaining sources of exposure in and around the home. Consideration should be given to the lead content of paint, dust, and soil in inner-city structures and outdoor areas that children may frequent.

Various obstacles exist in trying to ameliorate lead exposure in homes and other buildings. Communities that embark on lead poisoning prevention projects will be faced with many issues such as inadequate lead hazard identification and remediation, liability insurance, rental property issues, financial incentives for lead abatement or control, inadequate public information, poor coordination of public agencies, and potential for exposure at public schools and child care facilities. Communities may want to consider indicators such as the following:

1. Proportion (and number) of pre-1950 housing units in the

community; proportion (and number) of high-risk work sites in the community.

This indicator addresses the potential high-risk environments for children (i.e., homes that are likely to have lead-based paint or plaster) and adults (i.e., work sites with lead). In communities that find a substantial lead poisoning problem in children or adults, monitoring efforts should involve more than merely quantifying the number of high-risk sites. For instance, in addition to the proportion of pre-1950s housing, communities may want to map the location of high-risk housing and examine whether the location is correlated with lead poisoning cases among children. Surveys of residents can be conducted to learn more about whether lead-based paint has been abated (also see item 8 below). The local health department can provide information about the number of children who live in high-risk areas, so that prevention strategies can be developed. Information about high-risk work sites can be monitored in a similar way.

2. Proportion of housing units with identified lead hazards that have been remediated; proportion that are in the process of remediation; proportion that have been referred for legal enforcement.

Abatement of lead hazards in homes eliminates an important source of childhood lead poisoning. This indicator also measures the performance and coordination of federal agencies (e.g., HUD and EPA) with local housing and regulatory agencies, private owners, and other community stakeholders.

3. Proportion of local housing programs, weatherization programs, rehabilitation programs, and local building codes that include provisions for lead hazard control.

Lead hazards are more common in older housing; therefore, programs that target such housing should include provisions for lead hazard control. Programs that do not do so represent a "missed opportunity" for prevention and for addressing potential environmental hazards.

4. Proportion of lead inspectors, risk assessors, supervisors, project designers, and abatement workers certified through accredited training courses.

This measure is relevant to the safety of workers and their families as well as the identification and remediation of lead hazards in homes and other buildings. The presence of training courses and certification processes provides two opportunities for communities to monitor and influence the quality of technical training and the skill level and knowledge of technicians working in the community.

5. Environmental lead exposure as measured by sources such as the Toxic Release Inventory, Air Quality Management Districts, public water supply sources, contaminated food, and consumer product listings.

Community sources of lead exposure may include construction waste, lack of recycling, poor air quality, hazardous consumer products, and contaminated soil and water. Data relevant to these concerns are collected routinely in many communities by a number of state and local authorities. A periodic review of the diverse measures provides an opportunity to identify trends, problems, emerging problems, and signs of progress, and generally to determine if these sources are lead poisoning hazards to the community.

To prevent occupational lead poisoning, communities may have to address issues such as inadequate outreach, education, and technical assistance; lack of appropriate regulations, compliance and legislation; and lack of financing. Possible indicators in these areas follow.

6. Number of citations of companies by OSHA or state agencies for noncompliance with lead standards.

This indicator should be used with caution since OSHA investigations are initiated in response to employee complaints. If employees are unaware of the presence of lead in their workplace, feel that a complaint will jeopardize their job, or are unaware of the OSHA complaint option, no complaint will be filed. Thus, this indicator may not accurately reflect the extent of workplace hazards. However, communities may be able to use this measure in concert with other measures to monitor the performance of work site and environmental regulatory agencies.

7. Per capita state and federal matching funds devoted to work site training, technical assistance, and enforcement.

One approach to monitoring performance is to review and compare the number and complexity of tasks (e.g., work site training, technical assistance, and enforcement), the resources allocated to those tasks, and the outcomes of the tasks. Information about public-sector funding for work site training, technical assistance, and enforcement activities provides a starting point for such inquiries. However, it is difficult to track the allocation and use of funds from state coffers in local programs. Communities should approach this measure with some caution.

One of the barriers to providing adequate outreach, education, technical assistance, and regulatory activities is the lack of funding.

Social Environment

Many sectors of the community, in addition to the medical, public health, and environmental sectors, can influence and be influenced by lead poisoning prevention activities. For example, social service agencies play a potentially important liaison role between community members who need lead prevention services and service providers. When communities are not successful in prevention efforts, the demands on social service agencies, the health care system, and the educational system for services may increase (i.e., children and adults with lead-related conditions). Community resources can be used more efficiently when coordination exists between community agencies and organizations and when information is disseminated appropriately. To facilitate coordination and dissemination activities, communities may want to monitor the following indicators:

1. Per capita funding from state and local governments that is dedicated to education of the public and the medical community regarding lead poisoning.

As mentioned above, one approach to monitoring performance is to review and compare the number and complexity of tasks (e.g., educational activities for the public and medical community), the resources allocated to those tasks, and their outcomes. Information about funding for educational activities provides a starting point for such inquiries. Again, however, it is difficult to track the allocation and use of state funds in local programs. Communities should approach this measure with some caution.

There are many opportunities for providing effective prevention messages in the social environment. For instance, parents and caretakers can be educated about the risk posed by lead paint and the increased risk of lead poisoning for children with poor nutrition (i.e., infrequent meals, calcium deficiency, and iron deficiency) during physician visits and, in a less formal way, during visits to related businesses (hardware stores, supermarkets, science museums, etc.).

2. Existence of periodic lead-related disease meetings between different public agencies at the state and local levels (e.g., health departments; the Special Supplemental Food Program for Women, Infants, and Children [WIC]; Head Start) and meetings that include private health care community representatives.

This measure suggests one way in which information might be disseminated across agencies and organizations. However, it does not measure the quality of the information that is provided or the effectiveness of the strategy.

SAMPLE SET OF INDICATORS

Although all of the indicators discussed above are relevant to monitoring lead poisoning prevention efforts in communities, the nine measures listed below represent a minimal proposed set of indicators. Communities can supplement this list according to their interests and circumstances.

1. Proportion of children (under 6 years of age) who have blood lead testing as recommended by CDC.

These data are not currently available but could be collected in a community survey.

2. Proportion and number of tested children and adults with an elevated blood lead level.

About 35 states require that blood lead test levels be reported to a state authority by medical laboratories. However, reporting requirements vary from state to state. Medical laboratories may be required to report only positive lead test results.

3. Proportion of children and adults with elevated blood lead levels who receive follow-up services (monitoring, treatment, and reduction of exposure) in accordance with CDC guidelines.

These data may be available through a state's designated agency for lead reporting. Obtaining them may, however, require a review of medical records or a survey of health care providers.

4. Proportion (and number) of pre-1950 housing units in the

community; the proportion (and number) of high-risk work sites in the community.

The housing authority in a community should be able to provide this information. The health department and environmental agency may be able to provide supplementary information.

5. Proportion of housing units with identified lead hazards that have been remediated; proportion that are in the process of remediation; proportion that have been referred for legal enforcement.

The local housing authority and the local environmental agency should be able to provide data.

6. Proportion of local housing programs, weatherization programs, rehabilitation programs, and local building codes that include provisions for lead hazard control.

The local housing authority and the local environmental agency should be able to provide data. This information is also available through a survey of such programs.

7. Proportion of lead inspectors, risk assessors, supervisors, project designers, and abatement workers certified through accredited training courses.

The local housing authority and the local environmental agency should be able to provide data.

8. Environmental lead exposure as measured by sources such as the Toxic Release Inventory, Air Quality Management Districts, public water supply sources, and contaminated food and consumer product listings.

The state environmental and health agencies should be able to provide such information.

9. Number of citations of companies by OSHA or state agencies for noncompliance with lead standards.

OSHA or state agencies can provide this information.

The proposed indicator set includes measures of population-based risk factors (elevated blood lead in children, high-risk sites); medical care delivery (health care treatment and follow-up services); measures of lead in the environment (OSHA citations, air quality, toxic release inventory, water quality, foods); and prevention or risk reduction measures (blood testing, housing units under abatement, training). These measures also address the two major populations at highest risk for lead intoxication (children and workers) and a variety of exposure routes (air, water, and food; work sites; paint in older buildings; toxic releases).

The population-based health measure indicates whether the community as a whole has a problem with lead exposures. Children with elevated blood levels (>10 μg/dL) are directly indicative of a chronic, low-level, but still serious problem. Those with a higher blood lead level (>20 μg/dL) signal the need for immediate treatment and indicate a possible chronic, low-level problem in the population from which the people with the most serious problems come. Measures of air and water lead levels also relate to the community as a whole.

A number of the measures indicate the performance of broad sectors in the community. The proportion of children who have blood lead testing is a measure of the combined efforts of private physicians and health care plans, public health departments, and schools in providing the highly recommended clinical preventive service. The indicator on contaminated food and related products reflects the performance of federal, state, and local food and consumer regulatory agencies as well as product manufacturers and importers.

Other measures are more specific for particular segments of the community. The number of housing units with lead abatement completed is a direct measure of the performance of public and private housing agencies and regulatory agencies (at the national, state, and local levels). OSHA citations relate to employers who use lead in production and, indeed, can indicate specific employers that are cited. Similarly, EPA Toxic Release Inventories address the total amount of lead released by manufacturing companies into the community's environment and identify the specific companies involved. Certification of lead abatement inspectors, contractors, and workers relates to a specific group that is responsible for both the safety of lead workers and minimizing lead exposure in the immediate environment.

REFERENCES

American Academy of Pediatrics. 1993. Lead Poisoning: From Screening to Primary Prevention. *Pediatrics* 92:176–183.

California Department of Health Services. 1995. The Lead-Exposed Worker. *OLPPP/HESIS Medical Guidelines*. Berkeley: California Department of Health Services, Occupational Lead Poisoning Prevention Program and Hazard Evaluation System and Information Service. October.

CDC (Centers for Disease Control). 1988. *The Nature and Extent of Lead Poisoning in Children in the United States: A Report to Congress.* Atlanta, Ga.: U.S. Department of Health and Human Services.

CDC. 1991. *Preventing Lead Poisoning in Young Children. A Statement by the Centers for Disease Control—1991.* Atlanta, Ga.: U.S. Department of Health and Human Services.

IOM (Institute of Medicine). 1995. *Lead: A Public Health Policy Case Study.* K.A. Brix, D.R. Mattison, and M.A. Stoto, eds. Washington, D.C.: National Academy of Sciences.

IOM and National Institute of Public Health. 1996. *Lead in the Americas: A Call for Action.* C.P. Howson, M. Hernandez-Avila, and D.P. Rall, eds. Washington, D.C.: National Academy Press.

NCHS (National Center for Health Statistics). 1984. Blood Lead Levels for Persons Ages 6 Months to 74 Years: United States, 1976–1980. Data from the National Health and Nutrition Examination Survey. *Vital and Health Statistics.* Series 11, No. 233. Pub. No DHHS(PHS) 84-1683. Washington, D.C.: U.S. Department of Health and Human Services.

OSHA (Occupational Safety and Health Administration). 1995. OSHA Lead Standard. 29 CFR 1910.1025 (k) (l) (i) (o), App. C (7-1-95 Edition). Washington, D.C.: U.S. Department of Labor, Office of Occupational Medicine.

Pirkle, J.L., Schwartz, J., Landis, J.R., and Harlan, W.R. 1985. The Relationships Between Blood Lead Levels and Blood Pressure and its Cardiovascular Risk Implications. *American Journal of Epidemiology* 121(2):246–258.

USDHHS (U.S. Department of Health and Human Services). 1991. *Healthy People 2000: National Health Promotion and Disease Prevention Objectives.* DHHS Pub. No. (PHS) 91-50212. Washington, D.C.: Office of the Assistant Secretary for Health.

USDHHS. 1995. *Healthy People 2000: Midcourse Review and 1995 Revisions.* Washington, D.C.: USDHHS.

U.S. Preventive Services Task Force. 1996. *Guide to Clinical Preventive Services.* 2nd ed. Baltimore: Williams and Wilkins.

TABLE A.4-1 Field Model Mapping for Sample Indicator Set: Environmental and Occupational Lead Poisoning

Field Model Domain	Construct	Sample Indicators	Data Sources	Stakeholders
Disease, Health Care	Reduce the impact of lead-related morbidity	Proportion of children who have blood lead testing as recommended by CDC	Community surveys required	Health care providers Health care plans State health agencies Local health agencies Community organizations Special health risk groups Parents and care givers General public
		Proportion and number of tested children and adults with an elevated blood lead level	Laboratory reports, medical record reviews	
		Proportion of children and adults with elevated blood lead levels who receive follow-up services in accordance with CDC guidelines	State health department or other designated agency, medical record reviews	
Physical Environment	Identify and remediate sources of lead exposure	Proportion (and number) of pre-1950 housing units in the community; proportion (and number) of high-risk work sites in the community.	State and local agencies (e.g., environment, housing and community development)	State health agency State environmental agency State housing agency State and federal occupational safety agencies Local health agencies

continued on next page

TABLE A.4-1 *Continued*

Field Model Domain	Construct	Sample Indicators	Data Sources	Stakeholders
Physical Environment (*continued*)	Remediate lead hazards through legal mechanisms (regulatory and court actions)	Proportion of housing units with identified lead hazards that have been remediated; proportion that are in the process of remediation; proportion that have been referred for legal enforcement	State and local agencies	Local government Landlords, homeowners Business, industry Employees General public
	Improve coordination of community programs to address lead hazards	Proportion of local housing programs, weatherization programs, rehabilitation programs, and local building codes that include provisions for lead hazard control	State agencies, survey of programs	
		Proportion of lead inspectors, risk assessors, supervisors, project designers, and abatement workers certified through accredited training courses	State agencies, survey of programs	

	Periodic review of environmental lead data from sources such as Toxic Release Inventory, Air Quality Management Districts, etc.	Federal, state, and local environmental quality agencies
	Number of citations of companies by OSHA or state agencies for noncompliance with the lead standards	State or federal occupational safety agencies

NOTE: CDC, Centers for Disease Control and Prevention; OSHA, Occupational Safety and Health Administration.

A.5

Prototype Indicator Set: Health Care Resource Allocation

BACKGROUND

Since the 1950s, the share of gross national product devoted to personal health care has increased from 6 percent to 14 percent in the United States. This major annual investment has achieved substantial gains in the treatment of many diseases and has almost certainly contributed to improvements in life expectancy (Bunker et al., 1995). However, the United States still lags many other countries in critical measures of population health and of health system performance. For example, about 40 million Americans lack health insurance (Summer, 1994). Given that the United States spends almost 50 percent more per capita on health care than many other developed countries, the principal barrier cannot be a lack of resources to meet these needs. Rather, the United States faces a challenge of how to allocate its resources more efficiently to improve the health of the entire population.

Efficiency in health care entails achieving greater value—improved health status and increased satisfaction for a given expenditure. Although much work remains to be done to define value in health care, evidence of several types of inefficiency can be found in our current system.

First, there are numerous examples of the provision of ineffective or unwanted care (i.e., waste). The Prostate Patient Outcome Research Team, for example, found that many surgical interventions were being recommended by physicians based on symptom level alone, rather than on the degree to which the symptoms actually bothered patients or an understanding of the risks and benefits of surgery (Wasson et al., 1993). Providing balanced information led to substantial reductions in the rate of surgery. Investigators from RAND found that many of the diagnostic tests and surgical procedures that are performed are inappropriate (e.g., Park et al., 1989). The use of hospitals when alternative, less costly, and less intrusive sites of care are equally effective represents a similar problem—the unnecessary consumption of resources.

A second form of inefficiency can be found in failures to provide care that is known to be effective (i.e., lost opportunities). The failure to provide low-cost interventions of well-documented efficacy and effectiveness would represent an inefficiency of the community health system. From this perspective, the failure to provide childhood immunizations, adequate prenatal care, or appropriate screening for the early diagnosis of cervical cancer would all be evidence of an inefficient allocation of health care resources.

A third form of inefficiency is found when one examines differences in expenditures for the performance of specific health care-related tasks in a defined population (i.e., process inefficiency). Given an equal outcome, the treatment provided at a lower cost to the consumer is more efficiently delivered. This raises questions about both the amount of resources used and the prices paid for those services. Evidence of differences in the prices paid to providers for health care services is substantial for hospital services (e.g., Pennsylvania Health Care Cost Containment Council, 1995), for physician services (Welch et al., 1996), and for the provision of specific high-cost procedures that entail both physician and hospital care. Such evidence has led many purchasers to contract with specific "centers of excellence" that can provide high-quality care at a lower price—an improvement in efficiency from the payer's perspective. Consideration of price also leads quickly into highly charged questions about what represents a reasonable profit or operating margin. What is a fair return for a hospital? What is a reasonable income for a physician? What is a fair profit for a health plan?

Finally, one can consider outcome inefficiency, or expending more resources than necessary to achieve a given health outcome in a defined population. An approach to defining populations based in the current market-driven reforms of the health care system is the effort led by the National Committee for Quality

Assurance to evaluate enrollees' experience of managed care plans. HEDIS, the Health Plan Employer Data and Information Set (NCQA, 1993), encompasses measures in several categories, including quality of care for both prevention services and treatment, utilization of services, members' access to and satisfaction with services, and organization and operation of the health plan. Measures, chosen to produce information that promotes quality improvement within health plans, are reviewed and revised on a periodic basis.

A second population-based approach is reflected in the geographic analyses that have documented large variations in per capita health care resources, utilization, and expenditures across U.S. communities (e.g., Wennberg, 1996). Although there are clearly differences in population characteristics across geographic areas, the differences observed in the use of health care services have not been explained by detectable differences in the need for services (Wennberg, 1996), nor by any evidence that greater resource use is associated with improved health outcomes or satisfaction with care. A comparison of population-based outcomes of acute myocardial infarction (AMI) demonstrated that lower rates of post-AMI intervention were associated with both improved survival and improved control of symptoms (Guadagnoli et al., 1995).

Another demonstration of inefficient resource allocation is evident in a comparison of Medicare beneficiaries in Miami and Minneapolis. Although health care spending for Medicare beneficiaries residing in Miami is twice that for residents of Minneapolis (i.e., $5,922 per beneficiary compared to $2,966, after adjustment for differences in age, sex, race, and price), mortality rates are identical (i.e., 47 per 1,000 beneficiaries). A recent survey also found that residents of Miami are less satisfied with their care (Wennberg, 1996; J. Knickman, personal communication, 1996).

"FIELD" SET OF PERFORMANCE INDICATORS

The field model encourages a shift of focus from individual patients or enrolled populations to the community as a whole. Moreover, the model explicitly raises the question of whether the marginal investment in personal health care would not achieve a greater benefit if invested in other sectors of the community. The potential stakeholders for such an effort include all segments of the community. A community-based focus also draws attention to two problems that are easily ignored when the focus remains at the level either of the individual patient or of enrolled populations.

The first is the problem of the uninsured or other disadvantaged populations who may have difficulty receiving basic services. The second is the issue of the responsibility of local health care institutions to the community itself (Kaufman and Waterman, 1993; Showstack et al., 1996).

The committee used the field model as a framework to guide the selection of potential indicators of inefficient allocation of health care resources. The committee also recognized the importance of cross-community or longitudinal comparisons as guides to the interpretation of resource indicators. For many of the indicators, the absolute level of resources required to meet population health needs is unknown.

Benchmarking to other communities that are similar in terms of measures of need and yet appear to meet those needs with fewer resources provides a plausible and rational justification for resource reallocation (Fisher et al., 1992). The selection of performance indicators of health care resource allocation was thus guided both by the field model and by the possibility of applying an approach based on benchmarking.

Four domains of the field model are particularly useful for developing measures of potential need for health care within a community: disease, health and function, prosperity, and well-being. The committee suggests that data from its proposed community profile be assembled on the target community and on potential benchmark communities. Within the remaining domains, potential indicators are identified below.

Individual Behavior

The field model highlights the influence of factors in the environment on individual behavior. Examining the proportion of inpatient deaths that occur in the absence of a completed advance directive acknowledges that hospitals and physicians have an important role in influencing this specific individual behavior. Patients with advance directives are significantly more likely to participate in end-of-life decisions and to limit medical treatment when facing a terminal disease (Weeks et al., 1994). The committee proposed this measure of potential inefficiency because of the potentially high costs that may be incurred in terminal illness in which care continues only because an advance directive was not completed (Emanuel, 1996).

A second measure of the impact of factors in the environment that influence individual behavior is the rate of cigarette smoking.

Smoking is a significant underlying risk factor for many adverse health conditions (McGinnis and Foege, 1993). Physicians and many other individuals and organizations in the community can influence individuals' smoking behavior.

Social Environment

The excess capacity of the U.S. hospital system is well recognized, but the challenges of downsizing are substantial. A barrier to reallocation of resources from acute care to other sectors is the widespread assumption that greater levels of investment in health care are beneficial. The evidence of benefit from greater spending on personal health care is limited (Bunker et al., 1995), and there is some evidence to the contrary (Guadagnoli et al., 1995). The prevalence of this assumption is difficult to measure directly. However, the media portrayal of health care and public health services represents a potential construct for examining social assumptions regarding the value of health care spending. The data are not currently available.

Physical Environment

The physical environment of health care may provide some evidence of inefficiency. Two examples considered by the committee focus on regionalization. Substantial evidence documents the improved outcomes and lower costs that are achieved when patients receive coronary artery bypass graft surgery in high-volume regional centers (Luft et al., 1990; Hannan et al., 1991). Similarly, because most high-risk deliveries should be identified before birth, inadequate regionalization of high-risk obstetrical care can be identified by the number of low birth weight infants born in centers without appropriate facilities to handle them.

Communities may want to examine the number of avoidable hospitalizations by measuring ambulatory care sensitive (ACS) hospitalizations, an indirect measure of underutilization of outpatient services and poor primary care management (IOM, 1993). Studies correlating ACS hospitalizations with other factors are complex, but a raw count of inpatient hospitalizations for conditions that are known to be manageable in an outpatient setting (e.g., diabetes, asthma) might be adequate for communities. Data may be available through HEDIS and through state comprehensive hospital discharge databases (e.g., the Washington State Commission Hospital Abstract Reporting System), where available.

Health Care

Within the domain of health care, the committee identified three constructs of particular importance in judging the efficiency of resource allocation: (1) underprovision of basic, cost-effective services (i.e., missed opportunities); (2) overprovision of unnecessary services (i.e., waste); and (3) excess capacity (i.e., outcome inefficiency). The specific measures proposed for each of these constructs can feasibly be obtained from sources listed in the accompanying table.

Inadequate prenatal care. A reasonable indicator of inadequate prenatal care is the percentage of births to women who did not receive any care during the first trimester. The data for this measure are readily available through state vital statistics.

Inadequate primary care. The percentage of the population without a regular source of care, other than emergency departments, can be ascertained through the Behavioral Risk Factor Surveillance System (BRFSS) or may be available through other surveys as well. Communities may consider measuring selected relevant clinical outcomes. For example, COMAH (Clinical Outcome Measure Adjusted HEDIS) indicators are being pilot tested in the state of Washington (J. Krieger, personal communication, 1996). These indicators attempt to measure "root issues" such as respiratory flow for asthmatics, immunization levels for children, and blood sugar levels for diabetics.

Inadequate public health capacity. Public health is an essential component of the national health system. *Healthy People 2000* (USDHHS, 1991) includes an objective calling for 90 percent of the population to be served by a local health department that effectively caries out the core public health functions of assessment, policy development, and assurance. Essential services to fulfill those core functions have been defined as (Baker et al., 1994):

- Monitor health status to identify and solve community health problems.
- Diagnose and investigate health problems and health hazards in the community.
- Inform, educate, and empower people about health issues.

- Mobilize community partnerships and action to identify and solve health problems.
- Develop policies and plans that support individual and community health efforts.
- Enforce laws and regulations that protect health and assure safety.
- Link people to needed personal health services and assure provision of health care when otherwise unavailable.
- Assure a competent workforce for public health and personal care.
- Evaluate effectiveness, accessibility, and quality of personal and population-based health services.
- Research for new insights and innovative solutions to health problems.

Efforts are being made to develop tools that communities can use to evaluate the adequacy of the public health system in their local areas. A set of 10 public health practices have been used as a basis for developing survey instruments for assessing local health department effectiveness in performing the core functions (Miller et al., 1994; Turnock et al., 1994). Interpretation of the results of such surveys must take into account the extent to which segments of the community outside the health department contribute to meeting overall public health needs.

Additional measures that may be of interest to communities are (1) per capita expenditures, by county and state, for public health activities; and (2) public health expenditures as a percentage of total health care expenditures, by state. Estimates for fiscal year 1993 indicate that national spending for core public health functions amounted to $11.4 billion, or 1.3 percent of total health expenditures in the United States (Public Health Foundation, 1994).

Benchmarked rate of discretionary surgery. Small area variation studies have long been used to identify areas for which high rates reflect likely overuse of discretionary procedures such as coronary artery bypass surgery, cholecystectomy, cesarean section, or surgery for back pain.

Benchmarked rate of hospital and intensive care unit (ICU) utilization. The use of acute care hospitals to treat many acute and chronic conditions is increasingly questioned in terms of both the risks associated with hospitalization and the high costs of care in that setting. If possible, this indicator should be measured at the population rather than the institutional level. In addition, communities may want to examine the utilization of hospitals and ICUs for specific diagnoses.

Underuse of generic pharmaceutical agents. The growing availability of computerized pharmacy records will make it possible to monitor the proportion of eligible prescriptions that are written for generic drugs of generally equal effectiveness but substantially lower cost (Walzak et al., 1994).

Benchmarked supply of hospital beds, specialists, and primary care providers. Existing data from the American Hospital Association and physician organizations such as the American Medical Association (AMA) and the American Osteopathic Association can be used to determine the local supply of beds and physicians, while Medicare data or a state's hospital discharge data set can be used to adjust for border crossing and differences in age and sex across areas. A recently published analysis by researchers at Dartmouth provides such data for 1993 for all regions of the United States (Wennberg, 1996). Such analyses provide a potential source of data for benchmarking the level of personal health care resources within a community to numerous other communities that may achieve similar health outcomes with fewer resources.

SAMPLE SET OF INDICATORS

The 13 measures listed below represent a set of sample indicators that can be compiled by many communities throughout the United States:

1. Percentage of inpatients age 65 and over who die without an advance directive.

This measure would require a review of selected medical charts. The existence of an advance directive should be noted in the chart of patients with terminal conditions.

2. Percentage of health plan enrollees who smoke.

This measure would require a review of medical charts as well. Surveys at the community level may exist or could be developed.

3. Number of hospitals with a low volume of coronary artery bypass graft (CABG) surgery.

Data for this indicator might be obtained from a state's hospital discharge data system or from Medicare databases.

4. Number of infants weighing less than 1,500 grams born in hospitals without an advanced care nursery.

These data are available from vital statistics, through the state or local health agency.

5. Number of inpatient hospitalizations for asthma and diabetes.

These data are available from hospitals or from a state's hospital discharge data system.

6. Percentage of births without first trimester prenatal care.

Information about prenatal care is available on birth certificates and from vital statistics at the state or local health department.

7. Percentage of individuals without a usual source of care.

This information is collected through the state-level Behavioral Risk Factor Surveillance System. Surveys at the community level may exist or could be developed.

8. Performance ratio for 10 essential public health practices.

This indicator requires a survey of "public health" providers, including state and local government agencies, voluntary nonprofit community agencies, hospitals, physicians, clinics, community and migrant health centers, universities, federal agencies, foundations, and others. A survey protocol is available for use by communities (Miller et al., 1994).

9. Ratio of discretionary surgeries to benchmark rates.

This information can be compiled from hospital discharge or Medicare data. Communities also may consider conducting surveys.

10. Percentage of prescriptions for generic drugs, by class of drug.

Computerized pharmacy records can provide information, once the community has identified agents for which substitution should be possible and has specified brand names that fall within the class.

11. Ratio of hospital beds to benchmark rates.
The American Hospital Association compiles this information.

12. Ratio of medical specialists to benchmark rates.
The local medical community and the AMA can provide these data.

13. Ratio of primary care physicians to benchmark rates.
Again, the local medical community or the AMA is a source of data.

The proposed indicator set includes measures of individual behavior (advance directives and smoking), physical environment (low-volume CABG and obstetrical hospitals, avoidable ACS hospitalizations), and health care (missed opportunities, waste, and excess capacity). Most of the measures are tied to hospital data, reflecting its availability and reliability. One measure of public health efficiency (indicator 8) is included. Communities may also want to look for ways in which to incorporate measures of process efficiency and outcome efficiency. For example, communities may want to conduct surveys to learn about such process measures as whether purchasers of health care services are organized and whether consumers have adequate information.

REFERENCES

Baker, E.L., Melton, R.J., Stange, P.V., et al. 1994. Health Reform and the Health of the Public: Forging Community Health Partnerships. *Journal of the American Medical Association* 272:1276–1282.

Bunker, J.P, Frazier, H.S., and Mosteller, F. 1995. The Role of Medical Care in Determining Health: Creating an Inventory of Benefits. In *Society and Health.* B.C. Amick, S. Levine, A.R. Tarlov, and D.C. Walsh, eds. New York: Oxford University Press.

Emanuel, E.F. 1996. Cost Savings at the End of Life. What Do the Data Show? *Journal of the American Medical Association* 275:1907–1914.

Fisher, E.S., Welch, H.G., and Wennberg, J.E. 1992. Prioritizing Oregon's Hospital Resources: An Example Based on Variations in Discretionary Medical Utilization. *Journal of the American Medical Association* 267:1925–1931.

Guadagnoli, E., Hauptman, P.J., Ayanian, J.Z., Pashos, C.L., McNeil, B.J., and Cleary, P.D. 1995. Variation in the Use of Cardiac Procedures after Acute Myocardial Infarction. *New England Journal of Medicine* 333:573–578.

Hannan, E.L., Kilburn, H., Bernard, H., O'Donnell, J.F., Lukacik, G., and Shields, E.P. 1991. Coronary Artery Bypass Surgery: The Relationship between In-hospital Mortality Rate and Surgical Volume after Controlling for Clinical Risk Factors. *Medical Care* 29:1094–1107.

IOM (Institute of Medicine). 1993. *Access to Health Care in America.* M. Millman, ed. Washington, D.C.: National Academy Press.

Kaufman, A., and Waterman, R.E., eds. 1993. *Health of the Public: A Challenge to Academic Health Centers. Strategies for Reorienting Academic Health Centers Toward Community Health Needs.* San Francisco: University of California, Health of the Public Program.

Luft, H.S., Garnick, D.W., Mark, D.H., and McPhee, S.J. 1990. *Hospital Volume, Physician Volume, and Patient Outcomes: Assessing the Evidence.* Ann Arbor, Mich.: Health Administration Press.

McGinnis, J.M., and Foege, W.H. 1993. Actual Causes of Death in the United States. *Journal of the American Medical Association* 270:2207–2212.

Miller, C.A., Moore, K.S., Richards, T.B., and Monk, J.D. 1994. A Proposed Method for Assessing the Performance of Local Public Health Functions and Practices. *American Journal of Public Health* 84:1743–1749.

NCQA (National Committee for Quality Assurance). 1993. *Health Plan Employer Data and Information Set and User's Manual, Version 2.0 (HEDIS 2.0).* Washington, D.C.: NCQA.

Park, R.E., Fink, A., Brook, R.H., et al. 1989. Physician Ratings of Appropriate Indications for Three Procedures: Theoretical Indications vs. Indications Used in Practice. *American Journal of Public Health* 79:445–447.

Pennsylvania Health Care Cost Containment Council. 1995. *A Consumer Guide to Coronary Artery Bypass Graft Surgery.* Volume IV, 1993 Data. Pennsylvania's Declaration of Health Care Information. Harrisburg: Pennsylvania Health Care Cost Containment Council.

Public Health Foundation. 1994. *Measuring State Expenditures for Core Public Health Functions.* Final report to the U.S. Department of Health and Human Services, Office of Disease Prevention and Health Promotion. Washington, D.C.: Public Health Foundation.

Showstack, J., Lurie, N., Leatherman, S., Fisher, E., and Inui, T. 1996. Health of the Public: The Private-Sector Challenge. *Journal of the American Medical Association* 276:1071–1074.

Summer, L. 1994. The Escalating Number of Uninsured in the United States. *International Journal of Health Services* 24(3):409–413.

Turnock, B.J., Handler, A., Hall, W., Potsic, S., Nalluri, R., and Vaughn, E.H. 1994. Local Health Department Effectiveness in Addressing the Core Functions of Public Health. *Public Health Reports* 109:653–658.

USDHHS (U.S. Department of Health and Human Services). 1991. *Healthy People 2000: National Health Promotion and Disease Prevention Objectives.* DHHS Pub. No. (PHS) 91-50212. Washington, D.C.: Office of the Assistant Secretary for Health.

Walzak, D., Swindells, S., and Bhardwaj, A. 1994. Primary Care Physicians and the Cost of Drugs: A Study of Prescribing Practices Based on Recognition and Information Sources. *Journal of Clinical Pharmacology* 34:1159–1163.

Wasson, J., Fleming, C., Bruskewitz, R., et al. 1993. The Treatment of Localized Prostate Cancer: What Are We Doing, What Do We Know, and What Should We Be Doing? *Seminars in Urology* 11(1):23–26.

Weeks, W.B., Kofoed, L.L., Wallace, A.E., and Welch, H.G. 1994. Advance Directives and the Cost of Terminal Hospitalization. *Archives of Internal Medicine* 154:2077–2083.

Welch, W.P., Verrilli, D., Washington, D.C., Katz, S.J., and Latimer E. 1996. A Detailed Description of Physician Services for the Elderly in the United States and Canada. *Journal of the American Medical Association* 275:1410–1416.

Wennberg, J., ed. 1996. *The Dartmouth Atlas of Health Care.* Chicago: American Hospital Press.

TABLE A.5-1 Field Model Mapping for Sample Indicator Set: Health Care Resource Allocation

Field Model Domain	Construct	Sample Indicators	Data Sources
Disease, Health and Function, Prosperity, Well-being		See community health profile	Use to select benchmark communities[a]
Individual Behavior	Use of advance directives	Percentage of inpatients 65 and over who die without an advance directive[b]	Chart review of selected records
	Health risk behavior	Percentage of health plan enrollees who smoke	Chart review, HEDIS
Physical Environment	Inadequate regionalization of surgery	Number of hospitals with low volume of CABG surgery	Statewide hospital discharge database, Medicare databases
	Inadequate regionalization of high-risk care	Number of infants weighing <1,500 grams born in hospitals without an advanced care nursery	Vital statistics
	Avoidable hospitalizations	Number of inpatient hospitalizations for asthma and diabetes	Statewide hospital discharge database, hospital records
Health Care	Underprovision of basic services	Percentage of births without first trimester care	Vital statistics, state health department
		Percentage of individuals without a usual source of care	BRFSS

		Performance ratio for 10 essential public health practices	Survey needed
	Overprovision of services or waste	Ratio of discretionary surgeries to benchmark rates[c]	Statewide hospital discharge database, Medicare databases
		Percentage of prescriptions for generic drugs, by class of drug[d]	Computerized pharmacy records
	Excess health care capacity	Ratio of beds to benchmark rates	AHA data
		Ratio of medical specialists to benchmark rates	AMA, AOA, or local data
		Ratio of primary care physicians to benchmark rates	AMA, AOA, or local survey

NOTE: AHA, American Hospital Association; AMA, American Medical Association; AOA, American Osteopathic Association; BRFSS, Behavioral Risk Factor Surveillance System; HEDIS, Health Plan Employer Data and Information Set.

[a]Many of the measures in this indicator set are most easily interpreted by cross-sectional or longitudinal comparisons. Cross-sectional comparisons between one community and a similar benchmark community that appears to have equal resources (income) and outcomes (mortality), yet a lower-cost health system, represent one possibility. Longitudinal comparisons would allow individual communities to aim for improvement, regardless of their baseline rates on these numbers.

[b]Evidence that advance directives are effective in themselves at reducing expenditures does not exist. They may, however, be a necessary precondition to other cost-saving interventions.

[c]Surgical procedures prescribed by physicians in the absence of adequate provision of information to patients (potentially unwanted surgeries) include CABG, carotid endarterectomy, cholecystectomy, and back surgery. Small area analysis is only an indirect measure. Direct measure requires survey of information provision systems in a community.

[d]Development of this measure will require (1) identifying agents for which substitution should be possible, (2) defining brand names that fall within that class, and (3) obtaining computerized pharmacy records for analysis.

A.6

Prototype Indicator Set: Infant Health

BACKGROUND

During childhood, infancy is the most vulnerable period. Important determinants of infant health operate even before a child is conceived. A woman's general health, her socioeconomic and family circumstances, and her intentions regarding pregnancy all influence the health of the children she bears. During pregnancy, maternal health, nutrition, lifestyle, and socioeconomic and physical environments have an even more immediate influence on infant health. Once children are born, their healthy physical and psychosocial development continues to be subject to a variety of influences.

The most widely used indicator of infant health is the infant mortality rate: deaths of children less than 1 year of age per 1,000 live births. In the United States in 1993, the infant mortality rate was 8.4 (Gardner and Hudson, 1996). Most infant deaths occur in the neonatal period (within 28 days of birth), and low birth weight infants—those weighing less than 2,500 grams (5 pounds, 8 ounces)—are at greatest risk (McCormick, 1985; Paneth, 1995). The risk of death is especially high for infants born weighing less than 1,500 grams (3 pounds, 5 ounces). Low birth weight is also associated with increased risk of long-term health impairments (Hack et al., 1995). Thus, prevention of low birth weight is an important goal. The target set by *Healthy People*

2000 is for a low-birth weight rate of no more than 5 percent of live births (USDHHS, 1991).

In the United States, 7.3 percent of babies born in 1994 weighed less than 2,500 grams, and about 1.3 percent weighed less than 1,500 grams (Ventura et al., 1996). The incidence of low birth weight varies by race and ethnicity. Among African Americans, 13.2 percent of infants born in 1994 weighed less than 2,500 grams. In addition, factors such as poverty, lower levels of maternal education, unintended pregnancy, and delayed prenatal care are associated with increased rates of low birth weight (Hughes and Simpson, 1995). Many low birth weight infants require costly medical care. An estimate for 1988 (which does not capture the impact of new technologies) suggests added medical care costs of $15,000 per low birth weight infant during the first year of life (Lewit et al., 1995).

Low birth weight can occur because of an early, preterm birth or slow growth during a normal period of gestation (Paneth, 1995). Steps such as cessation of maternal smoking and adequate maternal nutrition have been shown to reduce the risk of slow fetal growth (USDHEW, 1973; IOM, 1990). The risk of mortality is higher for preterm births, but evidence for interventions that can reduce their occurrence is mixed (Paneth, 1995). Some evidence suggests that vaginal or intrauterine infections may be contributing to preterm births (Fiscella, 1996; Goldenberg and Andrews, 1996). Early and continuing prenatal care can help identify risks for low birth weight and may help ensure that both mothers and infants receive care that can improve survival even if low birth weight cannot be averted (Alexander and Korenbrot, 1995). Prenatal care can also provide benefits to mothers and infants that do not translate into changes in birth weight.

After the neonatal period, infant health is influenced strongly by family resources. A loving and caring home with educated parents makes an important contribution to healthy infant development and, therefore, future capacity to become a well-functioning adult (Carnegie Task Force on Meeting the Needs of Young Children, 1994). Among factors affecting physical health, injury is a leading preventable cause of mortality and morbidity. Parental knowledge of and attention to injury prevention have documented benefits for children (Bass et al., 1993; Gielen et al., 1995). Immunization also is a well-recognized means of protecting health and is a marker for adequate use of well child care (Rodewald et al., 1995). Promoting healthy psychosocial development is also important. For example, factors influencing the home environment, such as increased parental workforce participation that creates a need for nonparental child care, can have important consequences for infant well-being.

Children are the future of a community, and their well-being depends on a variety of factors. Protecting and improving infant health is a complex task that involves individual families plus health care, public health programs, and social programs that support families. Communities may also want to address factors such as educational attainment and employment of parents. Coordination of these various efforts can encourage optimal use of resources on behalf of infants.

"FIELD" SET OF PERFORMANCE INDICATORS

Each of the domains of the health field model addresses relevant determinants of infant health, many of which suggest specific health improvement interventions. These domains can be used to organize a field set of potential performance indicators for community efforts to protect and improve infant health. Although some of the proposed indicators address concerns that are not easily operationalized as quantitative measures, they help illustrate issues that might benefit from additional effort to develop suitable measures or data sources.

Disease

Leading causes of death during the neonatal period (within 28 days of birth) are congenital anomalies, respiratory distress syndrome, consequences of preterm birth, and effects of maternal complications. In the postneonatal period (28 days to 1 year of age), the principal causes of death are sudden infant death syndrome (SIDS), congenital anomalies, injury, and infection (USDHHS, 1991). In the United States in 1993, the neonatal mortality rate was 5.3 deaths per 1,000 live births and the postneonatal rate was 3.1 (Gardner and Hudson, 1996).

Disease influences infant health directly and through its impact on the health of the mother before, during, and after pregnancy. Maternal conditions that pose particular risks for infant health include hypertension and diabetes (either preexisting or emerging during pregnancy), vaginal infection, and preeclampsia (CDC, 1993; Ananth et al., 1995; McGregor et al., 1995). Conditions such as these can lead to preterm delivery and to intrapartum fetal distress. Early detection and careful management of these diseases before and during pregnancy can reduce their negative effects. The adverse effect of some maternal infections (e.g., HIV, hepatitis B, group B streptococcus) occurs with their transmission to infants before or during birth. In some cases, treatment of the mother or early treatment of the infant can reduce these adverse effects.

When preterm delivery cannot be prevented, infants are at increased risk for a variety of conditions including respiratory distress syndrome, intraventricular hemorrhage, and necrotizing enterocolitis. Improved treatment has increased survival, but treatment itself carries risks for conditions such as bronchopulmonary dysplasia and retinopathy of prematurity (Horbar and Lucey, 1995). Although proper management of these conditions in the appropriate intensive care nursery setting can improve outcomes, these infants are at greater risk than full-term, normal weight infants for neurologic and other impairments at later ages.

The most significant diseases after the first month of life are infections of various sorts. Appropriate immunization provides protection against conditions such as diphtheria, tetanus, pertussis, polio, hepatitis B, and *Haemophilus influenzae* type b disease. Effective therapies are available to treat many other infections such as otitis media, pneumonia, and gastroenteritis. Infants in group day care have a higher incidence of common respiratory and gastrointestinal infections compared with babies not in day care settings. The causes of SIDS are not fully understood, but evidence suggests that placing infants on their back or side to sleep, not on their stomach, may reduce its incidence (Willinger, 1995).

Indicators that might be considered include the following:

1. Number (or rate) of neonatal infant deaths.
2. Number (or rate) of postneonatal deaths.

Infant deaths are widely used as an indicator of infant health. Although some deaths are due to injuries rather than disease and to factors for which preventive interventions are not presently available (e.g., congenital anomalies), changes in the number of deaths relative to the number of births may help a community determine whether conditions affecting infant health are improving or worsening. The overall infant mortality rate is included in the community health profile indicators proposed by the committee (see Chapter 5). Examining early and later infant deaths separately makes it easier to assess the differing factors that operate in these periods. In many communities, the number of deaths will be small, making it necessary to aggregate data over multiple years to calculate stable rates.

3. Percentage of babies born weighing less than 1,500 grams.
4. Percentage of babies born weighing less than 1,000 grams.

Low birth weight is a marker for high risk of death or serious morbidity in the near and longer term. Communities might also use these very low weight births as the basis for a review of factors in maternal health that could be contributing to preterm birth or slow fetal growth.

5. Hospitalizations of pregnant women per 100 deliveries.

Healthy People 2000 uses this measure as an indicator of severe complications of pregnancy and has set a national target of no more than 15 such hospitalizations per 100 deliveries (USDHHS, 1991). This indicator is intended to reflect the extent of serious problems in maternal health that might contribute to infant health problems. Communities would hope to reduce such health problems, but for some women, hospitalization will represent the most appropriate form of care. A state's hospital discharge record system, which includes an indication of community of residence (e.g., zip code), would facilitate collecting information on hospitalizations outside a given community.

6. Hospitalizations of infants for illness during the postneonatal period.

Hospitalizations of infants 28 days to 1 year of age would be an indicator of severe illness among infants in a community. A rate might be based on the number of hospitalizations per 1,000 births. Data for multiple years may be needed to have enough cases to calculate a stable rate.

Individual Response

An infant's response to its environment will have some influence on its health, but a much greater influence will be the behavior and responses of others. A mother's behavior and lifestyle will be of particular importance because of the close biological linkage of pregnancy and the traditionally dominant role of the mother in child care. Fathers and other family members, as well as care givers in settings such as day care, will also have an influence.

Good maternal nutrition before and during pregnancy plays an important role in promoting proper fetal growth (IOM, 1990), and consumption of appropriate nutrients appears to lessen the risk of some birth defects (e.g., adequate levels of folic acid may reduce the risk of neural tube defects). Smoking has been linked to 20–30 percent of low-weight births (primarily through growth retardation) and also increases the risk of fetal and infant death (Kleinman and Madans, 1985). Exposure to environmental tobacco smoke increases the risk of respiratory and ear infections in infants and may increase the risk of SIDS (EPA, 1992). Heavy alcohol use during pregnancy can result in physical and mental impairments, which are labeled fetal alcohol syndrome in their most severe form (IOM, 1996), and alcohol abuse among adults can lead to behavioral problems that pose a health risk for infants in their care. Other substance abuse can affect maternal health before pregnancy, fetal health during pregnancy, and infant health after birth (Chomitz et al., 1995). Exposure before or during pregnancy to intravenous drug use, multiple sexual partners, or continuing sexual partners with high risk for infection can increase the risk of acquiring infections such as HIV and various sexually transmitted diseases (STDs) that can endanger the health of the baby.

A woman's contraceptive practices can contribute to success in avoiding an unintended pregnancy, which is associated with poorer outcomes for the baby (IOM, 1995). Nearly 60 percent of pregnancies are unintended, either mistimed or unwanted. Once pregnancy occurs, early use of prenatal care services and having at least half of the recommended number of prenatal visits are associated with lower rates of low birth weight (Kotelchuck, 1994) and may serve as a marker for other healthful practices (Alexander and Korenbrot, 1995). Following birth, breast feeding is associated with reduced infant illness, particularly in the first three to six months of life.

Maternal employment has mixed implications for infant health. It can increase a family's economic resources and improve a mother's sense of well-being. At the same time, it generally creates a need for day care services, which can be costly or of questionable quality and may increase an infant's exposure to common infectious diseases. Within the family, child abuse or neglect and other forms of domestic violence also pose a threat to an infant's physical and psychological health, even if the baby is not the immediate victim.

Indicators that might be considered include the following:

1. Percentage of women giving birth who used tobacco during pregnancy.

2. Percentage of women giving birth who used illicit drugs during pregnancy.

Both smoking and illicit drug use during pregnancy contribute to slow fetal growth, but pregnant women can adopt (and be guided in adopting) more healthful behaviors. Smoking status is recorded on most states' birth certificates, and some states record the use of illicit drugs. Underreporting may, however, limit the accuracy of birth certificate data. A community focusing on infant health issues might make a special effort to collect the data needed for these indicators.

3. Percentage of pregnant women who obtain first-trimester prenatal care.

Early prenatal care gives women access to care and advice that can promote better birth outcomes, including detecting high-risk conditions that may require special attention. Individual decision making may have a greater influence on when prenatal care is started than on how many visits are made, which may reflect special health risks (many visits) or limited service (few visits), as well as individual behavior in seeking care. Whether prenatal care was initiated in the first trimester is generally recorded on the birth certificate.

4. Percentage of new mothers who breast feed their babies for at least four weeks.

Breast feeding provides infants with nutritional, immunologic, and psychosocial benefits. It also reduces the need to purchase or prepare formula for infants and therefore provides practical benefits to the family.

5. Percentage of pregnancies identified as unintended.

Unintended pregnancy is widespread and increases the health risks for the babies that are born (IOM, 1995). To reduce unintended pregnancy, women (and men) may need better information about family planning, better access to family planning services, and better skills in practicing family planning. Information on unintended pregnancy could help communities assess whether family planning services might be improved or whether specific services could be offered when unintended pregnancies have occurred.

6. Number of reported and number of substantiated cases of violence against pregnant women in the community.

7. Number of reported and number of substantiated cases of child abuse and neglect for children under 1 year of age.

Reporting and substantiation of cases are incomplete, but these data give an indication of the amount of family violence occurring in the community. In assessing changes over time in the numbers of cases, consideration must be given to whether they reflect true changes in the number of cases or changes in the completeness of reporting and substantiation of cases. Both issues should be important to the community. Changes in the numbers of infants and pregnant women in the community could also affect the apparent incidence of violence.

Genetic Endowment

The genetic endowment of the parents, as well as the infant, can affect infant health. Parental intelligence, ability, and health shape the environment into which the infant is conceived and born. Genetic factors play a role in some birth defects and also are responsible for disorders such as cystic fibrosis and sickle cell disease. These conditions range in severity from almost immediately fatal to having little impact on normal life span. Preconceptional counseling for couples with known genetic risks can guide decisions regarding pregnancy. Prenatal screening for conditions such as Down syndrome and neural tube defects can inform families that a serious disorder is likely, giving them an opportunity to prepare for the care that the child will need or to decide not to continue the pregnancy.

Many states now have birth defects registries, and all states have neonatal screening programs for at least some important genetic defects for which early intervention can reduce morbidity and mortality. Among these conditions are phenylketonuria (PKU), hypothyroidism, galactosemia, and sickle cell disease. Other genetic diseases such as cystic fibrosis and Tay-Sachs disease can now be detected at very early ages, but treatment cannot yet fully prevent the morbidity. For many genetic disorders, infants who survive will have special health care needs throughout their lives.

Indicators that might be considered include the following:

1. Number and type of birth defects identified in children born during the previous year.

A community might wish to monitor the number and types of

birth defects to determine whether specific risk factors can be identified and addressed. This information may also help determine the need for genetic counseling within the community. Particular attention should be focused on those birth defects that might be prevented through prenatal care or through control of toxic exposures. For example, instances of neural tube defects might suggest the need to improve folic acid supplementation before and during pregnancy. Evidence of fetal alcohol syndrome would support efforts to address alcohol abuse among women of childbearing age.

2. Number of infants with conditions for which neonatal testing is possible but for which no routine screening is offered. Communities might monitor the incidence of these conditions to assess whether a screening program at the local or state level could be beneficial. With earlier discharge after delivery, there may also be a need to ensure that infants receive screening tests that are already offered and that follow-up after testing is appropriate, since early treatment can mitigate some adverse effects.

Social Environment

The social environment exerts a strong influence on infant health, especially through factors such as education, social networks, employment, and income. For both the pregnant woman and the infant, a nurturing family environment and broader social supports can improve health. Family, friends, health care providers, and outreach workers may be sources of this support. Ensuring that other infant caretakers, such as relatives and day care workers, have adequate social supports and nurturing environments is also important to infant health.

General support in the community for the well-being of women and families sets the stage for a positive environment for infant health. Educational and employment opportunities for girls and women increase their capacity to provide for their infants. Maternal education has an enduring association with improved pregnancy outcomes and infant health. Employment policies shape opportunities for parental leave, as well as time available for prenatal care and for sick and well child care. Employment can create a need for day care services, and the quality of those services can have an effect on an infant's health. Day care can also create an economic burden. Poverty has been shown to have a distinct, adverse impact on infant health (CDC, 1995).

Programs that address economic disadvantage have included Aid to Families with Dependent Children (AFDC),[1] WIC (Special Supplemental Food Program for Women, Infants, and Children), and Medicaid. Changes in state and federal welfare programs that limit benefit periods and emphasize employment requirements will have an as yet undetermined impact on the financial resources available to families and on the demand for day care services. The cost and quality of those services may have implications for infant health.

Many of the points discussed in the domain of individual response are part of an infant's social environment because parental behavior, in large measure, defines the social environment. In this regard, nutrition, smoking, domestic violence, and other behavioral factors influence the social environment.

Indicators that might be considered include the following:

1. Of pregnant women and women who have a child less than 1 year of age and who are eligible for AFDC, WIC, or related programs, percentage who are enrolled in those programs.

Programs such as WIC and AFDC provide nutritional and income support to low-income families in the community. WIC participation has been associated with improved pregnancy outcomes (Mayer et al., 1992).

2. Percentage of low-income pregnant adolescents served by home visiting programs.

3. Percentage of families with preterm or low birth weight infants or with infants with chronic illness or disabilities served by home visiting programs.

Programs addressed by these two indicators can provide a range of assistance that, for mothers or families at special risk, contributes to better pregnancy outcomes and better infant health (Olds and Kitzman, 1993). A community would want to ensure that programs are culturally appropriate for the families they serve.

---

[1]In August 1996, as this report neared completion, federal legislation—the Personal Responsibility and Work Opportunity Reconciliation Act of 1996 (P.L. 104-193)—substantially modified many public assistance programs. Under this legislation, Aid to Families with Dependent Children (AFDC) is replaced by a new program designated Temporary Assistance to Needy Families (TANF).

4. Percentage of mothers less than 18 years of age who are enrolled in school.

Pregnancy during adolescence can interrupt a mother's completion of high school, which can have long-term adverse implications for her health and that of her child and for her economic opportunities in the future (Zill, 1996). In some communities, special child care services are available to help teenage mothers return to school.

5. Percentage of children less than 1 year of age living in single-parent homes.

In general, single-parent homes have more limited financial resources, which can make it more difficult to meet the needs of an infant. Therefore, the health of these children may be at special risk.

6. Percentage of women with children less than 1 year of age who are employed outside the home.

A mother's employment could have positive or negative implications for a child's health. Added financial resources might be beneficial but could be offset by the cost of day care services. Similarly, some mothers may find that employment improves their personal well-being and, therefore, their ability to care for their child; other women may find that the added stress of employment and requirements for day care are a negative influence on them and their infants.

7. Percentage of employees who report that they can use paid leave for prenatal, well child, and sick child care.

For parents of infants and other children, the availability of paid leave time for health care visits can encourage appropriate and timely use of services. Employee perceptions, in contrast to employer policies, may provide a more realistic assessment of the practical availability of paid leave.

8. Percentage of employees with health insurance that covers at least 80 percent of the costs of prenatal care, delivery, and well child care.

Health insurance can reduce financial barriers to care needed to promote good infant health. Some employers, however, may offer plans that provide limited coverage for these services or may not offer any coverage for employees' families.

9. Percentage of infants in day care who are enrolled in programs licensed by the state or the community.

Day care services are provided in many forms, some of which include care by family members, in-home care by a paid but unlicensed care giver, and care in large group settings. Infants enrolled in large-group day care suffer more frequent respiratory and gastrointestinal infections than infants who are cared for without exposure to large numbers of other children, but such settings may offer benefits that must be weighed against this particular health risk. The proportion of infants receiving care in any specific setting or from specific providers may change frequently, making it difficult to monitor all sources of care. Comparing the proportion of infants with working mothers with the proportion of infants enrolled in licensed day care programs can suggest the number of infants cared for in other settings. To the extent that licensing promotes better-quality care, communities might want to encourage the use of such services. The capacity of licensed programs may limit the number of infants that can be cared for in that setting.

Physical Environment

In the womb, a developing fetus is affected by the mother's diet, exposure to toxic substances, and general health and well-being, issues that have largely been covered above. The physical environment of the birth process itself is also a source of vulnerability. Prolongation of labor, exposure to infection, and disruption of the blood supply can all lead to serious infant health outcomes. Following birth, the family's home and other physical settings, such as relatives' homes or day care, are the principal elements of the infant's physical environment.

As noted, exposure to environmental tobacco smoke has been shown to increase the likelihood of respiratory and ear infections in infants (EPA, 1992). Older housing with lead-based interior paint is a principal risk factor for toxic exposure to lead. Other products in newer homes (e.g., vinyl blinds) may also be a lead hazard. Serious injuries can occur from events such as falls, burns, and drowning, but preventive interventions can reduce some of the risks. For example, setting hot water heaters at a temperature of 120°F has been shown to reduce the risk of scald injuries to infants and young children (Erdmann et al., 1991). The risk of injury in automobile crashes can be reduced by proper use of car seats. In addition to these microenvironments, broader environmental hazards of toxic waste, air pollution, and water pollution also affect infant health.

Indicators that might be considered include the following:

1. Percentage of smokers living in homes with pregnant women or children less than 1 year of age.
2. Existence of a state or local ordinance restricting smoking in day care facilities.

Environmental tobacco smoke has been shown to be associated with low birth weight and increased rates of respiratory and ear infections, and it may increase the risk of SIDS. Information on smokers living with pregnant women or infants would suggest both the extent of infant exposure to tobacco smoke in the home and whether the need for a smoking cessation program emphasizing the health risks to infants is widespread. Day care is a setting in which an infant may spend an extended period of time; therefore, smoking restrictions would be a valuable way to limit exposure to this environmental hazard.

3. Percentage of infants living in houses built before 1950 that have not had lead abatement procedures carried out.

Deteriorating lead-based paint and lead-impregnated plaster are found in many older homes and create a risk of toxic lead exposures for their residents, particularly infants and small children. Lead abatement procedures can reduce the risk of toxic exposures.

4. Percentage of infants whose parents report that they are always transported in motor vehicles in properly installed child safety seats.

Safety seats can reduce the risk of serious injury and death, but studies show that they are often installed incorrectly, which limits their effectiveness (USDHHS, 1991).

Prosperity

Family income correlates highly with good health, and there is an enduring association between poverty and poor health throughout life including during infancy.

Indicators that might be considered include the following:

1. Percentage of infants living in families below the poverty level.

2. Percentage of infants living in families below 200 percent of the poverty level.

Families that are below the poverty level will have extremely limited financial resources for food, housing, and other essential aspects of daily living. For some families, assistance programs can mitigate some of the adverse effects of such limited financial resources. Even less extreme financial deprivation still poses a risk for infant health. Thus, communities might want to determine the proportion of infants in families with low but not poverty-level incomes.

Health Care

Many issues related to appropriate health care for mothers and infants have been alluded to above. Access to family planning services can help limit unintended pregnancy. Timely access to prenatal care services that include both suitable health behavior advice and prenatal care procedures has been shown to contribute to lower rates of low-weight births (Kogan et al., 1994; Kotelchuck, 1994). Guidance on the appropriate content of prenatal care can be provided by a source such as *Caring for Our Future: The Content of Prenatal Care* (U.S. Public Health Service, 1989). Many states and communities have established systems to screen pregnant women to ensure that high-risk pregnancies are cared for in facilities capable of dealing with problems that might arise. Mothers at high risk for delivering very low birth weight babies can be transferred to facilities with neonatal intensive care nursery services.

The appropriate application of neonatal intensive care can improve survival for those babies born prematurely or with serious health problems. Neonatal screening programs, discussed above, are an important health care service for dealing with treatable congenital defects. Screening can also identify problems such as hearing impairments. In addition, access is needed to well child care, including immunizations, and to sick child care in the event of illness. Within well child care, support for breast feeding can affect the likelihood that mothers initiate and continue this healthful process. The content of infant health care can be guided by sources such as the American Academy of Pediatrics and *Bright Futures* (Green, 1994).

Indicators that might be considered include the following:

1. Percentage of women 15 to 45 years of age who can identify a regular source of health care.

Women of reproductive age who do not have a regular source of health care may fail to receive preconceptional care that could promote a successful pregnancy and birth outcome. These women may also be more likely to delay the start of prenatal care or may have difficulty obtaining appropriate care during the course of their pregnancy. A mother's lack of a routine source of care might signal a risk that a routine source of infant care will not be established.

2. Percentage of women 15 to 45 years of age who report access to affordable family planning services.

This measure would reflect perceived availability of family planning services. Communities might want to examine ways to improve the availability of services to women who do not feel that they have access to them.

3. Percentage of mothers who gave birth during the past year who received the number of prenatal visits recommended by the American College of Obstetricians and Gynecologists.

This measure is similar to one proposed for inclusion in HEDIS 3.0 for Medicaid members (NCQA, 1996). The HEDIS measure adjusts the recommended number of visits downward if the initial prenatal visit is delayed or if an infant is born prematurely, both of which shorten the period during which visits could occur.

4. Percentage of infants weighing less than 1,500 grams at birth who are born in facilities designated as Level II or III perinatal care centers.

Such facilities have resources to provide specialized care for high-risk mothers and infants. Health care providers and hospitals should have procedures for identifying women at risk for low weight births and arranging for deliveries in appropriate facilities. Although it may not be possible for all such births to occur in Level II or III facilities, communities might want to examine whether the rate is as high as possible and address referral practices if it declines. HEDIS 3.0 (NCQA, 1996) proposes a measure of this type for Medicaid enrollees served by health plans.

5. Percentage of 1-year-olds who have received all age-appropriate immunizations recommended by the Advisory Committee on Immunization Practices.

Provider practices play an important role in ensuring that children are up to date on recommended immunizations. The committee's community profile includes immunization rates at 2 years of age, the age by which the initial series of recommended immunizations should be completed. In fact, however, recommendations call for most of these immunizations to be administered by 1 year of age (CDC, 1996). Currently this includes three doses of diphtheria–tetanus–pertussis (DTP) vaccine; three doses of *Haemophilus influenzae* type b (Hib) vaccine; two or three doses of polio vaccine; and two or three doses of hepatitis B vaccine. Unless an immunization registry is operating, a specialized data collection process would be needed.

Health and Function, Well-Being

It is difficult to assess the well-being and functional status of an infant. Because infants cannot report on their status, assessments must be based on observation by others. Measures of growth and developmental progress can be used as proxies. Although most children are basically healthy, as many as 10 percent of all children have two or more chronic physical conditions, and emotional and developmental problems affect an additional portion of the child population (Newacheck and Taylor, 1992). Early developmental progress may not, however, predict longer-term outcomes. Interventions may compensate for early deficits or latent problems may emerge.

An indicator that might be considered is

1. Percentage of 1-year-olds that have been identified as having a developmental delay, physical impairment, or chronic illness such as cystic fibrosis or kidney disease.

These children should be receiving appropriate care to promote optimal physical and psychosocial development. Criteria to be used to identify these children would require further specification.

SAMPLE INDICATOR SET

From this range of possible indicators, a more limited set is proposed for community-level performance monitoring. Reducing infant deaths is likely to be a priority for every community, but they will be rare enough that the infant mortality rate will not be a reliable measure in most communities unless data are aggregated over multiple years. Preventing or limiting long-term morbidity that has its origins in the prenatal or infant period is also likely to be a priority, and a variety of activities in the community could be expected to make contributions toward this end. For indicators that are adopted, communities will have to establish clear operational definitions and identify sources of relevant data. The committee proposes the following indicators.

1. Percentage of babies born weighing less than 1,500 grams.
2. Percentage of babies born weighing less than 1,000 grams.

Low birth weight is a marker for increased risk of morbidity and mortality. It reflects the combined effect of a variety of factors including the mother's health and lifestyle, the infant's genetic endowment, socioeconomic circumstances, and the quality of prenatal health care services. Therefore, responsibility and accountability are diffused throughout the community. Data on birth weight would be available from birth certificates. State vital records systems should be able to provide information on the basis on a mother's place of residence rather than the location of the birth. In communities with small numbers of births, data should be aggregated over multiple years to produce a stable measurement.

3. Of pregnant women and women who have a child less than 1 year of age and who are eligible for AFDC, WIC or related programs, percentage who are enrolled in those programs.

Programs such as WIC and AFDC provide nutritional and income support to low income families in the community, which can benefit the health of pregnant women and their infants. These public assistance programs are a response by federal, state, and local governments to needs created by economic deprivation. Program records at the state or local level should be able to provide data on the number of enrollees and are likely to have methods of estimating the percentage of those eligible who are enrolled. Alternatively, a community survey could be used to collect information.

4. Percentage of mothers less than 18 years of age who are enrolled in school.

Since higher levels of education are associated with better health, communities may want to encourage adolescent mothers to complete high school. Schools can play a major role by providing child care and programs designed specifically to meet the needs of mothers. A special community survey or follow-up program for teen births would probably be needed to obtain this information.

5. Percentage of employees who report that they can use paid leave for prenatal, well child, and sick child care.

With an increase in the proportion of infants with parents who work, employers have an important influence on access to necessary health care. Policies that provide paid leave time can reduce financial barriers to care that loss of paid work time might create. A community survey would probably be needed to obtain information from employees. A companion survey of employer policies might reveal discrepancies in the way policies are applied or the extent to which employees have been informed about those policies.

6. Percentage of employees with health insurance that covers at least 80 percent of the costs of prenatal care, delivery, and well child care.

Health insurance is another means of reducing financial barriers to appropriate health care. The terms of coverage reflect decisions by employers and insurers. This information would help communities determine the extent to which infants in families with working parents are, nevertheless, without insurance coverage because their family cannot afford available coverage or because employers do not offer it. A community survey or a survey of employers might be used to obtain this information.

7. Percentage of smokers living in homes with pregnant women or children less than 1 year of age.

Exposure to environmental tobacco smoke is an avoidable health risk for infants, even prenatally. Information on whether smokers live with pregnant women and small children can help a community formulate smoking cessation programs appropriate for that audience. This could include not only parents but also grandparents, siblings, and others. Health care providers might, for example, raise this issue with their patients. Data might be collected through special community-level sampling for a state survey for the Behavioral Risk Factor Surveillance System (BRFSS). Currently, the BRFSS includes questions on smoking, and it might be possible to add a question on household composition.

8. Percentage of infants weighing less than 1,500 grams at

birth who are born in facilities designated as Level II or III perinatal care centers.

Given current limitations in our understanding of how to prevent preterm (and therefore low-weight) births, it is important that high-risk births take place in facilities that can care for both the mother and the infant. Health care providers and hospitals play a primary role in directing women to appropriate facilities. With the development of a HEDIS 3.0 measure for Medicaid enrollees, health plans are likely to develop the capacity to provide this information. Other sources of data might be hospital discharge data systems.

9. Percentage of 1-year-olds who have received all age-appropriate immunizations recommended by the Advisory Committee on Immunization Practices.

The value of immunizations is clear, but currently few communities have a system to track immunizations or produce information that can help ensure that children are immunized on time. Recent data collection efforts have focused on the immunization status of 2-year-olds. Similar approaches might be used to obtain information on 1-year-olds. Because children can be immunized in many different places, it can be difficult to aggregate the information across a community to be sure every child is up to date. Some communities are developing immunization registries, which should make it possible to assess immunization status for any age group. Techniques being developed by health plans to produce HEDIS data for 2-year-olds could be adapted for 1-year-olds. Once systems are functioning, inadequately immunized children can be identified more easily and consistently, and responsibility for their immunization can be established and followed. Achieving improved immunization rates will require concerted cooperation across many segments of the community.

The indicators selected to provide an overall tool for assessing efforts in a community to improve infant health are a small segment of what might be a very large collection. These indicators bring together measures of health risk (birth weight, environmental tobacco smoke, and immunization) and actions in the community that can help reduce health risks (assistance programs, school enrollment, paid leave, insurance coverage, and referral for delivery). These indicators address infant health both directly and through the health of mothers.

They also address how various community stakeholders are

doing in providing prenatal and well infant care and setting reasonable policies at work to encourage the use of appropriate well infant and prenatal services. In addition, they point to a role for schools and social services in promoting the health of mothers and infants. Communities with specific infant health concerns or resources could find it useful to include indicators tailored to their particular circumstances.

REFERENCES

Alexander, G.R., and Korenbrot, C.C. 1995. The Role of Prenatal Care in Preventing Low Birth Weight. *The Future of Children* 5(1):103–121.

Ananth, C.V., Peedicayil, A., and Savitz, D.A. 1995. Effect of Hypertensive Diseases in Pregnancy on Birthweight, Gestational Duration, and Small-for-Gestational-Age Births. *Epidemiology* 6:391–395.

Bass, J.L., Christoffel, K.K., Widome, M., et al. 1993. Childhood Injury Prevention Counseling in Primary Care Settings: A Critical Review of the Literature. *Pediatrics* 92:544–550.

Carnegie Task Force on Meeting the Needs of Young Children. 1994. *Starting Points: Meeting the Needs of Our Youngest Children.* New York: Carnegie Corporation of New York.

CDC (Centers for Disease Control and Prevention). 1993. Prenatal Care and Pregnancies Complicated by Diabetes—U.S. Reporting Areas, 1989. *Morbidity and Mortality Weekly Report* 42:119–122.

CDC. 1995. Poverty and Infant Mortality—United States, 1988. *Morbidity and Mortality Weekly Report* 44:922–927.

CDC. 1996. Immunization Schedule—United States, January–June 1996. *Morbidity and Mortality Weekly Report* 44:940–943.

Chomitz, V.R., Cheung, L.W.Y., and Lieberman, E. 1995. The Role of Lifestyle in Preventing Low Birth Weight. *The Future of Children* 5(1):121–138.

EPA (Environmental Protection Agency). 1992. *Respiratory Health Effects of Passive Smoking: Lung Cancer and Other Disorders.* Pub. No. EPA-600/6-90/006F. Washington, D.C.: EPA, Office of Health and Environmental Assessment.

Erdmann, T.C., Feldman, K.W., Rivara, F.P., Heimbach, D.M., and Wall, H.A. 1991. Tap Water Burn Prevention: The Effect of Legislation. *Pediatrics* 88:572–577.

Fiscella, K. 1996. Racial Disparities in Preterm Births: The Role of Urogenital Infections. *Public Health Reports* 111:104–113.

Gardner, P., and Hudson, B.L. 1996. Advance Report of Final Mortality Statistics, 1993. *Monthly Vital Statistics Report* 44 (No. 7, supplement). Hyattsville, Md.: National Center for Health Statistics.

Gielen, A.C., Wilson, M.E., Faden, R.R., Wissow, L., and Harvilchuck, J.D. 1995. In-Home Injury Prevention Practices for Infants and Toddlers: the Role of Parental Beliefs, Barriers, and Housing Quality. *Health Education Quarterly* 22:85–95.

Goldenberg, R.L., and Andrews, W.W. 1996. Intrauterine Infection and Why Preterm Prevention Programs Have Failed. *American Journal of Public Health* 86:781–783.

Green, M., ed. 1994. *Bright Futures: Guidelines for Health Supervision of Infants, Children, and Adolescents.* Arlington, Va.: National Center for Education in Maternal and Child Health.

Hack, M., Klein, N.K., and Taylor, H.G. 1995. Long-Term Developmental Outcomes of Low Birth Weight Infants. *The Future of Children* 5(1):177–196.

Horbar, J.D., and Lucey, J.F. 1995. Evaluation of Neonatal Intensive Care Technologies. *The Future of Children* 5(1):139–161.

Hughes, D., and Simpson, L. 1995. The Role of Social Change in Preventing Low Birth Weight. *The Future of Children* 5(1):87–120.

IOM (Institute of Medicine). 1990. *Nutrition During Pregnancy.* Washington, D.C.: National Academy Press.

IOM. 1995. *The Best Intentions: Unintended Pregnancy and the Well-Being of Children and Families.* S.S. Brown and L. Eisenberg, eds. Washington, D.C.: National Academy Press.

IOM. 1996. *Fetal Alcohol Syndrome: Diagnosis, Epidemiology, Prevention, and Treatment.* K. Stratton, C. Howe, and F. Battaglia, eds. Washington, D.C.: National Academy Press.

Kleinman, J., and Madans, J.H. 1985. The Effects of Maternal Smoking, Physical Stature, and Educational Attainment on the Incidence of Low Birth Weight. *American Journal of Epidemiology* 121:832–855.

Kogan, M.D., Alexander, G.R., Kotelchuck, M., and Nagey, D.A. 1994. Relation of the Content of Prenatal Care to the Risk of Low Birth Weight: Maternal Reports of Health Behavior Advice and Initial Prenatal Care Procedures. *Journal of the American Medical Association* 271:1340–1345.

Kotelchuck, M. 1994. The Adequacy of Prenatal Care Utilization Index: Its U.S. Distribution and Association with Low Birthweight. *American Journal of Public Health* 84:1486–1489.

Lewit, E.M., Baker, L.S., Corman, H., and Shiono, P.H. 1995. The Direct Cost of Low Birth Weight. *The Future of Children* 5(1):35–56.

Mayer, J.P., Emshoff, J.G., and Avruch, S. 1992. Health Promotion in Maternity Care. In *A Pound of Prevention: The Case for Universal Maternity Care in the U.S.* J.B. Kotch, C.H. Blakely, S.S. Brown, and F.Y. Wong, eds. Washington, D.C.: American Public Health Association.

McCormick, M.C. 1985. The Contribution of Low Birth Weight to Infant Mortality and Childhood Morbidity. *New England Journal of Medicine* 312:82–90.

McGregor, J.A., French, J.I., Parker, R., et al. 1995. Prevention of Premature Birth by Screening and Treatment for Common Genital Tract Infections: Results of a Prospective Controlled Evaluation. *American Journal of Obstetrics and Gynecology* 173:157–167.

NCQA (National Committee for Quality Assurance). 1996. HEDIS 3.0 Draft for Public Comment. Washington, D.C.: NCQA.

Newacheck, P.W., and Taylor, W.R. 1992. Childhood Chronic Illness: Prevalence, Severity, and Impact. *American Journal of Public Health* 82:364–371.

Olds, D.L., and Kitzman, H. 1993. Review of Research on Home Visiting for Pregnant Women and Parents of Young Children. *The Future of Children* 3(3):53–92.

Paneth, N. 1995. The Problem of Low Birth Weight. *The Future of Children* 5(1): 19–34.

Rodewald, L.E., Szilagyi, P.G., Shiuh, T., Humiston, S.G., LeBaron, C., and Hall, C.B. 1995. Is Underimmunization a Marker for Insufficient Utilization of Preventive and Primary Care? *Archives of Pediatric and Adolescent Medicine* 149:393–397.

USDHEW (U.S. Department of Health, Education, and Welfare). 1973. *The Health Consequences of Smoking*. DHEW/HSM 73-8704. Washington, D.C.: USDHEW.

USDHHS (U.S. Department of Health and Human Services). 1991. *Healthy People 2000: National Health Promotion and Disease Prevention Objectives*. DHHS Pub. No. (PHS) 91-50212. Washington, D.C.: Office of the Assistant Secretary for Health.

U.S. Public Health Service. 1989. *Caring for Our Future: The Content of Prenatal Care*. A Report of the Public Health Service Expert Panel on the Content of Prenatal Care. Washington, D.C.: U.S. Department of Health and Human Services.

Ventura, S.J., Martin, J.A., Mathews, T.J., and Clarke, S.C. 1996. Advance Report of Final Natality Statistics, 1994. *Monthly Vital Statistics Report* 44 (No. 11, supplement). Hyattsville, Md.: National Center for Health Statistics.

Willinger, M. 1995. SIDS Prevention. *Pediatric Annals* 24:358–364.

Zill, N. 1996. Parental Schooling and Children's Health. *Public Health Reports* 111:34–43.

TABLE A.6-1 Field Model Mapping for Sample Indicator Set: Infant Health

Field Model Domain	Construct	Sample Indicators	Data Sources	Stakeholders
Disease	Reduce low birth weight and its adverse effects	Percentage of babies born weighing <1,500 grams Percentage of babies born weighing <1,000 grams	Birth certificates, vital statistics	Health care providers Health care plans State health agencies Local health agencies Community organizations Special health risk groups General public
Social Environment	Reduce the health impact of economic and nutritional deprivation	Percentage of eligible women and infants enrolled in AFDC, WIC, or related programs	Program records; community survey	State health agencies Local health agencies Social service agencies Local government Special health risk groups
	Encourage better education for adolescent mothers	Percentage of mothers less than 18 years of age who are enrolled in school	Community survey; program records	Local government Education agencies, institutions Community organizations General public
	Reduce workplace barriers to use of health care services	Percentage of employees who report that they can use paid leave for prenatal, well child, and sick child care	Community survey; employer survey and insurance licensing authority	Local government Business, industry General public

	Reduce financial barriers to health care services	Percentage of employees with health insurance that covers at least 80 percent of costs of prenatal care, delivery, and well child care	Community survey; employer survey	Health care plans Local government Business, industry General public
Physical Environment	Reduce exposure to environmental tobacco smoke	Percentage of smokers living in homes with pregnant women or children <1 year of age	Community survey	General public
Health Care	Ensure access to specialty care for high-risk births	Percentage of infants weighing <1,500 grams at birth born in facilities designated level II or III perinatal care centers	Health plan records; hospital discharge records	Health care providers Health care plans State health agencies Local health agencies Special health risk groups General public
	Ensure timely preventive care	Percentage of 1-year-olds who have received all recommended immunizations	Immunization registry or medical charts	Health care providers Health care plans State health agencies Local health agencies General public

NOTE: AFDC, Aid to Families with Dependent Children; WIC, Special Supplemental Food Program for Women, Infants, and Children.

A.7

Prototype Indicator Set: Tobacco and Health

BACKGROUND

Tobacco consumption poses many health risks. Despite a steady decline since 1964 in the proportion of the adult population that smokes, about 20 percent of all deaths in the United States are associated with tobacco use, making its prevention the single most effective way to reduce mortality (CDC, 1993b; McGinnis and Foege, 1993). Some of these deaths are nonsmokers affected by exposure to tobacco smoke and residential fires. In addition, smoking during pregnancy increases risks for prematurity, low birth weight, and infant deaths. Smoking-related illness is estimated to account for 7 percent of total medical care expenditures (CDC, 1994b) and for a disproportionate share of time lost from work and diminished productivity in the workplace.

Over the past 40 years, as evidence has accumulated on the extensive adverse health effects of tobacco use, tobacco products have been sold with little restriction. During this period, death rates for some conditions, such as lung cancer and chronic obstructive pulmonary disease (COPD), have actually risen (Gardner and Hudson, 1996). Continued sale and use of tobacco reflect both the addictive nature of nicotine and the political and economic influence of the tobacco industry. This makes the use of tobacco an excellent indicator of society's capacity to control a health problem in the face of strong counterpressures from industry and from those in the population who smoke.

Currently, about 25 percent of adults (CDC, 1996c) and 16 percent of adolescents (CDC, 1996a) smoke regularly. Because more than 80 percent of current smokers began as preteens or teenagers (CDC, 1994a), increasing efforts are being made to reduce youth access to tobacco by enforcing restrictions on the sale of tobacco products to minors. State education agencies also require public schools to teach the hazards of tobacco use, even in states that grow and process tobacco. Encouraging current tobacco users to quit is also a priority. Largely in response to the ill effects of environmental tobacco smoke, restrictions on public indoor smoking are increasingly widespread. California and Massachusetts have both increased excise taxes on cigarettes to encourage reduced consumption and to fund a variety of activities (e.g., media campaigns, school-based programs) aimed at reducing levels of tobacco use.

Healthy People 2000 (USDHHS, 1991) includes several objectives that target preventing and reducing tobacco use. More recently, both the U.S. Preventive Services Task Force (1996) and the Smoking Cessation Guideline Panel (1996), which was assembled by the Agency for Health Care Policy and Research (AHCPR), have issued recommendations that health care practitioners routinely provide cessation counseling to tobacco users and counseling to children and adolescents aimed at preventing initiation. In addition, the current draft of HEDIS 3.0 (NCQA, 1996) proposes that health plans report on the percentage of adult smokers who received advice to quit.

Tobacco use and its health effects can be measured in several ways. Morbidity and mortality from tobacco-related diseases can be measured, but these conditions often occur decades after smoking begins, so they are not immediately sensitive to changes in tobacco use. Data on the association between tobacco use and these diseases, however, make it possible to predict future levels of morbidity and mortality that would result from reduced tobacco use. Therefore, the intermediate measure of tobacco use can serve as a proxy for those health outcomes. Such measures include the numbers of people who currently use tobacco, who quit, and who start using tobacco.

It is also possible to measure efforts being made to reduce tobacco use through prevention and cessation. In addition, efforts to increase tobacco use through marketing and blocking tobacco control policies can be assessed. The current competition between these forces within communities will influence future tobacco use and the morbidity and mortality associated with it.

"FIELD" SET OF PERFORMANCE INDICATORS

The domains of the field model suggest a variety of indicators that might be used to examine a community's efforts to reduce the level of tobacco use and thereby improve health status. These efforts would include both increasing the cessation rate among current smokers and other users of tobacco products and reducing the number of young people who begin using tobacco products.

Disease

Tobacco use contributes to illness and death from a variety of causes. Estimates have been made that up to 30 percent of all cancer deaths and 21 percent of cardiovascular disease deaths are tobacco related (McGinnis and Foege, 1993). Specific conditions such as lung cancer and COPD are attributed almost entirely to prolonged smoking (CDC, 1989). Acute bronchitis is aggravated and prolonged in smokers, increasing the time lost from work or school. Use of smokeless tobacco is associated with oral cancers.

Nonsmokers who are exposed to environmental tobacco smoke also experience health problems. Approximately 3,000 lung cancer deaths per year among nonsmokers have been attributed to environmental tobacco smoke (EPA, 1992). Young children exposed to tobacco smoke in the home suffer more respiratory illness and otitis media than other children (EPA, 1992). About 10 percent of infant deaths and 20–30 percent of low-weight births are attributable to maternal tobacco use (Kleinman and Madans, 1985). Smoking is also linked to 25 percent of deaths in residential fires (U.S. Consumer Product Safety Commission, 1993).

Although the health consequences of tobacco use are indisputable, measures of many types of morbidity and mortality are not optimal indicators for monitoring efforts to reduce the health impact of tobacco use. Many years can be required for changes in tobacco use to be reflected in levels of morbidity and mortality. Communities can, however, use current levels of tobacco-related morbidity and mortality to demonstrate the community-level impact of this major health problem and, therefore, the importance of reducing the levels of tobacco use.

Indicators to consider include the following:

1. Number of deaths in the community due to lung cancer, cardiovascular disease, emphysema, chronic bronchitis, and respiratory infections; percentage of these deaths attributable to smoking.

In general, these conditions account for the greatest number of deaths attributable to smoking. The Centers for Disease Control and Prevention (CDC) has developed computer software that can be used to estimate smoking-attributable morbidity, mortality, and costs (SAMMEC) (Shultz et al., 1991). Even though these are leading causes of death, the number of cases at the community level may be small in any one year.

2. Percentage of infants born weighing less than 2,500 grams whose mothers report smoking during pregnancy.

Low birth weight is associated with increased risks for morbidity and mortality. Reducing the prevalence of smoking during pregnancy is a readily identifiable goal that would contribute to improved pregnancy outcomes and longer-term infant health.

Individual Response

Tobacco use is a learned behavior that typically begins before adulthood. For example, data show that among adults ages 30–39 who had ever been daily smokers, 82 percent began by 18 years of age (CDC, 1994a). Recent data also show that 25 percent of white high school students have used smokeless tobacco in the previous month (CDC, 1996a). Many different forces encourage young people to initiate and continue tobacco use (IOM, 1994), and it may never be possible to quantify the relative contribution of each. Some of the behavioral and personal influences include academic achievement, personality, and self-image. Other important influences are found in the social environment. Once use is initiated, the chemical addictive effect of nicotine quickly becomes a powerful motivator for continued use and a barrier to efforts to quit. Of adults who are current smokers, 69 percent are interested in quitting (CDC, 1996c), but only 2.5 percent succeed in quitting permanently each year (CDC, 1993a). Smokers with higher levels of education and income appear more successful in stopping. Data on the sociodemographic characteristics of smokers in a community could help guide cessation efforts.

Indicators to consider include the following:

1. Percentage of the adult population who smoke regularly.

This measure can be followed over time to track trends and can also be examined by age, race, and gender to identify those groups in which smoking behavior is changing. It might be revised to capture all tobacco use, including smokeless tobacco products. More difficult to measure accurately, but potentially important, is the quantity of tobacco used. Self-reports of tobacco use appear to understate consumption when compared to data on tobacco sales, but a consistent level of understatement makes it possible to track trends from such survey data (Hatziandreu et al., 1989). The importance attached to monitoring the prevalence of smoking is reflected in the recent decision by the Council of State and Territorial Epidemiologists to add it to the list of "conditions" reportable by states to the CDC (1996b).

2. Percentage of births for which mothers report smoking during pregnancy.

Mothers reported smoking during pregnancy in 15 percent of births in 1994 (Ventura et al., 1996). These data are obtained from birth certificate reports, but not all states report the smoking status of mothers. As with survey reports, birth certificate data may understate true levels of smoking.

3. Percentage of youth ages 11–18 who initiate smoking each year.

It is estimated that in the United States as many as 3,000 young people, most less than 18 years of age, begin smoking each day (Pierce et al., 1989). Because most smokers begin using cigarettes by age 18, prevention efforts will be focused on this population. Tracking initiation of smoking will reflect the effectiveness of those efforts.

4. Percentage of smokers who quit for more than six months in each year.

Among most smokers who try to quit, relapse is common; only 5.7 percent reported being able to quit for at least one month during the previous year (CDC, 1993a). The longer cessation continues, however, the greater is the long-term benefit to health. Increasing the number of smokers who quit and decreasing the length of their lifetime use of tobacco not only have personal health benefits but also diminish the number of smoking role models.

Genetic Endowment

There is some evidence from twin studies that genetic factors influence initiation and continuation of tobacco use (IOM, 1994). There may also be genetically influenced susceptibilities to tobacco-related illness. No performance indicators are proposed for this domain.

Social Environment

The social environment is the most critical piece in the tobacco puzzle. As noted, various social influences encourage the initiation of tobacco use by as many as 3,000 young people each day (Pierce et al., 1989). Some of these factors include friends who smoke, parental smoking, and advertising, which portrays smoking as an attractive adult behavior. These factors help shape perceived social norms regarding smoking. Advertising and marketing also appeal to normal tendencies of adolescents to rebel against authority. In addition, numerous studies have documented the ease with which even young teenagers can purchase cigarettes, despite laws in every state prohibiting sales to minors (see IOM, 1994; CDC, 1996a).

Strong forces are also operating to control, prevent initiation of, and encourage cessation of tobacco use. Increasingly, state and local laws restrict smoking in public spaces and workplaces, and more rigorous efforts are being made to enforce laws prohibiting tobacco sales to minors. These steps help create not only a legal but also a social environment that discourages tobacco use. By reducing the opportunity to smoke, public and workplace restrictions can help reinforce individuals' efforts to quit.

School and community health education programs and antitobacco media campaigns try to communicate both the ill effects of tobacco use and the benefits of cessation. School-based prevention programs have been shown to at least delay initiation of tobacco use (see U.S. Preventive Services Task Force, 1996). An examination of California's antismoking media campaign indicates that it has contributed to reduced levels of tobacco consumption and might have had a greater impact with higher levels of funding (Hu et al., 1995). Other steps to discourage tobacco use that are being taken, often at the state level, include increased excise taxes, price controls, litigation against the tobacco industry, and additional restrictions on advertising and marketing. In some states, however, preemptive state legislation may prevent local governments from implementing more stringent controls on matters such as placement of cigarette vending machines or enforcement of prohibitions on sales to minors (IOM, 1994).

Indicators that might be considered include the following:

1. Effectiveness of local enforcement of laws prohibiting tobacco sales to minors.

Enforcement of these laws is a reflection of a community's commitment to preventing tobacco use among youth. Some communities have demonstrated a drop in reported teenage smoking two years after implementing strict enforcement programs (see IOM, 1994). A community might monitor enforcement on the basis of the proportion of adolescents (e.g., ages 11–18) who report being asked for proof of age, the proportion of test purchases that elicit a request for proof of age, or the proportion of test sales that are completed.

2. Extent to which tobacco use prevention is incorporated into school curricula and activities.

All states encourage or require health curricula in public schools to address the dangers of tobacco use. Objective 3.10 in *Healthy People 2000* (USDHHS, 1991) calls for the inclusion of tobacco use prevention in school health curricula at all grade levels, and CDC (1994d) has issued guidelines for the content and implementation of school programs. The extent to which prevention messages are delivered and the adequacy of training teachers receive to teach tobacco use prevention, particularly to the early adolescent, vary. The best programs not only inform students of the ill effects of tobacco but also equip them to resist social pressures to use tobacco and seek to identify and assist those who use tobacco to quit successfully. In judging whether programs are appropriate, however, competing demands for curriculum time and other school resources should be taken into consideration.

3. Number of tobacco use cessation programs available in the community; their success rate (proportion of participants with at least six months of cessation following completion of the program).

Cessation programs are part of a community's resources to assist tobacco users who want to quit and to improve the prospects of successful quitting. Programs range from group efforts to individual counseling and hypnosis, and they vary greatly in their effectiveness, depending not only on the methods used but also on the skills of the program leaders. The need for additional programs might be suggested by a measure such as an increase in average waiting time to participate.

4. Existence of local or state ordinances to control the placement of tobacco advertising; if ordinances exist, the effectiveness with which they are enforced.

Federal law currently prohibits state and local regulation of the content of tobacco advertising, but court rulings have upheld regulation of its placement (Garner, 1996). Some states and municipalities have implemented ordinances that prohibit tobacco advertising near schools and playgrounds, at sports arenas, and on public transit systems. Highlighting the opportunity offered by such ordinances, and advocating for them in their absence, may be a way to reduce the impact of tobacco advertising and to express community support for reducing tobacco use. Criteria would have to be established to judge the effectiveness of enforcement.

5. Existence of local tobacco control organizations or coalitions.

The many national, state, and community organizations that are dedicated to reducing tobacco use initiate and support efforts at the community level to address issues such as youth tobacco use, environmental tobacco smoke, and public policies. If such organizations are operating, communities might want to assess their effectiveness in local tobacco control efforts. Their presence and effectiveness serve as an indicator of the extent of community support for tobacco control. Measuring the effectiveness of these groups would require specifying what they should be expected to accomplish.

Physical Environment

Smoking creates hazards in the physical environment in the form of environmental tobacco smoke (ETS) and fires. As noted above, ETS is estimated to cause as many as 3,000 lung cancer deaths per year, as well as to increase the severity of respiratory infections and otitis media in children. Smoking is also associated with residential fires. Estimates for 1990 link smoking to 44,000 fires, 1,200 deaths, and 3,360 injuries (U.S. Consumer Product Safety Commission, 1993).

Community efforts to reduce exposure to ETS can include restricting smoking in public places, work sites, and restaurants.

Both government and voluntary action are possible. Fire hazards might be reduced by enforcing requirements for installation of smoke detectors, but the benefit will be limited if residents and landlords do not keep installed detectors in working order.

Indicators might include the following:

1. Extent to which state or local ordinances control environmental tobacco smoke in the community.

Many states, counties, and municipalities have ordinances to control environmental tobacco smoke. Local ordinances will have to be assessed in the context of state laws, which may be sufficiently strict that local measures are not needed or, alternatively, may preempt the authority of local government to enact more stringent controls.

2. Number of residential fires in the community in the past year attributable to smoking; number of deaths and disabilities that resulted from these fires.

In any given community, the numbers of fires, deaths, and disabilities will be small, but they can serve as sentinel events that attract public attention to this hazard of tobacco use.

Prosperity

Direct and indirect costs associated with smoking have been estimated at $68 billion in 1990 (OTA, 1993). Near-term improvements in the efficiency or effectiveness of treatment of tobacco-related disease are likely, so the greatest impact on health care costs will come from reducing the levels of disease by reducing tobacco use.

For individuals who use tobacco, consumption of one pack of cigarettes per day costs about $700 per year, and additional costs can be incurred for health care and time lost from work. The disproportionately high smoking rates for lower socioeconomic populations increase the relative impact of the cost of tobacco on financial resources.

Tobacco use generates income for growers, manufacturers, and those who advertise, market, and sell tobacco products. In addition, excise taxes on sales of tobacco products generate revenue for federal, state, and local governments. A recent analysis suggests, however, that even complete elimination of tobacco from the economy would not result in a net national loss of jobs, although there would be losses in the southeastern states that grow and process tobacco (Warner et al., 1996).

Indicators that might be considered include the following:

1. Annual per capita retail cost of tobacco consumption for tobacco users.

The per capita cost of tobacco use is a product of the numbers of tobacco users, the quantity of tobacco consumed, and the current pricing of tobacco products, including excise taxes. For some individuals or families, expressing use in economic terms may provide a better incentive to quit or reduce consumption so that the money can be used for other purposes. To employ this measure, communities would need an estimate of the number of tobacco users in the population. State excise tax records might serve as a source of information on consumption.

2. Average annual value of retail sales of tobacco products per retail outlet.

This measure would provide an indication of the contribution of tobacco sales to retail income in the community. Where tobacco sales are a major source of income, communities might expect less support for efforts to reduce tobacco use. Data on excise tax receipts might be a basis for estimating the value of retail sales.

Health Care

The health care system can contribute to preventing tobacco use, promoting cessation of use, and treating tobacco-related illnesses. Most health care resources are used in treating illness, and cure is generally not possible for more serious conditions such as lung cancer and emphysema. Many tobacco-related health risks can be reduced when people stop using tobacco products, and studies have demonstrated that tobacco cessation counseling by health care providers can increase cessation rates (see U.S. Preventive Services Task Force, 1996). In one study, 5 percent of smokers quit as a result of their doctor's spending less than one minute encouraging them to do so (Russell et al., 1979). Cessation rates have been shown to increase as the time devoted to counseling increases (Smoking Cessation Guideline Panel, 1996). On a national basis, even a 5 percent annual cessation rate among smokers who have a health care visit would translate into about 1.6 million fewer smokers each year and, over the long term, a substantial reduction of disease burden.

Health care providers can also promote the use of nicotine replacement therapy as an adjunct to counseling. Health plans can be encouraged to support tobacco use cessation programs as well as purchase of the nicotine patch or nicotine gum to assist in cessation. Providers also have the opportunity to counsel children and adolescents against initiating tobacco use, but studies have not yet been done to demonstrate its effectiveness.

As noted above, recommendations have been issued that health care providers routinely ask about tobacco use and provide counseling for cessation or prevention (Smoking Cessation Guideline Panel, 1996; U.S. Preventive Services Task Force, 1996). *Healthy People 2000* calls for 75 percent of health care providers to routinely advise cessation, but only 37 percent of adult smokers reported receiving such advice in the previous year (CDC, 1993c) and only 25 percent of persons ages 10–22 reported any mention of smoking by a health care provider (CDC, 1995a). A specific effort was made to support the inclusion in HEDIS 3.0 of measures that would encourage providers to offer such counseling (Center for the Advancement of Health, 1996).

Indicators for a community might include the following:

1. Percentage of tobacco users whose health care providers ask about tobacco use; percentage whose providers deliver cessation counseling; percentage whose providers assist in the cessation process when interest in quitting is expressed.

Provider counseling promotes cessation of tobacco use, yet many physicians do not determine if their patients use tobacco. With the new edition of HEDIS (NCQA, 1996), however, health plans would be asked to report the proportion of their adult members (age 21 and older) who smoke and who received advice to quit.

2. Percentage of nonsmoking youth who are counseled by a health care provider not to begin tobacco use.

The impact of physicians counseling nonsmoking youth not to initiate use has not been measured, but such counseling has been recommended (Smoking Cessation Guideline Panel, 1996; U.S. Preventive Services Task Force, 1996). Clinicians are also advised to support the implementation and operation of school-based prevention programs, which have been shown to delay the initiation of tobacco use.

3. For the major health care plans serving the community's population, the percentage of covered lives with partial or complete coverage for participation in tobacco cessation programs.

Lack of insurance coverage for such programs may serve as a disincentive to participate. Variability in the success of cessation programs has deterred health plans from offering even partial coverage. Smoking cessation treatment has, however, been shown to be a cost-effective intervention (Cummings et al., 1989; Marks et al., 1990; Fiscella and Franks, 1996), and coverage for tobacco assessment, counseling, and treatment has been recommended (Smoking Cessation Guideline Panel, 1996).

Health and Function

Tobacco affects the domain of health and function primarily through the morbidity and disability that result from the predictable health consequences of tobacco use.

Indicators might include the following:

1. Number (or percentage) of people in the community who are partially or completely disabled as a result of tobacco-related illness.

Current and former smokers may experience debilitating conditions such as emphysema, chronic bronchitis, lung cancer, and cardiovascular disease. This impairment of health and function will tend to increase the demand for health care in the community and may increase the need for nursing home or other forms of long-term care. Over time, reductions in tobacco use will be reflected in lower rates of impairment from these conditions.

Well-Being

Tobacco users identify a sense of relaxation and reward when using tobacco. This has been associated with the effects of nicotine consumption. This perception of well-being is a powerful motivating force for continued tobacco use. Advocates for tobacco use cessation can only offer, over the long term, increased capacity for active living and an immediate improvement in some of the acute effects of tobacco such as aftertaste, headaches, and reduced lung capacity. These conflicting elements of well-being are at the heart of the problems of tobacco and health, and indicators that can assess them need to be developed.

SAMPLE INDICATOR SET

Selecting a primary set of indicators from the larger field set is simplified in this case because some indicators listed above are included in the committee's proposed community profile (see Chapter 5). Therefore, communities could expect to have such data even without a special effort to address tobacco use and its health consequences.

For the additional indicators, the community will have to identify appropriate sources of data. Because standard measures are not generally available for these indicators, comparisons with other communities or state and national data are not likely to be appropriate. An important exception is the new HEDIS measure on providers advising smokers to quit (NCQA, 1996), which could be applied for proposed indicator 9, below. The selected indicators, including those from the community profile, are listed below with comments on data and measurement issues and on implications for accountability.

Indicators that would be available from a community profile include the following:

1. Number of deaths in the community due to lung cancer, cardiovascular disease, emphysema, chronic bronchitis, respiratory infections; percentage of these deaths attributable to smoking.

These measures largely fall under the community profile indicator on leading causes of death (indicator 12 in Appendix 5A). Deaths due to fires could also be included. Data on cause of death are available from death certificates and compiled by state vital statistics offices. Estimating the percentage of those deaths attributable to smoking would require further analysis using tools such as the specialized software developed by CDC (Shultz et al., 1991).[1] In some communities, the number of deaths from specific

[1]The CDC SAMMEC II software (Shultz et al., 1991) will produce estimates of smoking-attributable mortality for the following specific causes of death, identified by ICD-9-CM diagnostic code:

- *Neoplasms:* lip, oral cavity, pharynx (ICD-9-CM codes: 140–149); esophagus (150); pancreas (157); larynx (161); trachea, lung, bronchus (162); cervix uteri (180); urinary bladder (188); kidney, other urinary (189)
- *Cardiovascular disease:* rheumatic heart disease (390–398); hypertension (401–405); ischemic heart disease (410–414); pulmonary heart disease (415–417);

causes may be small, so analysis will require aggregation of data over two or more years. Smoking-related fire deaths would be identified separately and would be so rare that no trend analysis would be possible. Because of the long-term nature of the relationship between smoking and most of these health outcomes, numbers of deaths serve more to inform the community of the opportunity for health improvement than to measure current performance.

2. Percentage of the adult population (age 18 and older) who smoke regularly.

In most national surveys, "smoking" refers to the use of cigarettes. For a community health improvement effort, this indicator might be modified to cover all forms of tobacco use. Specific definitions of smoking and other forms of tobacco use will be needed. The National Health Interview Survey, for example, distinguishes those who smoke every day from those who smoke some days (CDC, 1994c). Because this measure provides a near-term indication of the effects of smoking cessation efforts, it is a good proxy for anticipated long-term changes in smoking-related health outcomes. In terms of accountability, it captures the collective effect of actions across the community. Special sampling in a state survey for the Behavioral Risk Factor Surveillance System might be a source of community-level estimates.

3. Extent to which state or local ordinances control environmental tobacco smoke in the community.

Using this indicator will require establishing a definition of "control" of ETS. Communities might focus on ordinances for specific settings such as government buildings, private workplaces, and restaurants. The extent of these ordinances, the degree of compliance, and the degree to which they are enforced generally reflect the community's commitment to tobacco use prevention. In some instances, however, a community's desire to

---

cardiac arrest, other heart disease (420–429); cerebrovascular disease (430–438); atherosclerosis (440); aortic aneurysm (441); other arterial disease (442–448)

- *Respiratory disease:* respiratory tuberculosis (010–012); pneumonia, influenza (480–489); bronchitis, emphysema (490–492); asthma (493); chronic airway obstruction (496)
- *Pediatric conditions:* short gestation, low birth weight (765); respiratory distress syndrome (769); respiratory conditions-newborn (770); sudden infant death syndrome (798.0)

restrict smoking may conflict with state laws that limit local authority in this area.

Additional indicators proposed for monitoring community action to prevent the health consequences of tobacco use include the following:

4. Number of residential fires per year attributable to smoking.

Residential fires are another undesirable outcome of smoking. Unlike deaths from lung cancer and other causes, which are a long-term outcome, fires are a more immediate consequence of smoking. In addition to the small number of deaths and serious injury that occur, fires carry economic costs for individuals and the community. Data should be available from the fire department or a similar public safety agency.

5. Percentage of youth, ages 11–18, who initiate smoking each year.

Most smokers begin using cigarettes before age 18, making the adolescent population the focus of efforts to prevent tobacco use. Smoking initiation rates in this population will be an indicator of the success of prevention efforts. Depending on the community, it may be useful to track smoking initiation by gender or race, or among younger and older teens. If the population is large enough, age-specific rates could be used to monitor changes in the average age of smoking initiation. School-based surveys are a prominent candidate for data collection but will miss those teenagers who have dropped out of school. The Youth Risk Behavior Surveillance System (see CDC, 1995b) and other national surveys might be a source of validated questions for a community survey. Smoking initiation is a product of many factors, so specific accountability cannot be established, but school-based prevention programs and enforcement of age restrictions on sales of tobacco products would be important priorities.

6. Effectiveness of local enforcement of laws prohibiting tobacco sales to minors.

This indicator could be operationalized more specifically with measures such as

- Existence of a program by the local health department or other appropriate agency for routine checks on sales to minors.

- Percentage of test sales in which an underage purchase was completed.

These measures target actual sales practices, and data should be available from the agency responsible for enforcement. Survey data on the proportion of adolescents who report being asked for proof of age when purchasing cigarettes might also be sought. The extensive recommendations regarding enforcement of sales restrictions from the report *Growing Up Tobacco Free* (IOM, 1994) could suggest other measures that communities might want to use (e.g., on vending machine access, merchant licensing, merchant fines). Data could come from agencies charged with enforcing the ordinances. This indicator addresses accountability on the part of both merchants and enforcement agencies.

7. Extent to which tobacco use prevention is incorporated into school curricula and activities.

This indicator could be operationalized with measures such as

- Percentage of schools including tobacco use prevention in the curriculum of every grade level.
- For each grade level, percentage of health curriculum hours devoted to tobacco use prevention.

This indicator specifically addresses the role of schools in contributing to efforts to prevent tobacco use. The commitment of the local school system to this endeavor is also a good indicator of community support for the prevention of tobacco use. The necessary data should be available from school districts. These measures do not address the appropriateness of the curriculum content or the effectiveness with which it is presented. Guidelines issued by CDC (1994d) suggest some basis for making those judgments, but specific measures would have to be developed.

8. Number of tobacco use cessation programs available in the community; their success rate (proportion of participants achieving at least six months of cessation following completion of the program).

The number of cessation programs reflects, in a very general manner, capacity available in the community to provide assistance to smokers who want to quit. A specific definition of a cessation "program" would be needed to count how many there are. Measures of participation demonstrate the use of available services but may be hard to interpret. Some smokers may participate repeatedly and without success; others may quit successfully without any program participation. Success rates go beyond capacity and participation to measure program performance. They should be based on recent program attendance—for example, completion of a program 6–18 months previously. Data might come from community surveys or, perhaps, cessation program records if six-month follow-up information can be obtained from most participants. In terms of accountability, success rates target cessation programs directly, but responsibility for the number of programs is less specific. Hospitals, health plans, and organizations in the community such as the American Lung Association might be expected to offer programs, but market forces will influence the number of commercial programs.

9. Percentage of tobacco users whose health care providers ask about tobacco use; percentage whose providers deliver cessation counseling; percentage whose providers assist in the cessation process when interest in quitting is expressed.

Counseling from health care providers of all types promotes cessation of tobacco use but is not offered routinely to all patients who use tobacco. HEDIS reporting on cessation counseling for adults would generate data on the performance of providers in health plans but not for the community as a whole. The member survey used to generate HEDIS data might provide a model for a comprehensive community survey. "Assistance" in cessation, which will require a formal definition, could include follow-up counseling, self-help materials, referral to a cessation program or to more intensive individual counseling, or nicotine replacement products. This measure directly addresses the responsibilities of health care providers.

10. Percentage of nonsmoking youth who are counseled by a health care provider not to begin tobacco use.

This measure, which addresses prevention and complements the previous one on cessation, also focuses on health care provider responsibilities. A school-based survey, which has been suggested as a source of data for other measures, might be used here as well. Because the effectiveness of provider counseling has not been tested, the use of this indicator should be reassessed as additional evidence becomes available.

11. For the major health care plans serving the community's

population, the percentage of covered lives with partial or complete coverage for participation in tobacco cessation programs.

Health plan coverage for tobacco cessation programs may encourage participation. Data for this indicator would have to come from health plan records or possibly state records. The kinds of programs for which coverage would be expected would have to be specified. Consideration should be given to including coverage for nicotine replacement products approved by the Food and Drug Administration. As framed, the indicator would not measure the coverage available under indemnity plans. In terms of accountability, the indicator addresses health plans and purchasers of health services, particularly employers and Medicaid programs, whose choice of plans affects the availability of coverage for specific services.

The proposed indicator set includes measures of outcomes (smoking related deaths, house fires), risk factors (smoking prevalence, smoking initiation), and community actions aimed at reducing tobacco use and, thus, its long-term health impact. Tobacco use is a habit that is acquired within a couple of years but can take many more years to change. The mix of short- and long-term factors is reflected in the inclusion of risk measures that address both smoking initiation and smoking status. In interpreting trends in the smoking status indicator, it is important to consider whether changes reflect recent smoking cessation among those who began smoking in the past or are due to new cohorts of smokers who have substantially higher or lower rates of smoking than older adults. Similarly, there are both short- and long-term effects of smoking. The indicators on house fires and tobacco-related deaths reflect this range of possible effects.

The smoking outcome measures (indicators 1 and 4) and risk factors (indicators 2 and 5) indicate the performance of the community as a whole, in conjunction with regional and national trends in preventing and controlling tobacco use. Other proposed indicators suggest (groups of) responsible entities in the community that might be held accountable for tobacco control measures. The measures relating to laws and regulations (ETS ordinances, tobacco sales to minors) indicate political will in the community to take legal measures to control tobacco use. Responsibility for enacting the appropriate ordinances and regulations, an initial step without which the proposed indicators have no meaning, may however lie at the state rather than the community level.

Both of the measures are also written to indicate the ability of the community to enforce these ordinances and regulations, either by official, governmental means or by the actions of those directly responsible such as employers and merchants.

Other measures reflect specific actions that entities in the community can take to influence tobacco use. Indicator 7, for instance, measures school-based efforts (curriculum and other efforts) to prevent initiation of tobacco use. It reflects the capacities and actions of school boards, administrators, and teachers, as well as the community's willingness to accept these efforts. Indicator 8 addresses smoking cessation programs in the community. Such programs might be provided by voluntary health agencies such as the American Lung Association (ALA); public health departments; managed care organizations, hospitals, or other health service providers; or some combination of the above (e.g., a hospital might sponsor a program and provide space, the ALA might provide the staff, and the health department might advertise its availability). A small number of smoking cessation programs in the community does not mean that any one of these parties is responsible; rather, it points to an opportunity for the community that can be met only if some of the relevant parties work together.

The indicators regarding counseling by health care providers (indicators 9 and 10) and coverage for cessation programs (indicator 11) measure actions that can be taken by the health care delivery system to reduce tobacco use. Indicators 9 and 10 directly measure provider behavior, which is the product not only of an individual's immediate actions but also of other influences such as professional training, expectations of colleagues and patients, and health system policies regarding tobacco counseling. Indicator 11, on health plan coverage for cessation programs, is an important measure in its own right and might provide an incentive for the development of smoking cessation programs in the community.

REFERENCES

CDC (Centers for Disease Control and Prevention). 1989. *Reducing the Health Consequences of Smoking: 25 Years of Progress—A Report of the Surgeon General.* DHHS Pub. No. (CDC)89-8411. Washington, D.C.: U.S. Department of Health and Human Services.

CDC. 1993a. Smoking Cessation During Previous Year Among Adults—United States, 1990 and 1991. *Morbidity and Mortality Weekly Report* 42:504–507.

CDC. 1993b. Cigarette Smoking-Attributable Mortality and Years of Potential Life Lost—United States, 1990. *Morbidity and Mortality Weekly Report* 42:645–649.

CDC. 1993c. Physician and Other Health-Care Professional Counseling of Smokers to Quit—United States, 1991. *Morbidity and Mortality Weekly Report* 42:855–857.

CDC. 1994a. *Preventing Tobacco Use Among Young People: A Report of the Surgeon General.* DHHS Pub. No. 94-0111-P. Washington, D.C.: U.S. Department of Health and Human Services.

CDC. 1994b. Medical-Care Expenditures Attributable to Cigarette Smoking—United States, 1993. *Morbidity and Mortality Weekly Report* 43:469–472.

CDC. 1994c. Cigarette Smoking Among Adults—United States, 1993. *Morbidity and Mortality Weekly Report* 43:925–930.

CDC. 1994d. Guidelines for School Health Programs to Prevent Tobacco Use and Addiction. *Morbidity and Mortality Weekly Report* 43(RR–2).

CDC. 1995a. Health-Care Provider Advice on Tobacco Use to Persons Aged 10–22 Years—United States, 1993. *Morbidity and Mortality Weekly Report* 44:826–830.

CDC. 1995b. Youth Risk Behavior Surveillance—United States, 1993. *Morbidity and Mortality Weekly Report* 44(SS–1).

CDC. 1996a. Tobacco Use and Usual Source of Cigarettes Among High School Students—United States, 1995. *Morbidity and Mortality Weekly Report* 45:413–418.

CDC. 1996b. Addition of Prevalence of Cigarette Smoking as a Nationally Notifiable Condition—June 1996. *Morbidity and Mortality Weekly Report* 45:537.

CDC. 1996c. Cigarette Smoking Among Adults—United States, 1994. *Morbidity and Mortality Weekly Report* 45:588–590.

Center for the Advancement of Health. 1996. Development of Tobacco-Related Performance Indicators for Managed Care. Washington, D.C. (mimeo)

Cummings, S.R., Rubin, S.M., and Oster, G. 1989. The Cost-Effectiveness of Counseling Smokers to Quit. *Journal of the American Medical Association* 261:75–79.

EPA (Environmental Protection Agency). 1992. *Respiratory Health Effects of Passive Smoking: Lung Cancer and Other Disorders.* Pub. No. EPA-600/6-90/006F. Washington, D.C.: EPA, Office of Health and Environmental Assessment.

Fiscella, K., and Franks, P. 1996. Cost-Effectiveness of the Transdermal Nicotine Patch as an Adjunct to Physicians' Smoking Cessation Counseling. *Journal of the American Medical Association* 275:1247–1251.

Gardner, P., and Hudson, B.L. 1996. Advance Report of Final Mortality Statistics, 1993. *Monthly Vital Statistics Report* 44 (No. 7, supplement). Hyattsville, Md.: National Center for Health Statistics.

Garner, D.W. 1996. Banning Tobacco Billboards: The Case for Municipal Action. *Journal of the American Medical Association* 275:1263–1269.

Hatziandreu, E.J., Pierce, J.P., Fiore, M.C., Grise, V., Novotny, T.E., and Davis, R.M. 1989. The Reliability of Self-Reported Cigarette Consumption in the United States. *American Journal of Public Health* 79:1020–1023.

Hu, T., Sung, H., and Keeler, T.E. 1995. Reducing Cigarette Consumption in California: Tobacco Taxes vs an Anti-Smoking Media Campaign. *American Journal of Public Health* 85:1218–1222.

IOM (Institute of Medicine). 1994. *Growing Up Tobacco Free: Preventing Nicotine Addiction in Children and Youths.* B.S. Lynch and R.J. Bonnie, eds. Washington, D.C.: National Academy Press.

Kleinman, J., and Madans, J.H. 1985. The Effects of Maternal Smoking, Physical Stature, and Educational Attainment on the Incidence of Low Birth Weight. *American Journal of Epidemiology* 121:832–855.

Marks, J.S., Koplan, J.P., Hogue, C.J.R., and Dalmat, M.E. 1990. A Cost-Benefit/Cost-Effectiveness Analysis of Smoking Cessation for Pregnant Women. *American Journal of Preventive Medicine* 6:282–289.

McGinnis, J.M., and Foege, W.H. 1993. Actual Causes of Death in the United States. *Journal of the American Medical Association* 270:2207–2212.

NCQA (National Committee for Quality Assurance). 1996. HEDIS 3.0 Draft for Public Comment. Washington, D.C.: NCQA.

OTA (Office of Technology Assessment). 1993. *Smoking-Related Deaths and Financial Costs: Office of Technology Assessment Estimates for 1990.* Washington, D.C.: U.S. Congress.

Pierce, J.P., Fiore, M.C., Novotny, T.E., Hatziandreu, E.J., and Davis, T.M. 1989. Trends in Cigarette Smoking in the United States: Projections to the Year 2000. *Journal of the American Medical Association* 261:61–65.

Russell, M.A.H., Wilson, C., Taylor, C., and Baker, C.D. 1979. Effect of General Practitioners Advice Against Smoking. *British Medical Journal* 2(6184):231–235.

Shultz, J.M., Novotny, T.E., and Rice, D.P. 1991. Quantifying the Disease Impact of Cigarette Smoking with SAMMEC II Software. *Public Health Reports* 106:326–333.

Smoking Cessation Guideline Panel. 1996. *Smoking Cessation: A Guide for Primary Care Clinicians.* Clinical Practice Guideline, No. 18. AHCPR Pub. No. 96–0693. Rockville, Md.: U.S. Department of Health and Human Services.

U.S. Consumer Product Safety Commission. 1993. *Practicality of Developing a Performance Standard to Reduce Cigarette Ignition Propensity. Overview.* Washington, D.C.: U.S. Consumer Product Safety Commission.

USDHHS (U.S. Department of Health and Human Services). 1991. *Healthy People 2000: National Health Promotion and Disease Prevention Objectives.* DHHS Pub. No. (PHS) 91-50212. Washington, D.C.: Office of the Assistant Secretary for Health.

U.S. Preventive Services Task Force. 1996. *Guide to Clinical Preventive Services.* 2nd ed. Baltimore: Williams and Wilkins.

Ventura, S.J., Martin, J.A., Mathews, T.J., and Clarke, S.C. 1996. Advance Report of Final Natality Statistics, 1994. *Monthly Vital Statistics Report* 44 (No. 11, supplement). Hyattsville, Md.: National Center for Health Statistics.

Warner, K.E., Fulton, G.A., Nicolas, P., and Grimes, D.R. 1996. Employment Implications of Declining Tobacco Product Sales for the Regional Economies of the United States. *Journal of the American Medical Association* 275:1241–1246.

TABLE A.7-1 Field Model Mapping for Sample Indicator Set: Tobacco and Health

Field Model Domain	Construct	Sample Indicators	Data Sources	Stakeholders
Disease	Reduce the impact of tobacco-related mortality	Deaths due to lung cancer, cardiovascular disease, respiratory diseases; percentage of these deaths attributable to smoking	Death certificates	Health care providers Health care plans State health agencies Local health agencies Business, industry Community organizations Special health risk groups General public
Individual Response	Reduce the prevalence of smoking	Percentage of adults who smoke regularly Percentage of youth who initiate smoking each year	Community surveys Community or school-based surveys	State health agencies Local health agencies Education agencies and institutions Community organizations Special health risk groups General public
Social Environment	Reduce youth access to tobacco	Effectiveness of enforcement of local laws prohibiting tobacco sales to minors	Local (or state) government enforcement agencies	State health agencies Local health agencies Local government Business, industry General public

continued on next page

TABLE A.7-1 *Continued*

Field Model Domain	Construct	Sample Indicators	Data Sources	Stakeholders
Social Environment (*continued*)	Promote prevention of initiation of tobacco use	Extent to which tobacco use prevention is incorporated into school curricula and activities	School systems	Local Government Education agencies and institutions General public
	Promote cessation of tobacco use	Number of cessation programs available; success rate (percentage of participants achieving at least 6 months of cessation)	Community surveys; cessation program records	Health care providers Health care plans Business, industry Community organizations General public
Physical Environment	Reduce exposure to environmental tobacco smoke	Extent to which ordinances control environmental tobacco smoke	Local (or state) government enforcement agencies	State health agencies Local health agencies Local government Business, industry General public
	Reduce loss of life and property from fires	Number of residential fires attributable to smoking	Public safety agencies	

Health Care	Promote health care provider counseling on cessation of tobacco use	Percentage of tobacco users whose health care providers ask about tobacco use; provide cessation counseling; assist cessation efforts	Community surveys	Health care providers Health care plans Local health agencies Business, industry General public
		Percentage of nonsmoking youth counseled by a health care provider not to begin tobacco use	Community or school-based surveys	Health care providers Health care plans Local health agencies General public
	Reduce financial barriers to participation in cessation programs	Percentage of health plans' covered lives with partial or complete coverage for participation in tobacco cessation programs	Health plan records	Health care plans State health agencies Local health agencies Business, industry General public

A.8

Prototype Indicator Set: Vaccine-Preventable Diseases

BACKGROUND

Each year in the United States, several thousand adults and smaller numbers of children develop infectious diseases that are highly preventable with the appropriate use of existing vaccines. Currently recommended childhood immunizations protect against measles, mumps, rubella, diphtheria, tetanus, pertussis, poliomyelitis, *Haemophilus influenzae* type b (Hib), hepatitis B, and varicella. Vaccines for influenza and pneumococcal pneumonia are recommended primarily for older adults and younger people with special health risks.

Immunization targets set by *Healthy People 2000* (USDHHS, 1991) call for 90 percent of 2-year-old children to have received all recommended vaccine doses and for 60 percent of persons aged 65 and over to have received a pneumococcal vaccination and an annual influenza vaccination. Estimates for 1994 indicate that 72 percent of 2-year-old children are fully immunized (CDC, 1996c). Among adults 65 years of age and older living in households in 1993, only 28 percent had received pneumococcal vaccine and 52 percent an annual influenza immunization (CDC, 1995a).

State laws requiring up-to-date immunization for school entry have led to nearly complete immunization coverage by the time children are 5 or 6 years of age. Most states have also adopted immunization requirements for participation in state-licensed day care and are adding requirements for measles and hepatitis B immunizations for adolescents. Colleges are also requiring evidence of up-to-date immunization. For most preschool children, adolescents, and older adults, however, no universal gateway comparable to school entry ensures that immunizations are up to date.

Delayed immunization for preschool children and for adults has been linked to personal and family characteristics and to barriers and deficiencies in the health care delivery system (e.g., Orenstein et al., 1990; NVAC, 1991, 1994; Schulte et al., 1991; Freed et al., 1993; Szilagyi et al., 1993, 1994; IOM, 1994; CDC, 1995c; Frank et al., 1995; Wood et al., 1995). Family factors include lack of knowledge about immunization requirements, low socioeconomic status, low maternal education, and larger family size. In the health care system, providers may miss opportunities to immunize from practices such as not checking immunization status and not immunizing during minor illnesses. Barriers are created by requirements such as appointments for immunization and a comprehensive physical exam prior to immunization.

The recognition that incomplete immunization poses an avoidable health risk has prompted a variety of efforts at national, state, and local levels to raise immunization rates. Activities include establishing collaborations that can promote responsibility and accountability for immunization, improving provider practices and communication with the public, and developing better information resources. Although the focus is generally on increasing immunization rates, communities also need to ensure that they can achieve their current levels of coverage for future cohorts.

The committee included vaccine-preventable diseases among the health issues used to illustrate the development of performance indicators because of the high morbidity, mortality, and costs associated with these conditions and the availability of vaccines as an effective but underused preventive intervention. The incidence of illness and death is much higher among the elderly, but preventable morbidity or mortality among children should be unacceptable in a community. This is also an issue that touches many segments of a community, including children and their families, the elderly, health departments, private and public health care services, schools, and employers.

"FIELD" SET OF PERFORMANCE MEASURES

By using the domains of the field model, it is possible to identify many measures that might serve as performance indicators for a community's efforts to improve immunization levels and reduce the incidence of vaccine-preventable diseases.

Disease

Reducing as much as possible the cases and deaths attributable to vaccine-preventable diseases is the health outcome of primary interest. In the United States, from 20,000 to 40,000 influenza-associated deaths have occurred annually during recent epidemics (CDC, 1995b), and excess hospitalizations have been estimated to reach 172,000 during severe epidemics (Barker, 1986). Annual costs associated with epidemics have been estimated to exceed $12 billion (Nichol et al., 1994). Pneumococcal infections lead to another 40,000 deaths each year (CDC, 1989). Past successes in immunizing children have made the incidence of most "childhood" illnesses much lower, but they have not been eliminated. In a resurgence of measles from 1989 to 1991, approximately 55,000 cases were reported (CDC, 1993a). In 1994, nearly 4,600 cases of pertussis were reported, 2,500 of which occurred in children less than 5 years of age (CDC, 1996b).

Although vaccines are effective in reducing the incidence of illness and the severity of cases that do occur, they cannot always prevent all cases. The vaccine for measles, mumps, and rubella, for example, is not usually given to children less than 12 months of age, which leaves younger children susceptible to these diseases. The effectiveness of influenza vaccine can vary from year to year, depending on how well the mix of antigens matches the circulating virus strains. Pneumococcal vaccine, which is usually administered only once, is formulated to protect against 23 (but not all) strains of pneumococcus.

Estimates of the numbers of cases and deaths depend on the accuracy of diagnosis and the completeness of reporting. Because the incidence of most childhood illnesses is low, communities will probably have to monitor numbers of cases rather than incidence or mortality rates. Influenza and pneumococcal infections are more common. Death certificates can provide mortality data by cause of death, but pneumococcal pneumonia may be underreported because some deaths will be attributed to pneumonia without a specific diagnosis.

Indicators that a community might consider monitoring include the following:

1. Incidence (number of cases) of vaccine-preventable disease in children less than 5 years of age.

This preschool population is the primary target of recent immunization improvement programs. The vaccine-preventable diseases are measles, mumps, rubella, polio, diphtheria, tetanus, pertussis, hepatitis B, Hib, and varicella.

2. Incidence (number of cases) of hepatitis B among persons aged 15–29 years.

Hepatitis B can be transmitted by sexual contact and exposure to blood and from pregnant mothers to their infants. Despite recommendations that preschool children and adolescents receive the hepatitis B vaccine, immunization rates are currently lower than for other vaccines (CDC, 1996b).

3. Incidence of pneumonia and influenza.

4. Pneumonia and influenza death rates for persons aged 65 years and older.

Potential problems in obtaining accurate data for these indicators have been noted above.

Genetic Endowment

Genetic factors that impair the immune system can increase susceptibility to disease and limit the immune response generated by a vaccine. Such individuals would be among those in the community who are at higher risk for infection and, during disease outbreaks, might be the focus of special immunization efforts (for those vaccines that would be effective) or other forms of preventive care. An indicator for the influenza immunization rate among the population that is at higher risk is included in the following section.

Individual Behavior, Social Environment, Health Care

Because vaccines effectively prevent disease, immunization rates can seen as both a process measure and a meaningful proxy for health outcomes. As has been noted, many factors combine to influence whether immunizations are received at appropriate times. In terms of the field model, these factors include individual behavior (e.g., seeking available services), the social environment (e.g., economic barriers to immunization services, insufficient information about the need for immunization), and health care services (e.g., missed opportunities for immunization during health care visits). Among children, underimmunization is also a marker for shortcomings in other forms of well child care, including screening for anemia, lead toxicity, and tuberculosis (Rodewald et al., 1995).

Immunization rates can be used as community performance indicators, but they raise some conceptual and measurement issues. Rates of preschool immunization are usually presented as a composite of rates for at least four vaccines, three of which require multiple doses. With a summary rate such as this, a child who has missed a single dose of one vaccine is not distinguishable from a child who has received no vaccinations. In addition, focusing on immunization status at a particular age (e.g., 24 months) does not reveal the timeliness of immunizations at younger ages.

Obtaining the data needed to calculate immunization rates—immunization status of individuals at specific ages and size of the population at those ages—may pose a challenge for communities. Retrospective rates can be calculated when children enter school, but these rates do not reflect current immunization levels among 2-year-olds. Many health plans can provide data on members, but the accuracy of the data will depend on their completeness. Missing information on immunizations received from other sources (e.g., a public clinic) will lead to underestimates. To obtain data on a community as a whole, a periodic survey or immunization registry may be needed, but the cost of these approaches may be a constraint.

Indicators that might be used include the following:

1. Immunization rate for children at 24 months of age.

This is the broadest assessment of preschool immunization performance in the community. The measure is also included among the community profile indicators proposed by the committee.

2. Immunization rate at 24 months of age for children enrolled in day care.

The day care setting poses special risks for very young children because it increases the likelihood that they will be exposed to infectious agents. Up-to-date immunization improves protection for the immunized child and can also reduce some infection risks for unimmunized children.

3. Retrospective immunization rate at 24 months of age for grade school entrants.

This measure can provide a 24-month immunization rate if no other data collection system is available. The limitation is that the rate is approximately three years old when it is calculated.

4. Average number of underimmunized days per child for children 24 months of age.

This measure can indicate whether there are extended periods of underimmunization, but the detailed information needed to construct it may not be available in communities that do not have an immunization registry.

5. Percentage of children under 24 months of age with up-to-date immunization status.

This measure could be used to monitor adherence to the immunization schedule over the first two years of life. It might be operationalized as immunization rates for children at specific ages (e.g., 6 months, 12 months). It would require data most easily produced by an immunization registry.

6. Immunization rate for adolescents at 13 years of age.

The current immunization schedule (CDC, 1996a) calls for administering four vaccines at 11–12 years of age if all recommended doses have not yet been received. These vaccines are hepatitis B, tetanus–diphtheria, measles–mumps–rubella (MMR), and varicella. Proposed as an indicator for HEDIS 3.0 (NCQA, 1996) is the percentage of enrolled 13-year-olds who received a second dose of MMR by age 13.

7. Influenza immunization rate for all persons.

8. Percentage of Medicare enrollees who received an influenza immunization during the previous calendar year; percentage who have ever received a pneumococcal pneumonia immunization.

Even though Medicare benefits include coverage for both of the above immunizations, immunization rates remain low. Medicare claims files might be a source of data for this indicator, but they will not reflect immunizations provided in settings in which fee-for-service claims are not generally submitted (e.g., hospitals, public health clinics, managed care organizations). The immunization rate for the Medicare population is included in the community health profile proposed by the committee.

9. Influenza immunization rate for persons at high risk living in the community (the "noninstitutionalized" population).
10. Influenza immunization rate for persons in nursing homes.

Influenza can pose an especially high risk of serious illness and death in both of these populations. Determining the size of a community's population at high risk (the denominator needed for the rate in item 9) may prove difficult, however.

Social Environment

Factors in the social environment can affect both risk of illness and immunization rates. Language and other cultural differences may hinder access to all forms of health care or may have a specific impact on willingness to accept immunization. Low socioeconomic status is frequently associated with inadequate health care, including delays in receiving immunizations. Low-income families often have not had a regular source of care, which can make it difficult to maintain accurate immunization records. Programs serving these families (e.g., WIC), can be a base for interventions targeting immunization. Lack of health insurance can create economic barriers to immunization, but similar barriers may exist with health insurance policies that do not cover the cost of preventive services such as immunization. Medicare coverage for influenza immunizations was not available until 1993.

Lack of easy access to current information on the immunization status of children in a community has spurred interest in state or local immunization registry systems. Such systems promise health care providers easy access to up-to-date immunization records. Communities (through health departments, health plans, or other means) could use registry information to identify categories of children whose immunization rates are low or to inform families of specific children who are due for immunizations. Registries will benefit a community most if all children are included and all providers contribute immunization records, but the cost of creating and maintaining a registry should not be overlooked.

Indicators that a community might want to monitor include the following:

1. Immunization rate at 24 months of age for children currently enrolled in Medicaid.
2. Immunization rate at 24 months of age for children enrolled in WIC.

Children enrolled in Medicaid or WIC are an identifiable population that generally is at higher risk for underimmunization. Because enrollment in Medicaid is often not continuous, the numerator and denominator for the Medicaid rate would require clear definition. Some children enrolled at 24 months of age may not have been enrolled at ages when immunizations were due, and other children not currently enrolled might have been enrolled at those ages.

3. Among children with commercial health insurance coverage, percentage with full coverage for childhood immunizations.

The cost of vaccines and the fees charged to administer them have contributed to delayed immunization even for children who have health insurance. Full coverage ensures that immunizations will be paid for by the insurer whether or not a deductible requirement has been met. In some states, this indicator will be less relevant because free vaccines are available to all children, regardless of health insurance status.

4. Number and percentage of health insurance policies that cover influenza immunizations for persons at high risk.

The population at high risk must be defined clearly, and criteria for counting health insurance policies would be required. Policies that provide full coverage should be distinguished from those that require payment of a deductible.

5. Existence in the community of a computerized immunization registry that provides automated appointment reminders; if a registry exists, percentage of children in the community included.

At present, few communities have registries. This indicator should become more useful in the future as registry development proceeds. If a statewide registry is developed, a community would still want to know what proportion of its children were included.

6. Existence in the community of an active childhood immunization coalition involving health service providers, the lo-

cal health department, parents, and interested community organizations.

A community may benefit from the creation of a coalition that brings together individuals and groups interested in improving immunization rates. A coalition can help coordinate separate activities that may be under way and provide leadership for activities that may be needed to reach parts of the community not being served by independent efforts (Hubbert and Peck, 1993).

Physical Environment

The physical environment influences vaccine-preventable disease and immunization rates primarily through the problems that long distances and lack of transportation pose for access to immunization services. These factors may be a special concern in rural areas. In urban areas, transportation problems might be considered a function of the socioeconomic rather than the physical environment. No performance indicators related to this domain are suggested.

Health Care

Because immunization is a health care service, the practices of individual and institutional health care providers (health plans, hospitals, clinics, etc.) play a large part in determining immunization rates in a community. Missed opportunities to administer immunizations could be reduced by steps such as reviewing immunization status at all visits, giving all scheduled vaccines during a visit, and vaccinating during visits for mild illnesses. Adoption of the Standards for Pediatric Immunization Practices (CDC, 1993b), which are aimed at reducing missed opportunities and other provider-based barriers to immunization, has recently been shown to improve immunization rates in a public health clinic (Pierce et al., 1996). Increasingly, health plans are applying continuous quality improvement tools to assess immunization practices, identify missed opportunities and incomplete immunization records, and guide the development of new policies and procedures (e.g., Leatherman et al., 1995; Carlin et al., 1996).

Community-level performance indicators that might be monitored include the following:

1. Immunization rate at 24 months of age for children enrolled in managed care organizations.

2. Immunization rates for influenza and pneumococcal disease for persons aged 65 and older who are enrolled in managed care organizations.

In much of the country, managed care organizations (MCOs) are serving an increasing proportion of the population, including Medicare enrollees. Their membership is a defined subpopulation served primarily by a defined set of providers. Many MCOs have or are developing information systems that can generate data on immunization status. To give an accurate measure, MCO records must include information on immunizations that a member receives from other sources.

3. Percentage of health care providers who have a policy to give immunizations to children seen at a visit for minor illness or injury.

4. Percentage of health care providers who have a policy to give simultaneous vaccinations.

5. Percentage (or number) of hospitals that have a policy to immunize children who are seen in emergency rooms for minor illnesses or injuries.

6. Percentage of health care providers who have a policy to screen the medical chart for immunization history whenever a child is seen.

Adoption of these four policies would address leading reasons for missed opportunities to vaccinate. Policies must, however, be put into practice to have an impact on immunization rates. Obtaining data would probably require a survey of providers in the community. Companion measures might be created to reflect the proportion of a community's children served by providers with such policies.

7. Percentage of health care providers who do regular, sample chart audits to determine the immunization status of pediatric or adult patients.

Currently, many providers lack automated information systems that can generate information on the immunization status of their patients. Regular chart audits are one way to identify patients whose immunizations are not up to date.

8. Percentage of health care providers who refer patients to public clinics for immunizations.

Referring patients to another location such as a public clinic delays the immunization process and can make it more burdensome for families.

Health and Function

The vaccines for pneumonia and influenza are recommended primarily for older adults, but both illnesses also occur among working-age adults and result in time lost from work or other usual activities. A community might want to monitor lost work time as an indicator of the impact of these conditions on overall health status.

1. Number of work days missed due to pneumonia or influenza.

A means of obtaining this information would have to be developed. Employers might be able to report on short-term disability claims.

SAMPLE INDICATOR SET

From the preceding list of potential indicators, eight are proposed as the primary set that a community might use to monitor *community-level* performance. The proposed set is a mix of structure, process, and outcome measures reflecting the collective contribution of multiple entities that a community might expect to be accountable. Their selection reflects the committee's best judgment, but individual communities must consider available resources, including the availability of data. Comments are included on other uses of the measure (e.g., as a *Healthy People 2000* objective), data and measurement issues, and suggestions as to where accountability for performance might lie.

Five of the eight proposed indicators are probably measured most easily through a community or state computerized immunization registry. Immunization registries are expensive, but other than periodic chart review on a community-wide basis, they are the only way to make the regular assessments of current immunization status that can inform efforts to improve immunization rates and health status. One of the indicators may require cooperation from employers to obtain necessary data.

If a community does not have the resources for a registry or if employer involvement is limited, other indicators for which data may be more readily available should be considered (e.g., reported disease rates, death rates, health care provider policies). Small numbers of cases will, however, limit the usefulness of morbidity and mortality rates. Indicators based on policies are capacity measures that do not give a direct assessment of process and may not be sensitive to changes in health status. A community is advised to use the most appropriate indicators within the resources available to the stakeholders involved in the performance monitoring process. Starting with some indicators and developing additional ones over time is better than waiting until data can be collected on the ideal indicator.

1. Immunization rate for children at 24 months of age.

High community immunization rates can promote further reductions in morbidity and mortality from several vaccine-preventable diseases. As noted, *Healthy People 2000* has set a target for 90 percent of 24-month-old children to have all age-appropriate immunizations. To use this measure, it will be necessary to specify what combination of immunizations will constitute a "complete series" at that age. As the immunization schedule changes, the composition of a complete series will change. Data may be available from a computerized immunization registry or could be obtained from a community survey or review of a sample of public and private medical records (which would require linking records for those children who received immunizations from more than one source). Retrospective rates can be calculated by reviewing immunization records of children entering school. This approach is inexpensive, but it does not produce information on the current immunization status of preschool children. Consideration should be given to calculating rates for any subpopulations in the community that are a focus of concern. This indicator reflects the overall ability, and accountability, of the community to ensure that children receive appropriate immunizations.

2. Immunization rate at 24 months of age for children currently enrolled in managed care organizations.

This indicator provides accountability for a specific segment of the health care sector. To compare data over time or across MCOs, however, consistent data collection methods and definitions of the population included in the denominator of the rate must be used. The current draft of HEDIS 3.0, which would apply to both Medicaid and commercial enrollees, specifies that the denominator includes children reaching 2 years of age during the reporting period who have been continuously enrolled for the 12 months preceding that birthday (NCQA, 1996). The numerator includes children with at least four doses of diphtheria–tetanus–pertussis vaccine, three doses of polio vaccine, one dose of MMR vaccine between the first and second birthday, one dose of Hib vaccine between the first and second birthday, and two doses of hepatitis B vaccine. The 1997 reporting year will add an indicator for administration of the varicella vaccine, but this will not be included in the combined measure. A community may want to consider whether the continuous enrollment provisions and the specified vaccine doses are appropriate, but changes in the measure would add to an MCO's reporting burden.

3. Immunization rate at 24 months of age for children currently enrolled in Medicaid.

The Medicaid population can be one of a community's most vulnerable groups. For this population, facilitating access to immunization and other health services is particularly important. Although Medicaid removes financial barriers to health care, other barriers may be created by transportation, cultural differences, limited education, and provider access. Because many states have moved, or are planning to move, their Medicaid population to managed care plans, many children should be served by providers who can support this indicator through their HEDIS reporting. Primary accountability may rest jointly with Medicaid providers and the local public health agency. A broader measure, which would require more diverse data collection, might examine the immunization status of children who were enrolled in Medicaid at any time up to their second birthday. In that case, responsibility and accountability for up-to-date immunization might extend to additional health care providers.

4. Existence in the community of a computerized immunization registry that provides automated appointment reminders; if a registry exists, the percentage of children in the community included.

Public and private funding is encouraging states and local areas to create computerized immunization registries that can generate appointment reminders (Faherty et al., 1996). Because they are intended to provide information on all children and all immunizations received, registries should be a valuable tool to support efforts to increase immunization rates and have the potential to support other health services for children. To produce accurate data, they will have to update on a continuing basis information on the child population (births and children moving into or out of the registry area) and on immunizations administered by all providers. As a new approach to improving immunization rates, registries should be evaluated for their effectiveness (and cost-effectiveness), so that communities can make informed choices in allocating available resources. In terms of accountability, this indicator reflects the cooperation that is necessary among health departments, public and private health care providers, and others to develop, implement, and maintain a registry.

5. Among children with commercial health insurance coverage, percentage with full coverage for childhood immunizations.

This indicator was chosen because the cost associated with childhood immunizations has created a barrier for some families. In communities with a substantial capitated MCO presence, this indicator may be less appropriate because coverage for preventive services such as immunizations is usually included. In addition, state programs that offer free vaccine to all children make specific terms of health insurance coverage less influential. The information required for this indicator may not be readily available in a community. Some information may be available from the state insurance licensing authority on provisions of policies offered in the state, but the licensing authority will not have information on self-insured companies and probably will not have community-specific data on numbers of children covered. It may be necessary to contact the employers that employ and insure the largest number of community residents or to obtain information through a community survey. Information provided by this indicator can be used to establish accountability by employers and insurers for reducing financial barriers to immunization.

6. Percentage of Medicare enrollees who received an influenza immunization during the previous calendar year; percentage who have ever received a pneumococcal pneumonia immunization.

This indicator corresponds to Objective 20.11 in *Healthy People 2000*, which calls for 60 percent immunization rates for older persons living in the community. Data should be available from Medicare claims files for fee-for-service patients requiring vaccine in an outpatient setting. These data may understate immunization rates if a large percentage of Medicare enrollees in the community are enrolled in capitated managed care plans that do not file claims for the individual services provided or are vaccinated as inpatients. The proposed inclusion in HEDIS 3.0 of a measure on influenza immunization for Medicare members would help overcome these limitations. Hospitals and other public and private health care providers that give immunizations share responsibility for the rates in the community.

7. Pneumonia and influenza death rates for persons age 65 and older.

Healthy People 2000 has targeted reducing the epidemic-related death rates in the older population. Immunization is an important tool for reducing these rates, but as noted, the available vaccines are effective against only a portion of the infectious agents that cause these diseases. Data on cause of death are obtainable from death certificates. The number of deaths in a single year may be small for some communities, so calculation of stable rates may require aggregating data over multiple years. Where numbers of deaths are small, caution is required in comparing data over time or with other communities.

8. Existence in the community of an active childhood immunization coalition, involving health service providers, the local health department, parents, and interested community organizations.

Such a coalition may be able to provide the leadership needed to organize and coordinate the actions of health service providers, health departments, and other groups in the community to reach out to families with young children who need immunizations, ensure that immunization services are available and accessible, and—in conjunction with a immunization registry—see that children get the immunizations they need. It may also be able to advocate for better provider practices and insurance coverage. The effectiveness of such coalitions should be tested to ensure that the mechanism can achieve its intended aims. In addition, an issue-specific coalition should be closely linked to any broader health coalition in the community.

The proposed indicator set is intended to support a community effort to reduce morbidity and mortality from vaccine-preventable diseases. The indicators include measures of health outcomes (pneumonia and influenza deaths), risk factors (immunization coverage rates for all children, children in managed care organizations, Medicaid children, Medicare enrollees), and community actions that can help to improve immunization coverage in the long run (registries, health insurance coverage, immunization coalitions).

Only one direct health outcome measure is included (influenza and pneumonia death rates). Thanks largely to the success of immunization programs, vaccine-preventable diseases are rare in children. The small numbers of cases are unreliable indicators of the effectiveness of childhood immunization efforts. On the other hand, deaths from pneumonia and influenza remain common in older people, and data are readily available from vital statistics.

Because immunization is a proven effective means for preventing a number of diseases, most of the proposed indicators focus on immunization coverage rates (indicators 1, 2, 3, and 6) as measures of health risk. In terms of performance, the indicator for immunization coverage rates for all children covers the community as a whole. Three other measures (children in managed care organizations, Medicaid children, Medicare enrollees) address the performance of specific health care delivery sectors. The inclusion of an indicator for immunization rates for children in managed care organizations, as opposed to other health care providers, primarily reflects the greater availability of data from MCOs. In practice, all providers serving children in the community share responsibility for ensuring that those children are immunized. Comparing the overall immunization rate with the rates for MCOs or Medicaid gives an indirect indication of rates among children not included in either of the two specific systems. The residual group includes children both with and without health insurance coverage.

Two measures (registries and immunization coalitions) are indicators of a community's willingness and ability to organize itself to overcome barriers to immunization (due, perhaps, to factors based in domains of the field model other than health services). These indicators do not measure the performance of specific entities in the community because the community as a whole must make them happen. Coalitions, in particular, however, do provide an opportunity for community entities (such as health departments) to play leadership roles. Thus, the presence of a coalition suggests that some entity in the community is performing well in this regard.

REFERENCES

Barker, W.H. 1986. Excess Pneumonia and Influenza Associated Hospitalization During Influenza Epidemics in the United States. *American Journal of Public Health* 76:761–765.

Carlin, E., Carlson, R., and Nordin, J. 1996. Using Continuous Quality Improvement Tools to Improve Pediatric Immunization Rates. *Joint Commission Journal on Quality Improvement* 22:277–288.

CDC (Centers for Disease Control and Prevention). 1989. Pneumococcal Polysaccharide Vaccine: Recommendations of the Immunization Practices Advisory Committee (ACIP). *Morbidity and Mortality Weekly Report* 38:64–68, 73–76.

CDC. 1993a. Measles—United States, 1992. *Morbidity and Mortality Weekly Report* 42:378–381.

CDC. 1993b. Standards for Pediatric Immunization Practices. *Morbidity and Mortality Weekly Report* 42(RR-5):1–13.

CDC. 1995a. Influenza and Pneumococcal Vaccination Coverage Levels Among Persons Aged 65 Years—United States, 1973–1993. *Morbidity and Mortality Weekly Report* 44:506–507, 513–515.

CDC. 1995b. Prevention and Control of Influenza: Recommendations of the Advisory Committee on Immunization Practices (ACIP). *Morbidity and Mortality Weekly Report* 44(RR-3).

CDC. 1995c. Increasing Pneumococcal Vaccination Rates Among Patients of a National Health-Care Alliance—United States, 1993. *Morbidity and Mortality Weekly Report* 44:741–744.

CDC. 1996a. Immunization Schedule—United States, January–June 1996. *Morbidity and Mortality Weekly Report* 44:940–943.

CDC. 1996b. Monthly Immunization Table. *Morbidity and Mortality Weekly Report* 45:99.

CDC. 1996c. National, State, and Urban Area Vaccination Coverage Levels Among Children Aged 19–35 Months—United States. *Morbidity and Mortality Weekly Report* 45:145–150.

Faherty, K.M., Waller, C.J., DeFriese, G.H., et al. 1996. Prospects for Childhood Immunization Registries in Public Health Assessment and Assurance: Initial Observations from the All Kids Count Initiative Projects. *Journal of Public Health Management and Practice* 2(1):1–11.

Frank, R.G., Dewa, C.S., Holt, E., Hughart, H., Stobino, D., and Guyer, B. 1995. The Demand for Childhood Immunizations: Results from the Baltimore Immunization Study. *Inquiry* 32(2):164–173.

Freed, G.L., Bordley, W.C., and DeFriese, G.H. 1993. Childhood Immunization Programs: An Analysis of Policy Issues. *Milbank Quarterly* 71:65–96.

Hubbert, E.D., and Peck, M.G. 1993. *What Works II: 1992 Urban MCH Programs.* Omaha, Neb.: CityMatCH at the University of Nebraska Medical Center.

IOM (Institute of Medicine). 1994. *Overcoming Barriers to Immunization: A Workshop Summary.* J.S. Durch, ed. Washington, D.C.: National Academy Press.

Leatherman, S., Venus, P., Smalley, M.A., Hunt, G., McCarthy, D., and Peterson, E. 1995. Population Health Surveillance in a Managed Care Setting: A Continuous Quality Improvement Project to Increase Pediatric Immunization Rates Using Administrative Claims and Survey Data. Minneapolis: United Healthcare Corporation, Center for Health Care Policy and Evaluation. Draft.

NCQA (National Committee for Quality Assurance). 1996. HEDIS 3.0 Draft for Public Comment. Washington, D.C.: NCQA.

Nichol, K.L., Margolis, K.L., Wuorenma, J., and Von-Sternberg, T. 1994. The Efficacy and Cost Effectiveness of Vaccination Against Influenza Among Elderly Persons Living in the Community. *New England Journal of Medicine* 331:778–784.

NVAC (National Vaccine Advisory Committee). 1991. The Measles Epidemic. The Problems, Barriers, and Recommendations. *Journal of the American Medical Association* 266:1547–1552.

NVAC. 1994. *Adult Immunization.* A Report by the National Vaccine Advisory Committee. Washington, D.C.: U.S. Department of Health and Human Services.

Orenstein, W.A., Atkinson, W., Mason, D., and Bernier, R.H. 1990. Barriers to Vaccinating Preschool Children. *Journal of Health Care for the Poor and Underserved* 1:315–330.

Pierce, C., Goldstein, M., Suozzi, K., Gallaher, M., Dietz, V., and Stevenson, J. 1996. The Impact of the Standards for Pediatric Immunization Practices on Vaccination Coverage Levels. *Journal of the American Medical Association* 276:626–630.

Rodewald, L.E., Szilagyi, P.G., Shiuh, T., Humiston, S.G., LeBaron, C., and Hall, C.B. 1995. Is Underimmunization a Marker for Insufficient Utilization of Preventive and Primary Care? *Archives of Pediatric and Adolescent Medicine* 149:393–397.

Schulte, J.M., Brown, G.R., Zetzman, M.R., et al. 1991. Changing Immunization Referral Patterns Among Pediatricians and Family Practice Physicians, Dallas County, Texas, 1988. *Pediatrics* 87:204–207.

Szilagyi, P.G., Rodewald, L.E., Humiston, S.G., et al. 1993. Missed Opportunities for Childhood Vaccinations in Office Practices and the Effect on Vaccination Status. *Pediatrics* 91:1–7.

Szilagyi, P.G., Rodewald, L.E., Humiston, S.G., et al. 1994. Immunization Practices of Pediatricians and Family Physicians in the United States. *Pediatrics* 94:517–523.

USDHHS (U.S. Department of Health and Human Services). 1991. *Healthy People 2000: National Health Promotion and Disease Prevention Objectives.* DHHS Pub. No. (PHS) 91-50212. Washington, D.C.: Office of the Assistant Secretary for Health.

Wood, D., Donald-Sherbourne, C., Halfon, N., et al. 1995. Factors Related to Immunization Status Among Inner-City Latino and African-American Preschoolers. *Pediatrics* 96:295–301.

TABLE A.8-1 Field Model Mapping for Sample Indicator Set: Vaccine-Preventable Diseases

Field Model Domain	Construct	Sample Indicators	Data Sources	Stakeholders
Disease	Eliminate vaccine-preventable diseases	Pneumonia and influenza death rates for persons age 65 and older	Death certificates	Health care providers Health care plans State health agencies Local health agencies Business, industry Community organizations Special health risk groups General public
Individual Response	Ensure that Medicare enrollees are immunized appropriately	Percentage of Medicare enrollees who received an influenza immunization during the previous year; percentage who have ever received a pneumococcal pneumonia immunization	Immunization registry or medical charts	Health care providers Health care plans State health agencies Local health agencies Community organizations Special health risk groups General public
	Ensure that children are immunized appropriately	Immunization rate for children at 24 months of age		
Social Environment	Ensure that populations with special health risks are immunized appropriately	Immunization rate at 24 months of age for children currently enrolled in Medicaid	Immunization registry or medical charts	Health care providers State health agencies Local health agencies Special health risk groups

	Reduce financial barriers to immunization	Among children with commercial health insurance, percentage with full coverage for immunization	Employers, insurance licensing authority	Health care plans Local government Business, industry General public
	Provide leadership for immunization efforts	Existence in the community of an active childhood immunization coalition		Health care providers Health care plans State health agencies Local health agencies Local government Business, industry Education agencies and institutions Community organizations Special health risk groups General public
Health Care	Ensure that the health care system is organized to provide high immunization rates	Immunization rate for children at 24 months of age	Immunization registry or medical charts	Health care providers Health care plans State health agencies Local health agencies Business and industry Community organizations Special health risk groups General public
		Immunization rate at 24 months of age for children currently enrolled in managed care organizations	Immunization registry or medical charts	Health care providers Health care plans Business and industry General public

continued on next page

TABLE A.8-1 *Continued*

Field Model Domain	Construct	Sample Indicators	Data Sources	Stakeholders
Health Care (*continued*)		Existence in the community of a computerized immunization registry; if available, percentage of children in the community included	Immunization registry, birth records	Health care providers Health care plans State health agencies Local health agencies General public
	Ensure that Medicare enrollees are immunized appropriately	Percentage of Medicare enrollees who received an influenza immunization during the previous year; percentage who have ever received a pneumococcal pneumonia immunization		

A.9

Prototype Indicator Set: Violence

BACKGROUND

Violence is one of America's most challenging and concerning public health problems. More than 2 million Americans are victims of violent injury each year (USDHHS, 1995), and violence is increasingly identified as one of the major concerns cited by citizens in urban and nonurban communities around the country (Rosenberg and Fenley, 1991). Although the public fears random violence, most violent acts are committed by individuals well known to the victim.

Violence is an issue that involves society at large; its causes and consequences permeate all sectors of a community. The committee acknowledges that violence is an issue for which measurement strategies are not standardized and health professionals have poorly defined roles. The prototype indicator set is intended to move the discussion of violence forward, not to be a final word on the issue. The committee chose to include this issue because the health effects of violence are clearly a major area of public concern.

The violent death rate (including both homicide and suicide) in the United States exceeds that of all other industrialized nations and constitutes the fourth leading cause of years of potential life lost prior to age 65 in the United States. Homicide is the leading cause of death in African American males aged 15–34 and the second leading cause for young white men aged 15–24. Violence leads to many injuries as well as deaths, some of which require health care in hospital emergency rooms and other settings. In 1992, about 1 per 10,000 Americans suffered assault injuries (USDHHS, 1995).

The costs of violence are high—estimated at $54,000 per attempted or completed rape, $19,200 per robbery, and $16,000 per assault. A portion of these costs are financial, but the majority reflect pain, suffering, the risk of death, psychological damage, and reduced quality of life (NRC, 1993). Although violence affects all segments of American society, minorities are substantially more likely to be victims of violent crime. In 1990, for instance, African Americans were 41 percent and Hispanics 32 percent more likely than whites to be victims of violent crime (NRC, 1993).

Violent actions including rape, domestic violence, drive-by shootings, and terrorist attacks are highlighted daily in all forms of media. The issues of violence in our society are also highlighted in the content of television fiction and nonfiction programming. It is estimated that by age 18, children will have been exposed to 18,000 televised murders and 800 suicides; most will have seen 100,000 acts of violence on television by the sixth grade (Canterwall, 1992).

Substance use and psychosocial, family-mediated factors are major risk factors for violent behavior. Social factors associated with violence include concentration of poor families in geographic areas, income inequality, population turnover, community transition, family disruption, housing density and other aspects of social disruption, and opportunities for violence such as illegal markets in drugs and firearms (NRC, 1993). Dysfunctional family life (e.g., absent or divorced parents, turmoil and fighting between family members) is an early predictor of violence, especially for youth. Witnessing violence in the home and community is harmful to children and youth exposed to the violent event, even if they are not victims of the violence. Thus, as more violence occurs in homes, in neighborhoods, and in the media, greater percentages of the population are at risk to experience violence.

Criminal justice, health care, education, social services, and other community institutions can address the effects of violence and help prevent it. Strategies range from passing and enforcing strong gun control laws, to more punitive sentencing guidelines and building more jails, to community education and outreach programs aimed at violence prevention. Others focus on addressing the underlying causes of violence such as substance abuse and social disintegration.

Violence has been widely viewed as a health issue since the 1985 Surgeon General's Workshop on Violence and Health encouraged health professionals to address violence of all types. Violence is also one of the priority targets identified in *Healthy People 2000: National Health Promotion and Disease Prevention Objectives* (USDHHS, 1991). Specific objectives are included for homicide, suicide, weapons-related deaths, assault injuries, rape, adolescent suicide attempts, adolescent weapons carrying, and other issues. In 1995, "weapons" was changed to "firearms" and an additional objective was added regarding laws requiring the proper storage of firearms to minimize access and the likelihood of discharge by minors (USDHHS, 1995).

"FIELD" SET OF PERFORMANCE INDICATORS

As indicated above, the causes and consequences of violence are broad and diverse, and cover many domains of the field model. Thus, it is possible to measure many dimensions of violence, its consequences, and its risk factors that shed light on the efforts of various community entities to address it.

Health and Function, Disease

The direct effects of violence include physical injury, death, and psychological problems. These can be measured through vital statistics (indicators 1 and 2, below), hospital discharge data (indicator 3), or survey data (indicator 4).

1. Homicide rate per 100,000 people.

2. Firearm-related deaths per 100,000 people.

Both of these indicators, which are included in *Healthy People 2000*, can be calculated from vital statistics even at the local level. For small communities, however, the number of cases will be small and the number rather than the rate should be reported.

3. Number of emergency department visits related to violence, particularly gunshot wounds.

Data to measure this indicator may be available from hospital emergency department databases in states that E-code injury visits (i.e., Missouri and Nebraska). In areas that have not yet implemented E-coding of emergency department visits, information on the number of gunshot wounds may be available from police departments, since the reporting of such incidents is generally required by law. Police data, however, may underestimate the number of visits. A review of emergency room logs and records would provide this information.

4. **Number of assault injuries among people aged 12 and over.** This measure, which appears in *Healthy People 2000*, can be ascertained from police records, program data from rape crisis centers and shelters for victims of domestic violence, or population surveys.

Well-Being

Well-being can depend directly on the physical or psychological consequences of violence, but these dimensions are probably best measured directly. The one dimension that is not captured in health-related statistics is the effect on well-being of concerns about individual safety. A community might reduce fear of violence in three ways: (1) by reducing the actual risk of violence, (2) by helping people adapt to the possibility of violence by giving them information on how to alter their behavior to remain safe, and (3) by making information available regarding the true risks, which might be lower than people think. One way to measure this dimension is as follows:

1. **Restriction of activities due to fear of violence.** Although not now generally available, population surveys could include questions to determine whether people fear violence enough to change their behavior or to measure specific activity restrictions (e.g., not going out at night or alone, not going to certain neighborhoods).

Individual Response

Violence is a complex problem of human behavior, so there are many ways to measure "individual response" to the social and physical environments associated with it. Some possible measures are as follows:

1. **Suicide rate per 100,000.**
2. **Number of suicide attempts by adolescents aged 14 to 19.** Suicide is an important component of violence, which is re-

flected in the fact that both of these indicators are included in *Healthy People 2000.* The first indicator can be obtained from vital statistics even in small communities, but the number of cases may be small. If so, the number rather than the rate should be reported. Suicide attempts could be tracked through a hospital-based surveillance system for those cases serious enough to require inpatient or emergency care.

3. Number of rapes and attempted rapes.

Rape is an extreme form of sexual violence, and is addressed by *Healthy People 2000.* Data on reported rapes and rape attempts can be obtained through police reports and crime victim surveys, but these are thought to underestimate the true extent of the problem.

4. Prevalence of child maltreatment.

5. Prevalence of physical abuse of women by male partners.

6. Prevalence of elder abuse.

The three measures reflect the most common forms of domestic or family violence. Although there are mandatory reporting requirements for child abuse in most states, actual reports of domestic violence to police and child protective services probably reflect only a small portion of the events that take place. Furthermore, although there are multiple reports for some children, the available statistics have usually not been analyzed to indicate how many individual children have been involved. Unlike child abuse, health professionals and others are not required in most states to report cases of domestic or elder abuse, so data are likely to be even more incomplete. Domestic violence can be detected in population surveys, and indeed *Healthy People 2000* relies on survey data for baseline estimates for the first two of these indicators.

7. Number of confirmed child abuse cases reported to authorities; percentage of confirmed cases receiving child protective services and appropriate medical care.

8. Number of restraining orders to protect women from domestic violence.

9. Number of batterers tried by the court system; percentage convicted or referred to treatment.

The courts and child protective systems can provide information on two dimensions of violence. First, numbers of violence-related cases in the courts and in child protective services indicate something about the prevalence of violent acts in the community. Only a small proportion of violent events ever reach the courts and protective services, however, so if the percentage changes over time because of changed social norms about reporting, increased efficiency of the system, or other factors, changes in numbers of cases may not reflect changes in the prevalence of violence in the community. Data from the courts and protective services also can indicate something about the performance of those systems: Do investigators appropriately identify true cases of abuse, and does the system take the proper protective action? However, since reporting patterns may change over time (leading to higher or lower proportions of "true" cases among those reported) and courts and protective service determinations are not infallible, trends in the number or percentage of "positive outcomes" of these systems should be interpreted with caution. In addition, rates of substantiation or service referrals depend on the availability of resources for support services.

10. Incidence of physical fighting among adolescents.
11. Incidence of weapons carrying among adolescents.
12. Prevalence of substance abuse among youth and adults.

Violent behavior is more common among youth than at older or younger ages, so some of the measures of individual response ought to focus on youth violence. Substance abuse is a major contributor to violent behavior in a community, and can be measured through school-based as well as population surveys.

Health Care

Two types of measures can be used to address the role of health care in relation to violence: injuries resulting from violence that require health care and opportunities to prevent violence. Some possible measures are as follows:

1. Cost of care for intentional injuries (total and firearm injuries).

As indicated above, the costs of the physical and psychological consequences of violence are high. One measure of these costs might be obtained from emergency department and hospital discharge records, but this information is not available on a regular basis. Furthermore, such information must be interpreted carefully, since health care costs are only a small part of the costs of violence (NRC, 1993), and records for an initial hospital visit usually do not reflect follow-up treatment.

2. Number of people in substance abuse programs.

Because substance abuse is a major contributor to violence in a community, utilization of substance abuse programs is one way that a community can measure the contribution of the health sector to the prevention of violence. The number of people in such programs, however, may be due to both the availability of programs and the needs of the population. Ideally, it would be preferable to measure the proportion of those that need substance abuse programs that utilize them, but denominator data for this measure are generally not available. Thus, trends in utilization per se should be interpreted with caution.

3. Existence of protocols for health care professionals to identify, treat, and properly refer for further services individuals who attempt suicide; victims of sexual assault; and victims of spouse, elder, and child abuse.

4. Existence of child death review systems.

5. Proportion of children identified as neglected or physically or sexually abused who receive physical and mental evaluation with appropriate follow-up.

Injuries, including death, resulting from violence are not always easy to identify. Careful review of cases that present to health officials can help identify situations in which violence occurs, ensure that the victims and their caretakers receive the services they need, and provide an opportunity to prevent further violence in the future. These measures suggest actions that the health sector can take to respond to violence and contribute to its prevention.

Social Environment

As indicated above, the social factors associated with violence include concentration of poor families in geographic areas, income inequality, population turnover, community transition, family disruption, housing density and other measures of social disruption, and opportunities for violence such as illegal markets in drugs and firearms (NRC, 1993). Only some of these factors are amenable to public health or public policy interventions, at least in the short run, but communities might want to monitor all of them to help understand the causes of violence, and to target interventions to the areas in which they are most needed.

1. Concentration of poor families in geographic areas.

Of all of the underlying social factors associated with violence, this might be easiest to measure in communities because of income data available from the decennial census, even at the census block level. It would be important to measure not just level of income, but the concentration of poverty in small areas and disparities with other areas. It might also be possible to measure such items as vacant housing units and the proportion of families that own their own homes.

2. Opportunities for violence such as gangs, illegal markets, and firearms in the community.

Gangs, illegal markets, and firearms are typical of the situations in a community's social environment that provide opportunities for violence. Although the presence of such situations is difficult to represent in statistical terms, the use of focus groups and other observational techniques for documenting the existence of contributors to violence in a community would be an important measure of the performance of the police and criminal justice system and of local policymakers concerned with housing, economic development, and so on.

3. Use of community policing techniques.

"Community policing" is the policy by which police are assigned to specific neighborhoods and spend most of their time there solving problems before they lead to serious trouble. The premise of this policy is that if police are thought of as members of the community, they can contribute to an improved sense of security and intervene early to prevent violence and other crimes before they occur. Initial studies suggest that this approach can be effective (Fleissner and Heinzelmann, 1996).

4. Number of hours of violence-related programming on television most watched by children and youth.

Violence on television contributes to a social norm that condones or even glamorizes violence. As such, violence on television is a measure of the private sector's concern for the community, as well as the community's political will to control the forces that impact the health of its members.

5. Gun control laws.

The availability of guns in the community is an important proximal risk factor for violence. Gun control laws can address the sale, possession, storage, or use of guns and can address various types of weapons from assault rifles to concealable handguns.

6. Availability of shelters for battered women and their children.

Shelters provide opportunities for women in abusive relationships to remove themselves and their children from a situation in which violence is likely to continue or to increase. The availability of shelters, which can be represented by the number of beds or perhaps the number of women turned away in times of need (USDHHS, 1991), is one measure of the contribution of community-based, often religious, organizations that typically provide these shelters.

Physical Environment

1. Percentage of youth reporting carrying weapons to school.

The availability of weapons is an important situational factor in the causal chain leading to violence (NRC, 1993). From a public health perspective, reducing the number of weapons in the school environment is analogous to removing the vector that transmits disease. Data on youth possession of weapons, including guns, at school could be obtained from school records of children found with weapons or from school-based surveys.

Genetic Endowment

Although there are some preliminary reports of genetic predisposition to violent behavior, not enough is known at this time to suggest performance measures in this area.

Prosperity

As indicated above, a community's prosperity both depends on and affects violence. Violence carries high economic costs, not only in treating its direct effects, but in terms of pain and suffering, psychological damage, and reduced quality of life. Similarly, economic factors, especially income inequality, are important risk factors for violence. These factors, however, are difficult to measure on a community basis and are reflected in other measures proposed above, so no specific measures are proposed in this area.

SAMPLE SET OF INDICATORS

From the preceding list of potential indicators, the following 12 are proposed as a primary set that might be used to monitor the performance of the community as a whole and of specific segments within it. Their selection reflects the committee's best judgment, but individual communities must consider available resources, including the availability of data. Comments on other uses of the measures (e.g., in *Healthy People 2000*), data and measurement issues, and suggestions of where accountability may lie are presented for each of the measures. The relatively large number of indicators in this suggested set reflects the varied forms of violence, causal factors for violence, and possible preventive and remedial interventions.

Of the five measures of the physical consequences of violence, one (firearm-related deaths) can be obtained from vital statistics in every community. The others (assault injuries, rapes, abuse of women by partners, and suicides attempts) might be obtained from a combination of police reports (e.g., through the Uniform Crime Reports System [FBI, 1994]) and state-based hospital discharge data systems. Data from these sources are also available at the local level, but both may underrepresent the actual number of cases for a variety of reasons. A population survey will be necessary to measure one of the proposed indicators (restriction in activities due to fear of violence) and could supplement official records of the nonfatal consequences of violence.

1. Firearm-related deaths per 100,000 people.

This indicator is the most reliable and valid of the proposed set. It is easily obtainable in a timely manner from public health departments, but it may be difficult to use as a performance measure in small communities because the number of firearm-related deaths will usually be small. With small numbers, changes are difficult to attribute to any of the accountable entities in the community. This indicator measures not only the outcome of violence, but also something about the risk factors for violence in the community and interventions such as gun control laws to control these risks. This indicator is included in *Healthy People 2000*.

2. Number of assault injuries among people aged 12 and over.

Data for this indicator should be available from hospital discharge data, police records, and population surveys. Each source is likely to be incomplete, but together they should yield an accurate representation of the situation in the community. The E-coding of hospital discharge data (to indicate the cause of injuries) would help to identify assault cases, but it is not uniformly done throughout the country.

3. Number of rapes and attempted rapes.
4. Prevalence of physical abuse of women by male partners.
5. Number of suicide attempts by adolescents aged 14 to 19.

Data for these three indicators can be obtained from police and medical records, as well as from a population survey. Care must be taken to preserve the confidentiality of the individuals concerned.

6. Restriction of activities due to fear of violence.

This indicator, for which data must be obtained from a population survey, measures adverse effects on well-being that are not captured in health-related data. Although not now generally available, population surveys could include questions either to determine whether people fear violence enough to change their behavior or to measure specific activity restrictions (e.g., not going out at night or alone, not going to certain neighborhoods).

7. Number of hours of violence-related programming on television most watched by children and youth.

There are no standard measures of this indicator now, but the voluntary classification system agreed to by the television industry in 1996 will provide a starting point for definitions for measuring the amount of violence-related programming.

8. Percentage of youth reporting carrying weapons to school.

This measure reflects both individual response and the physical environment. Data can be obtained from school and police records and from student surveys. A version of this indicator appears in *Healthy People 2000.*

9. Number of confirmed child abuse cases reported to authorities; percentage of confirmed cases receiving child protective services and appropriate medical care.

Although not reported in a consistently reliable and valid manner, the number of confirmed child abuse cases in a community is an indicator of the level of violence in families. Data on the number of cases are available from child protective service systems (NCCAN, 1996). The number of confirmed cases reflects the ability of the health care and education systems, as well as others in the community, to detect possible cases as well as the true incidence of child abuse. The second part of this indicator—the percentage of abused children receiving appropriate social and medical services—measures the ability of these systems to respond to identified needs. Determining whether the services provided are adequate and appropriate is a judgment that must be made in each community, informed by scientific evidence about the kinds of programs that are effective.

10. Existence of protocols for health care professionals to identify, treat, and properly refer for further services individuals who attempt suicide; victims of sexual assault; and victims of spouse, elder, and child abuse.

This indicator measures the capacity of the health care system to appropriately identify, treat, and refer victims of violence for further treatment and other services that may prevent future occurrences. There are no specific quantitative measures of the availability of these protocols, so implementation of this indicator will depend on judgment relevant to local circumstances.

11. Use of community policing techniques.

The implementation of community policing can be measured by the number or proportion of police on community policing beats or by the number of blocks of the community covered by a community policing approach.

12. Gun control laws.

The effect of gun control laws on the actual possession or use of guns will be difficult to measure, but their effect might be seen, for instance, in the proportion of homicides or robberies in which guns were involved. Rather than a statistical measure, an analysis of the strength of national, state, and local gun control laws and their implementation would be an appropriate indicator for the law enforcement sector.

The measures include the primary forms of violence that have been the focus of the public health community's concern and interventions: child abuse (indicators 9 and 10), violence against women (indicators 3, 4, and 10), youth violence (indicators 5, 7, and 8), and gun-related violence (indicators 1, 8, and 12). The proposed set combines measures of the direct effects of violence (indicators 1–5), one measure of the long-term social consequences of violence (indicator 6), measures relating to predisposing factors for violence (indicators 7 and 8), measures of the quality of the treatment of its effects (indicators 9 and 10), and measures related to community efforts to prevent violence (indicators 11 and 12).

The direct measures of violence (indicators 1–6) reflect many factors in the community, and are indicative of the community's efforts as a whole to control violence. The indicators that measure the potential contributions of the schools (indicators 8 and 9), the media (indicator 7), the police and the criminal justice system (indicators 11 and 12), and the health care system (indicators 9 and 10), suggest specific actions for which these sectors in the community can be held accountable.

REFERENCES

Canterwall, B.S. 1992. Television and Violence: The Scale of the Problem and Where We Go from Here. *Journal of the American Medical Association* 267:3059–3063.

FBI (Federal Bureau of Investigation). 1994. *Crime in the United States, 1994.* Washington, D.C.: Government Printing Office.

Fleissner, D., and Heinzelmann, F. 1996. *Crime Prevention Through Environmental Design and Community Policing.* Research in Action Series. Washington, D.C.: U.S. Department of Justice, National Institute of Justice.

NCCAN (National Center on Child Abuse and Neglect). 1996. *Child Maltreatment 1994: Reports from the States to the National Center on Child Abuse and Neglect.* Washington, D.C.: U.S. Government Printing Office.

NRC (National Research Council). 1993. *Understanding and Preventing Violence.* A.J. Reiss, Jr., and J.A. Roth, eds. Washington, D.C.: National Academy Press.

Rosenberg, M.L., and Fenley, M.A., eds. 1991. *Violence in America: A Public Health Approach.* New York: Oxford University Press.

USDHHS (U.S. Department of Health and Human Services). 1991. *Healthy People 2000: National Health Promotion and Disease Prevention Objectives.* DHHS Pub. No. (PHS) 91-50212. Washington, D.C.: Office of the Assistant Secretary for Health.

USDHHS. 1995. *Healthy People 2000: Midcourse Review and 1995 Revisions.* Washington, D.C.: USDHHS, Public Health Service.

TABLE A.9-1 Field Model Mapping for Sample Indicator Set: Violence

Field Model Domain	Construct	Sample Indicators	Data Sources
Health and Function, Disease	Violence-related mortality and morbidity	Firearm-related deaths per 100,000 people	Vital statistics
		Number of assault injuries among people aged 12 and over	Police records, program data, population surveys
Individual Response	Frequency of sexual violence	Number of rapes and attempted rapes	Police records, surveys
	Frequency of domestic violence	Prevalence of physical abuse of women by male partners	State health department; police records
		Number of confirmed child abuse cases reported to authorities; percentage of confirmed cases receiving protective services and appropriate medical care	Child protective services data
	Prevalence of self-directed violence	Number of suicide attempts by adolescents aged 14–19	State health department, program data, hospital discharge databases
Well-being	General impact of violence in personal activities	Restriction of activities due to fear of violence	Survey required

Social Environment	Atmosphere that supports violence	Number of hours of violence-related programming on television most watched by children and youth	Television industry voluntary classification system
	Law enforcement prevention activities	Use of community policing techniques	Police department
	Legislative changes to decrease violence	Gun control laws	Police department, state and local statutes
Health Care	Professional awareness and support for victims of violence	Existence of protocols for health care professionals to identify, treat, and properly refer individuals who attempt suicide; victims of sexual assault; victims of spouse, elder, and child abuse	Surveys
Physical Environment	Environmental hazards	Percentage of youth reporting carrying weapons to school	State health department (*Healthy People 2000* indicator data), surveys, education department, school districts

B

Methodological Issues in Developing Community Health Profiles and Performance Indicator Sets

Michael A. Stoto

The focus of this report is on developing the conceptual framework for a community health improvement process (CHIP) by which communities can use health profiles and performance measures to marshal the forces in their communities to improve the health of populations. Because of this focus, much of the committee's attention to the development of community health profiles and performance indicator sets has been focused on content issues. When it comes to the implementation of these concepts in actual communities, however, a number of practical, methodological issues often arise. Because the development of measures must depend on local circumstances as well as the available data, this appendix cannot provide cookbook solutions to statistical issues. Rather, it discusses these issues so as to inform those wishing to develop performance measures in local communities.

To address these points, this appendix draws on positive and negative examples from *Healthy People 2000* (USDHHS, 1991), as discussed in "Public Health Assessment in the 1990s" (Stoto, 1992b). The objectives in *Healthy People 2000* are not performance measures per se, but that report is a major point of reference for many in public health and its objectives do provide starting points for CHIPs to consider. Most of the objectives in *Healthy People 2000* are carefully written, but others illustrate a number of methodological and statistical problems that should be avoided.

SPECIFICATION OF PERFORMANCE INDICATORS

Performance measures must be carefully specified so that they truly measure the performance of accountable entities rather than other changes in a community's health. If the results are to be interpreted with confidence, careful development and testing are needed to ensure that the objectives are operationalized in a clear and unambiguous way. For the HEDIS (Health Plan Employer Data and Information Set) measures, for instance, substantial time and effort was required to develop precise definitions that make sense in a variety of managed care settings and are obtainable from readily available data files (NCQA, 1993). Even a measure that seems simple, such as the proportion of children at age 24 months who have received all of the recommended immunizations, requires agreement on which immunizations are recommended at what time, decisions about whether to include children who have not been covered by the health plan since birth, and so on.

Performance measures must be written in a statistically operational form. When they are not, it can be difficult to tell what progress is being made, even if all of the information is in hand. For example, *Healthy People 2000* Objective 7.17 calls for local jurisdictions to have "coordinated, comprehensive violence prevention programs." Although a long list of attributes of coordinated and comprehensive programs is given in the text, no operational definition is provided by which to judge whether a particular jurisdiction's program is coordinated and comprehensive. It would be better to identify a small number of performance indicators connecting accountable entities to specific actions, as illustrated in the committee's prototype violence indicator set (Appendix A).

Problems of this sort often arise when one does not distinguish between general health issues and operational measures of these issues. Rarely are data available in the precise form policymakers prefer, so concessions must be made to data constraints. The presentation of the performance measures should reflect this compromise by separately identifying the issues to be monitored and the best available data or proxy variables for those issues and by stating targets in terms of the measurable quantities. For example, *Healthy People 2000* measures the initiation of cigarette smoking by children and youth as the proportion of cigarette smokers in the 20-24 age group. The actual measure is smoking prevalence, not initiation. This is appropriate, however, because prevalence rates are easier to obtain from population surveys and because initiation rather than cessation is thought to be the dominant force for young people.

Measures should be both valid and reliable and both sensitive and specific (Sofaer, 1995). Practical problems often require compromises in these respects. *Healthy People 2000* Objective 15.1 on coronary heart disease exemplifies the problem. The objective addresses the coronary heart disease mortality rate because this component of overall cardiovascular mortality is the most amenable to prevention efforts. The specific grouping of diagnostic codes used to define coronary heart disease is not, however, routinely available in vital statistics reports. In many communities, it might be more appropriate to measure progress in terms of readily available cardiovascular mortality rates, while bearing in mind that reduction beyond a certain point is unlikely.

Lacking population-based data on the incidence or prevalence of specific diseases, performance measure developers often think about using numbers of people receiving treatment for the disease in question. For instance, *Healthy People 2000* Objective 15.3 calls for a reversal in the increasing number of people with "end-stage renal disease (requiring dialysis or transplantation)." The baseline figures cited, however, count the number of people *receiving* dialysis or transplantation, not those *requiring* it. Thus, these trends reflect changes in diagnostic and treatment patterns as well as access through an expanding federal program, and it is doubtful whether future changes in the data can be attributed to the success of prevention activities as intended by *Healthy People 2000*. In certain circumstances, however, hospital treatment data can yield appropriate performance measures. For instance, an Institute of Medicine (IOM, 1993) report on measuring access to health care identifies a number of "ambulatory care sensitive conditions" for which hospital admissions should be avoidable if individuals have access to appropriate ambulatory care.

UNIT OF ANALYSIS

When a performance measure calls for action by a number of similar entities in the community such as schools, work sites, and health care plans, there are basically two ways to create performance measures. A community can measure the proportion of entities taking the action, as in Objective 3.11 of *Healthy People 2000*:

- Increase to at least 75 percent the proportion of worksites with a formal smoking policy that prohibits or severely restricts smoking at the workplace.

With a measure worded in this way, a small community with only four work sites could meet the goal if the three smallest sites had smoking policies. If, however, the one work site without a policy was very large, only a minority of the community would receive the benefits of nonsmoking policies. Alternatively, a community can measure the proportion of people affected by an action, as in Objective 1.8 of *Healthy People 2000*:

- Increase to at least 50 percent the proportion of children and adolescents in 1st through 12th grade who participate in daily school physical education.

In technical terms, the difference between these two types of measures is that the latter can be thought of as a weighted average, where the weights correspond to the number of students in each school. In practical terms, the first sort of measure can be obtained simply from a survey of a small number of work sites, schools, or similar entities. The second requires a population survey or at least some calculations based on numbers of people associated with each entity. The first type of measure also tends to suggest that the impetus for action is with the work site (or school), whereas the second focuses on the individual.

INTERPRETATION OF SURVEY DATA

Population-based health interview surveys provide many of the health status measures that are used in *Healthy People 2000* and are potentially available for performance measures. Trends in health interview data, however, can be difficult to interpret (Wilson and Drury, 1984). The U.S. National Health Interview Survey (Adams and Marano, 1995), an important source of data for the year 2000 objectives, measures the annual incidence of acute conditions and the prevalence of chronic conditions through a combination of open- and closed-ended questions about the presence of specific diseases and conditions. A common finding from these data has been that chronic illness and disability have been increasing at the same time that mortality (even for related diseases) has been falling. At least part of this increase does not reflect actual worsening in physical illness. Methodological explanations that may account for the trend include (1) improved survey design that may have increased the proportion of the population reporting diseases and conditions that exist; (2) improved access to medical care and better screening efforts that may have increased the proportion of the population diagnosed with and therefore aware of asymptomatic disease; and (3) changing role expectations and improved disability benefits that may have increased the proportion of the population reporting a work-related disability.

Complex questions are also difficult to monitor through population surveys. Consider, for example, *Healthy People 2000* Objective 5.8:

- Increase to at least 85 percent the proportion of people aged 10 through 18 who have discussed human sexuality, including values surrounding sexuality, with their parents and/or have received information through another parentally endorsed source, such as youth, school, or religious programs.

Although survey data could provide information on aspects of this objective, specific questions would have to be designed to assess the proportion of adolescents that meet the specific criteria implied.

COMPARISONS ACROSS TIME AND COMMUNITIES

To assess the meaning of performance measures, CHIPs can examine trends over time or can compare their results with an externally set benchmark or with other communities in the same state. Each of these comparisons can provide valuable insights, but this requires that measures be operationalized in a way that will permit meaningful comparisons. Health outcomes measures from hospitals or health care systems, for instance, should be risk adjusted so that they do not inadvertently attribute variations that are a function of population case mix or severity of illness to differential system performance (Sofaer, 1995). Even something as simple as population estimates for use as denominators in rates must be carefully examined. In Massachusetts, for example, adolescent fertility rates calculated using state demographic estimates were found differ substantially from those obtained when population estimates from national sources were used (D.K. Walker, personal communication, 1996). When comparing across states, denominator data for all should be from the same source.

Healthy People 2000 presents numerical targets for most of the national objectives, which can provide a starting point for local benchmarking. To determine meaningful local benchmarks, CHIPs must, in addition to standardizing for population composition, take into account differences from national values in baseline rates and trends in the measures in question. Benchmarks can also be set by comparison with other geographic areas or with epidemiological models that account for important risk factors in the population.

There are a number of statistical models that can help CHIPs set meaningful benchmarks. None of these can be used on a strictly mechanical basis, and all require significant subject matter judgment. These methods can, however, give some idea of what is likely to happen in the absence of further interventions or indicate the likely impact of interventions on outcomes. Thus, models can help to set or to fine-tune the benchmarks.

The most straightforward statistical model is simple trend analysis. Such models can predict the level of various objective measures—assuming that current trends continue—as well as provide statistical confidence intervals. Benchmarks should usually be somewhat more favorable than the results that trend analysis suggests will be achieved without any intervention (Stoto, 1989).

Models that identify the lowest possible morbidity and mortality rates observed in specific groups could also be useful in setting targets. Such groups could be other countries or geographic, racial, ethnic, or socioeconomic subpopulations of the United States. Woolsey (1981), for instance, has proposed a version of this. Hahn and colleagues (1990) have estimated the possible reduction in mortality rates that can be expected with the elimination of the most important risk factors for chronic disease.

Mathematical models that relate health outcomes to specific interventions for many specific diseases and health behaviors can also be helpful in setting benchmarks. For instance, the National Cancer Institute has developed a model to project cancer incidence and mortality under various cancer control programs such as prevention programs, screening, and treatment (Levin et al., 1986). Such models require more data than simple trend analyses and take time to develop and verify. In addition, there can be substantial uncertainties in modeling interventions and the interactions among them. The modeling process itself, however, helps to focus discussion and thinking, and leads to a range of plausible benchmark values. Similar models have been, or are being, developed for cardiovascular disease, AIDS, and other diseases (e.g.,

Weinstein et al., 1987). Using such models as appropriate, *Closing the Gap* (Amler and Dull, 1987) synthesizes much of what is known about the potential health effects of health promotion and disease prevention.

Simple extrapolation models and process models such as the one for cancer form two extremes of a spectrum. Extrapolation models that take into account age–period–cohort effects, projected demographic changes, and other factors (Brown and Kessler, 1988) fall between the two and offer some promise.

DATA FOR LOCAL AREAS

If performance monitoring is to achieve its potential for community health improvement, communities of all sizes—states, counties, municipalities, and other groups such as a company's employees and their families—must adopt their own objectives and measure progress toward them. Counties, cities, and smaller communities, however, often find that local-level data are unavailable or of poorer quality than national data. For instance, in assessing the ability of states to monitor the draft year 2000 objectives prepared in 1989, the Public Health Foundation (1990) found that, on average, states could monitor only 39 percent of the objectives, and the situation is clearly worse for smaller communities. Obtaining community-level data for specific racial, ethnic, and socioeconomic groups is even more difficult.

CHIPs will generally not be able to obtain appropriate data simply by disaggregating national survey data. No national survey is likely to have a large enough sample to provide reliable direct estimates for all of the subpopulations of interest. Furthermore, up-to-date community-level denominator data by race, ethnicity, and socioeconomic status are not generally available from the U.S. Census Bureau. Rather than a single national survey, survey methodologies that can be replicated easily at the community level need to be developed. The Behavioral Risk Factor Surveillance System (BRFSS), developed by the Centers for Disease Control and Prevention (CDC) but implemented by the states (Siegel et al., 1993), might serve as a model.

Even when data are available for small geographical areas, as they are for vital statistics, the events are infrequent, thereby making the rates unreliable. One approach to the problem of sparse data is to use measures that are stable at the local level as proxies for measures used in the national objectives. For instance, a local health department might choose to monitor infant health in terms of the proportion of low birth weight babies rather than the infant mortality rate. Because the proportion of babies born with low birth weight is higher than the proportion who die, this rate is more reliable for small areas. In choosing such proxy measures, however, it is important to verify that changes in the proposed measure truly reflect changes in the health characteristic to be monitored.

Another approach is to use formal statistical methods designed for small areas. These are not yet commonly used in public health assessment but are discussed below because they warrant further development.

ADMINISTRATIVE RECORDS

Because of the relative lack of survey data at the community level, many of the indicators proposed in Appendix A are derived from administrative records. Administrative data arise from the day-to-day management of a system such as a health care delivery organization, and they usually arise from the records needed to provide appropriate services to individual patients or clients. They frequently come from encounters with health care or service providers, but administrative data rarely include health status measures for any defined population. The administrative data cited in the prototype indicator sets include records from managed care organizations and other health care delivery systems. Administrative records from a variety of public and private organizations (e.g., local welfare agencies and private employers) can also provide valuable data for performance monitoring in CHIPs. Examples include hospital discharge data, including diagnoses, procedures completed, and perhaps even outcomes; public assistance records on immunization and other factors for covered children; and employment records that include health-related data.

With the widespread and increasing use of computerized record systems to manage service delivery in health care, government agencies, and private companies, the growth in the availability of administrative records can fill an important data gap at the community level. Administrative records can be more timely and less costly than special-purpose statistical data systems. On the other hand, administrative records usually relate to services provided to certain individuals, not to the overall need for services or to the health status of the entire population of a community (Hoaglin et al., 1982).

Use of administrative data may also be complicated by the

lack of an appropriate denominator. Indemnity insurers, for instance, often know only the number of "covered lives" in their plan and nothing about the characteristics of that population. With data of this sort, crude per capita rates are the only possible measures; determining the proportions of people in certain demographic groups or with certain health needs is not possible. With such data it is not possible, for instance, to assess the proportion of women age 50 and over who have had mammograms in the past two years.

For example, consider the following indicators from *Healthy People 2000*:

- Increase to at least 75 percent the proportion of adults who have had their blood cholesterol checked within the preceding 5 years (Objective 15.14).
- Reduce the prevalence of blood cholesterol levels of 240 mg/dL or greater to no more than 20 percent among adults (Objective 15.7).

On the national level, these proportions can be measured accurately through a population-based survey, the National Health and Nutrition Examination Survey (NHANES). On the local level, a CHIP might try to gather such data from health care records or perhaps even from records of employee screening programs.

With regard to the first of these two objectives, one is likely to find that data on the percentage of health plan members who have had their cholesterol checked is available only from managed care organizations, and probably only from those with good cholesterol screening programs. Thus, the data likely would be biased upward. The second of these two objectives can be calculated only for those whose serum cholesterol has been tested. Since this may not be a representative group, the proportion with high cholesterol levels may be greater than in the general population. Trends in these measures can yield information on the performance of the health plans that are covered, but only when interpreted with caution. An increase in the proportion of people screened for cholesterol would indicate a positive performance, as long as the population base did not change because of the addition of people more likely to have been screened for reasons unconnected to the plan. An increase in the proportion of those tested with high levels would be a negative result, unless it was the result of screening a large number of new, high-risk plan members.

STANDARDIZATION

Standardization methods are used to account for demographic changes in a single population over time. For instance, if there were no changes in the age-specific cancer rates between 1987 and 2000, aging of the population alone would cause the overall death rate to increase from 195.9 to 217.1 per 100,000, given the Census Bureau's median population projection for the United States. It is important to understand this sort of pattern when vital statistics are used as performance measures: an increase to only 200.0 per 100,000 would actually be an advance (Stoto, 1992a).

Standardization also serves a second, very different purpose, because some of the differences that exist between communities reflect differences in population composition rather than differences in underlying rates. Communities differ in the age, race, and sex composition of their population, so communities with the same age-, race-, and sex-specific death rates will have different crude death rates, both overall and cause specific. In setting benchmarks for performance measures, communities should look at the national target set in *Healthy People 2000* or some other source, as well as current rates of other communities. This comparison makes sense only if differences in the composition of the national and community populations are "removed." If all communities are adjusted to the same standard population, standardization provides a bridge from the national targets to state and local benchmarks.

For some purposes, however, standardization could lead to difficulties. Some CHIPs will want to consider setting priorities among health issues. Many factors go into such choices, but the current level of mortality associated with a disease or other health problem is a major one. Standardized rates present a different impression about the relative importance of various causes of death than unstandardized rates. For example, unintentional injuries have a somewhat higher mortality rate than cerebrovascular diseases when adjusted to the 1940 population (35.0 versus 29.7 per 100,000), but the crude cerebrovascular mortality rate is more than 50 percent higher than the crude unintentional injury mortality rate (61.2 versus 39.5 per 100,000).

The choice of a standard can make a substantial difference. Compare, for example, the overall cancer death rate standardized to the 1940 and the estimated 1990 populations. The greatest difference is in the level of the rates: the 1987 rate is fully 50 percent higher (199.9 compared to 132.9 per 100,000) when the 1990 population, rather than the 1940 population, is chosen as the standard. The choice of standard affects trends as well. With the 1990 standard, the cancer death rate increased by 6.2 percent between 1970 and 1987; with the 1940 standard, it increased by only 2.3 percent. Neither of these standards is "correct" in any absolute sense, but it is important to note that they are different. Whatever decision is made about adjustment and choice of standard, it is important that the decision be applied consistently to all of the mortality objectives.

In some cases, the examination of age-specific rates should not be avoided. If rates are to be standardized, many statisticians favor using the 1940 U.S. population as a standard, primarily because it would be consistent with the long-term practice of the National Center for Health Statistics and others in reporting mortality rates (Curtin, 1992). Using this standard would facilitate the efforts of states trying to monitor their own progress on the objectives. Others argue against adjusting, especially to the 1940 population, because it masks the public health impact of the levels seen in crude death rates. One compromise would be to standardize the rates to a more recent population, such as the U.S. population in 1990. This would give a better picture of the current public health impact of various diseases (as measured by the relative numbers of deaths) and would provide the analytic benefits of age adjustment. The difficulty with using a new standard is that special calculations would be needed to adjust past data for trend analyses.

STATISTICAL MODELS FOR SMALL AREAS

For measures that are highly variable at the state or local level, numerator data for three, five, or more years can be aggregated into one or a running series of calculated rates. Such measures are slower to show the impact of interventions because they include data from past years, but they may be stable enough to show meaningful trends. When rates are changing over time, aggregated rates will not be comparable unless all of the rates are based on the same number of years. Thus, standards are needed to judge whether the variability of rates and measures is sufficiently small for tracking purposes and to ensure that the results are comparable within states and the nation.

Kalton (1991) has proposed four statistical models for small area estimation that have potential for public health assessment.

"Synthetic estimation" uses information on the age, sex, and race distribution within a small area in combination with national race-, age-, and sex-specific rates of the outcome in question to estimate prevalence in the small area. Elston and colleagues (1991), for instance, have applied this approach to estimate the number of functionally dependent individuals for states and counties. Spasoff and colleagues (1996) have found, however, that synthetic estimates did not agree with estimates obtained through a community health survey in the same small area. "Regression estimation" uses information from a sample of small areas with complete data on a continuous outcome variable—the maternal mortality rate, for example—and other generally available predictor variables to estimate a regression equation and then uses these results to calculate predicted values of the maternal mortality rate in other communities for which the predictor variables are available. "Structure preserving estimation" techniques use the methods of discrete data analysis, such as iterative proportional fitting, to combine survey-based information on the age and sex structure for an outcome such as disability with census information on the number of individuals in a community to estimate the prevalence of disability in a small community. "Composite estimation" combines information from the community in question (which might have a high degree of variability, depending on the size of the population) with a model-based estimate, such as those described above, according to an empirical Bayes model. Manton and colleagues (1989), for instance, describe the use of such a model to stabilize cancer mortality rates for counties in the United States. Malec and colleagues (1993) have developed a similar method for use with binary variables in the National Health Interview Survey.

As Kalton (1991) points out, all of these approaches depend on a statistical model, so the choice of a good model and effective auxiliary variables is important. Unless the auxiliary variables are strongly related to the outcome variable in question, the small area estimates will vary little from one area to another. In practice, the choice of the model and auxiliary variables is limited by the data available. Thus, although these approaches may be useful for health planners in predicting health care needs, they will be helpful for public health assessment purposes only if auxiliary variables are available to accurately reflect changes over time and local differences from national levels.

REFERENCES

Adams, P.F., and Marano, M.A. 1995. Current Estimates from the National Health Interview Survey, 1994. *Vital and Health Statistics*, Ser. 10, No. 193. PHS 96-1521. Hyattsville, Md.: National Center for Health Statistics.

Amler, R.W., and Dull, H.B., eds. 1987. *Closing the Gap: The Burden of Unnecessary Illness*. New York: Oxford University Press.

Brown, C.C., and Kessler, L.G. 1988. Projections of Lung Cancer Mortality in the United States: 1985–2025. *Journal of the National Cancer Institute* 80:43–51.

Curtin, L.R. 1992. A Short History of Standardization for Vital Events. In *Reconsidering Age Adjustment Procedures: Workshop Proceedings*. M. Feinleib and A.O. Zarate, eds. Hyattsville, Md.: U.S. Department of Health and Human Services, National Center for Health Statistics.

Elston, J.M., Koch, G.G., and Weissert, W.G. 1991. Regression-Adjusted Small Area Estimates of Functional Dependency in the Noninstitutionalized American Population Age 65 and Over. *American Journal of Public Health* 81:335–343.

Hahn, R.A., Teutsch, S.M., Rothenberg, R.B., and Marks, J.S. 1990. Excess Deaths from Nine Chronic Diseases in the United States, 1986. *Journal of the American Medical Association* 264:2654–2659.

Hoaglin, D.C., Light, R.L., McPeek, B., Mosteller, F., and Stoto, M.A. 1982. *Data for Decisions: Information Strategies for Policymakers*. Cambridge, Mass.: Abt Books.

IOM (Institute of Medicine). 1993. *Access to Health Care in America*. M. Millman, ed. Washington, D.C.: National Academy Press.

Kalton, G. 1991. Methods of Small Area Estimation: A Review. In *Proceedings of Consensus Conference on Small Area Analysis*. DHHS Pub. No. HRS-A-PE 91-1(A). Washington, D.C.: Health Resources and Services Administration.

Levin, D.L., Gail, M.H., Kessler, L.G., and Eddy, D.M. 1986. A Model for Projecting Cancer Incidence and Mortality in the Presence of Prevention, Screening, and Treatment Programs. In *Cancer Control Objectives for the Nation, 1985–2000*. NCI Monograph #2. Bethesda, Md.: National Cancer Institute.

Malec, D., Sedransk, J., and Tompkins, L. 1993. Bayesian Predictive Inference for Small Areas for Binary Variables in the National Health Interview Survey. In *Case Studies in Bayesian Statistics*. C. Gatsonis, J.S. Hodges, R.E. Kass, and N.D. Singpurwalla, eds. New York: Springer-Verlag.

Manton, K.G., Woodbury, M.A., Stallard, E., Riggan, W.B., Creason, J.P., and Pellom, A.C. 1989. Empirical Bayes Procedures for Stabilizing Maps of U.S. Cancer Mortality Rates. *Journal of the American Statistical Association* 84:637–650.

NCQA (National Committee for Quality Assurance). 1993. *Health Plan Employer Data and Information Set and User's Manual, Version 2.0 (HEDIS 2.0)*. Washington, D.C.: NCQA.

Public Health Foundation. 1990. *A Report on the States' Ability to Measure Progress Towards the Year 2000 Objectives*. Washington, D.C.: Public Health Foundation.

Siegel, P.A., Frazier, E.L., Mariolis, P., Brackbill, R.M., Smith, C., and State Coordinators for the Behavioral Risk Factor Surveillance System. 1993. Behavioral Risk Factor Surveillance, Summary of Data for 1991: Monitoring Progress Toward the Nation's Year 2000 Health Objectives. *Morbidity and Mortality Weekly Report* 42(SS-4):1–21.

Sofaer, S. 1995. *Performance Indicators: A Commentary from the Perspective of an Expanded View of Health.* Washington, D.C.: Center for the Advancement of Health.

Spasoff, R.A., Strike, C.J., Nair, R.C., Dunkley, G.C., and Boulet, J.R. 1996. Small Group Estimation for Public Health. *Canadian Journal of Public Health* 87(2):130–134.

Stoto, M.A. 1989. Statistical Issues in Formulating the Health Objectives for the Year 2000. In *Proceedings of the 1989 Public Health Conference on Records and Statistics.* Washington, D.C.: National Center for Health Statistics.

Stoto, M.A. 1992a. Age Adjustment for the Year 2000 Health Objectives. In *Reconsidering Age Adjustment Procedures: Workshop Proceedings.* M. Feinleib and A.O. Zarate, eds. Hyattsville, Md.: U.S. Department of Health and Human Services, National Center for Health Statistics.

Stoto, M.A. 1992b. Public Health Assessment the 1990s. *Annual Review of Public Health* 11:319–334.

USDHHS (U.S. Department of Health and Human Services). 1991. *Healthy People 2000: National Health Promotion and Disease Prevention Objectives.* DHHS Pub. No. (PHS) 91-50212. Washington, D.C.: Office of the Assistant Secretary for Health.

Weinstein, M.C., Coxson, P.G., Williams, L.W., Pass, T.M., Stason, W.B., and Goldman, L. 1987. Forecasting Coronary Heart Disease Incidence, Mortality, and Cost: The Coronary Heart Disease Policy Model. *American Journal of Public Health* 77:1417–1426.

Wilson, R.W., and Drury, T.F. 1984. Interpreting Trends in Illness and Disability: Health Statistics and Health Status. *Annual Review of Public Health* 5:83–106.

Woolsey, T.D. 1981. Toward an Index of Preventable Mortality. *Vital and Health Statistics*, Ser. 2, No. 85. Washington, D.C.: U.S. Government Printing Office.

C

Using Performance Monitoring to Improve Community Health: Exploring the Issues

Workshop Summary[1]

SUMMARY

Performance monitoring is being used as a tool for evaluating the delivery of personal health care services and for examining population-based public health activities. The Institute of Medicine's Committee on Using Performance Monitoring to Improve Community Health is exploring how such efforts might be coordinated and directed toward improving the health of entire communities. The committee is considering the individual and interrelated roles that public health agencies, health care providers in the private sector, and various other stakeholders play in influencing community-wide health; how the performance of those roles can be monitored in a systematic manner; and how a performance monitoring system can foster collaboration among stakeholders and promote improvements in health status for all members of the community. An important task for the committee will be developing prototypical sets of indicators that communities can use to monitor specific health issues and the role that public health agencies, personal health care organizations, and other

[1]This appendix is an abridged version of a workshop summary published separately as *Using Performance Monitoring to Improve Community Health: Exploring the Issues* (Institute of Medicine [1996], J.S. Durch, ed.; Washington, D.C.: National Academy Press).

entities with a stake in these matters could be expected to play in addressing those issues. The study is funded by the U.S. Department of Health and Human Services and by The Robert Wood Johnson Foundation.

A May 1995 workshop reviewed a variety of public and private activities in health-related performance monitoring. An opening presentation focused on conducting and using an assessment of health status in New York City's Washington Heights/Inwood neighborhood. The subsequent presentation explored characteristics and limitations of health plan performance indicators and how they might be applied in a broader community context. The final presentation in this portion of the workshop reviewed the development of measures of public health practice for assessing the performance of local health departments and Illinois's application of such assessments in certification of its local health departments.

A set of presentations on Washington State and Seattle–King County included discussions of the state health department's focal role in public health policy; links between the University of Washington School of Public Health and the state's local health departments; the community-oriented approach of the private nonprofit Group Health Cooperative of Puget Sound; efforts to bring a health outcomes perspective to assessments of environmental health activities; the state's voluntary public–private collaboration in the development of health data systems; and an overview of the health assessment and monitoring program in Seattle–King County.

Final presentations reviewed activities of several federal agencies and national organizations, including work on clinical performance measures and health plan reporting; the national health promotion and disease prevention objectives of *Healthy People 2000*; tools to help communities and local health departments assess health needs and set objectives for improvement; and proposals for linking federal block grants in specific health areas to state performance commitments.

The presentations and discussion highlighted several points. Identifying shared interests that can promote collaboration in meeting health needs will be important. Throughout the workshop, consulting with the community was emphasized as an important means of learning about areas of concern, gaining a better understanding of the data collected, and building support within the community for the monitoring process. Public health agencies can often play a valuable role in initiating and sustaining community collaboration.

Applying performance monitoring to community health issues will require population-based data at the community level, but some communities will need to expand their capacity for data collection and analysis. A determinants-of-health framework helps demonstrate the need for information on clinical services plus environmental health and other factors such as education and social services that have an impact on health. Assembling data from a variety of public and private sources avoids duplication of effort in data collection and provides a more complete picture. Better evidence on the impact of many community health interventions on health status are needed. Schools of public health may be to able to assist performance monitoring efforts by conducting research on the effectiveness of interventions, providing analytic training for public health practitioners, and serving as source of expert advice for communities.

Any effort to propose a model for a performance monitoring system must take into account the social, political, economic, and organizational differences among states and communities, all of which influence capacity and willingness to address community health. An assessment of how well private sector health plans are serving their members and the community is seen by many as an appropriate element of the community monitoring process. Questions arise, however, about the extent to which health plans can and should be held accountable for the health status of all residents in the community. Also important is understanding how to achieve constructive change. Differences across communities and among the participants and audiences within communities emphasize the need for the committee to discuss performance monitoring in a way that is understandable from many perspectives.

INTRODUCTION

As part of its effort to collect information on current and planned performance monitoring activities, the Institute of Medicine (IOM) Committee on Using Performance Monitoring to Improve Community Health held a workshop on May 24–25, 1995. The workshop gave the committee the opportunity to meet with researchers studying performance monitoring and with representatives of public and private organizations conducting or developing performance monitoring activities. This report summarizes the workshop presentations and discussion. It does not present any formal recommendations or conclusions from the committee.

CONNECTING WITH THE COMMUNITY

Improving the health of communities requires looking beyond the contributions of medical care and providers of personal health care services. Similarly, measures of community health must be based on a broader population than those who have received medical care or who are members of a particular health plan. The first two presentations gave the committee an opportunity to learn about projects based on building links between the medical and the community perspectives.

Assessing a Community's Health[2]

Washington Heights/Inwood is a neighborhood of about 200,000 residents, predominantly lower income and Latino, in the northern part of Manhattan in New York City. It also is the home of Columbia Presbyterian Medical Center. In producing *Washington Heights/Inwood: The Health of a Community* (Garfield and Abramson, 1994), the Health of the Public Program at Columbia University used data gathering for an assessment of the community's health as a way to build better ties between the academic health center and the community.

The report, which has proved useful to many different groups, presents a broad range of information about the community, including health-related data (e.g., death rates and immunization rates) and health services measures (e.g., ambulatory care visits and inpatient insurance status). Also presented are data on characteristics of the community that can influence health, such as ethnicity, immigration status, household composition, per capita income, and educational attainment. For many measures, the report shows that Washington Heights/Inwood has relatively good health status. Household stability among the predominantly immigrant population may be a factor. The neighborhood is not without health problems, however. Of particular concern are violence, AIDS, and teen pregnancy.

The discussion also emphasized the need to consult with the likely audience for such reports to identify issues of interest and

[2]This section is based on a presentation by Richard Garfield.

potential sources of data, and to produce data and reports that are understandable to a broad audience. Involving the community and responding to its concerns may increase the community's interest in and acceptance of the findings, particularly negative ones.

Adapting Health Plan Performance Indicators for the Community[3]

The Center for the Advancement of Health in Washington, D.C., in connection with the California Wellness Foundation's Health Improvement Initiative, has considered how performance indicators developed for health plans might become a tool for accountability to stakeholders in communities served by health plans (see Sofaer, 1995). These stakeholders include consumers, employers, and public agencies, including regulators. The Center's expanded view of health emphasizes psychosocial and behavioral aspects of the delivery of health services and a public health perspective for the assessment of services to improve health.

The project identified several functions of performance indicators: specifying criteria for evaluation and values regarding health and health services; making explicit the expectations for some aspects of health care delivery; providing information for decisions on health services; supporting quality assessment and improvement; and, potentially, guiding the development of information systems. Further consideration focused on the normative, technical, strategic, and operational aspects of performance indicators. The normative element reflects value judgments made in selecting areas of performance (i.e., health outcomes) for which health plans or other organizations or individuals will be held accountable. Technical aspects of performance indicators include measurement issues such as the quality of the data being used and the validity and reliability of the indicators. Indicators must also permit meaningful comparisons across entities. Strategic concerns relate to the purposes indicators are expected to serve. The appropriate number, focus, and mix of indicators (e.g., outcomes versus structure or process) require consideration as does setting targets for desired performance at levels that will lead to meaningful improvements. Operational issues include the feasibility of obtaining data and approaches to disseminating results.

---

[3]This section is based on a presentation by Shoshanna Sofaer.

A review by the Center for the Advancement of Health and the Western Consortium for Public Health (1995) of many activities in the public and private sectors to develop and use performance indicators examined the extent to which the indicators addressed a range of consumer and community health concerns. They found a focus on the performance of individual providers and the use of health services. With programs such as the Health Plan Employer Data and Information Set (HEDIS), which the National Committee for Quality Assurance (NCQA, 1993) now sponsors, measures are moving beyond users of health services to entire enrolled populations in managed care plans.

Several "gaps" were noted among the indicators that were reviewed, including individuals' functional status, health-related quality of life, and behavioral and psychosocial aspects of illness and health care. Mental health and substance abuse services receive some attention, but they are often provided by separate specialty groups, making it difficult to identify problems in integrating psychosocial services with other forms of care. Determining appropriate indicators for multidimensional health problems is also a concern.

Regarding accountability, one concern is reaching agreement among stakeholders on where accountability for health outcomes can and should lie. In particular, the role that private sector health plans (and other medical care providers) should be expected to play in community-based health improvement efforts is a source of concern and debate. Currently, employers are a principal locus of oversight and influence in "operationalizing" accountability. It is not clear whether the plan selections made by individual consumers will have sufficient impact. Regulatory requirements are possible but may not be optimal. Some health plans are willing to accept limited responsibility for elements of community health but others may not yet be ready to so.

ASSESSING COMMUNITY PUBLIC HEALTH PRACTICE[4]

Federal, state, and local public health agencies have special responsibilities for protecting and improving community health. *The Future of Public Health* (IOM, 1988) defined their core functions as assessment of health status and health needs, policy development, and assurance that necessary health services are

---

[4]This section is based on a presentation by Bernard Turnock.

available. *Healthy People 2000: National Health Promotion and Disease Prevention Objectives* (USDHHS, 1991) included as Objective 8.14 that 90 percent of the population be served by local health departments that are effectively carrying out the core functions of public health. Work is now under way to develop measures of effective public health performance to assess progress toward this *Healthy People 2000* objective that states and communities can use to monitor and improve public health practice.

Developing Performance Measures for Public Health Practice

The workshop presentation focused on activities based at the University of Illinois at Chicago (see Turnock et al., 1994a, 1994b, 1995) and also drew on collaborative work with the University of North Carolina (UNC) (see Miller et al., 1994a, 1994b). The work at the University of Illinois at Chicago has focused on developing a measurement tool for the *Healthy People 2000* objective on the performance of local health departments. In contrast, the project at UNC is developing selfassessment tools for local health departments. These efforts, and a third project at the University of South Florida (see Studnicki et al., 1994), have been encouraged by the Public Health Practice Program Office of the Centers for Disease Control and Prevention (CDC).

Efforts to measure the performance of local public health departments have focused on process—public health practice—rather than on inputs, outputs (e.g., specific programs or services), or health outcomes. A set of 10 practices has been linked to the core public health functions of assessment, policy development, and assurance.

Using sources such as *APEXPH: Assessment Protocol for Excellence in Public Health* (NACHO, 1991) and *Healthy Communities 2000: Model Standards* (APHA et al., 1991), the University of Illinois at Chicago project selected a set of public health practice indicators and sent them to a panel of local health officials for review. After revisions, the indicators were sent to a national sample of local health departments for comments on issues such as whether the indicators were important descriptors of local public health practice and whether proposed measures were appropriate.

Most recently a set of 20 indicators that merge the results of the work at the University of Illinois at Chicago and UNC have been developed and tested. The indicators reflect standards for both performance and capacity to perform. For example, for assessment practices the selected indicators include whether there is a community health needs assessment process and whether adequate laboratory facilities exist to meet diagnostic and surveillance needs.

Using Public Health Performance Measurement

Information from monitoring public health performance has various applications. At the national level, the measurement tools being developed provide a way to monitor progress toward the *Healthy People 2000* objective of having 90 percent of the population served by local health departments effectively carrying out core public health functions. States and communities can use this kind of information to identify practice areas that need attention and to track changes in performance and the circumstances associated with those changes.

National Surveillance

Responses from the University of Illinois at Chicago's survey of local health departments indicated that, on average, those health departments performed about 50 percent of the activities associated with the 10 public health practices. Overall, health departments performed more practices related to the assurance function than those related to assessment or policy development. Survey responses suggest that, in terms of the *Healthy People 2000* objective, about 20–30 percent of health departments, serving about 40 percent of the population of the United States, had an "effective" level of performance (Turnock et al., 1994b).

Application in Illinois

In 1992 and 1994, the performance of local Illinois health departments was assessed using a set of 26 measures of public health practice (see Turnock et al., 1995). Between 1992 and 1994, the percentage of practices performed rose from an average of 55 percent to an average of 85 percent. Several changes contributed to the improved performance, including the state's requirement that local health departments conduct assessments based on the *APEXPH* model (NACHO, 1991) or on an Illinois version called IPLAN (Illinois Plan for Local Assessment of Needs). Community health assessment was implemented through a collaboration between the state and the local health departments. For most local health departments, community health needs assessment was a new and unfamiliar task for which they had few resources and little training. Resources provided by the state health department included orientation and training programs.

Comments on the Committee's Task

It was suggested that the public health practices framework applied to local health departments might prove useful to the committee in looking at the performance of a broader range of public and private entities that play a role in protecting and improving a community's health. Discussion by the committee pointed to the importance of state infrastructure for local health department performance and the need to be able to assess state as well as local capacity and performance. In addition, it was emphasized that differences among states in the nature of local health departments can affect which functions can be conducted at the local level and, therefore, their apparent level of "effectiveness."

MONITORING AND IMPROVING COMMUNITY HEALTH: A WASHINGTON STATE CASE STUDY

Understanding the political, economic, and social systems that influence the determinants of health will be crucial for the committee's consideration of sets of indicators for performance monitoring. Several workshop presentations explored how one state has been preparing its health system for a role in monitoring community health.

In Washington State, a major health reform initiative has led to substantial change in medical care and public health systems. In 1993, passage of the Health Services Act (HSA) authorized universal access to health insurance for all residents through managed competition funded by an employer mandate, individual contributions, and state-subsidized insurance premiums. The HSA also initiated the Public Health Improvement Plan, a biennial blueprint for the future public health system. The plan emphasizes the core functions of public health and population-based prevention rather than acute clinical care for individuals. The first version of the plan, published in 1994, articulated how the public health system would assure accountability for its contribution to health status improvement through a set of system capacity standards and health status outcomes (Washington State Department of Health, 1994).

In 1995, the legislature repealed large sections of the 1993 HSA. The new legislation contained some insurance reforms, portions of the previous health data system, and quality improvement initiatives. It increased state-sponsored health care for low income individuals and families and left intact the public health system reforms reflected in the Public Health Improvement Plan. Some activities under way before the legislative changes were emphasizing the value of prevention and the need for partnerships among public, private, and academic health systems.

Public Health in Washington State[5]

Washington's population of about 5 million is served by 33 local health jurisdictions that are independent of the state health department and provide few personal health care services. In the late 1980s, the state reestablished a Department of Health (DOH) separate from the combined Department of Social and Health Services. The broad perspective of public health and the concerns of local health departments had not fit well with the more targeted responsibilities of the various social service programs. The role of the state board of health was reaffirmed, along with its connection to local health departments. The DOH is a principal link between the state government and local health departments, but it also has a broader perspective on health that includes working with other state agencies (e.g., education) and with the private sector to provide for the health of the public. The department is also working with the private sector in developing improved data systems.

Two elements of Washington's experience were important for the IOM committee's work. First, the early and continuing emphasis on a systems approach required collaboration across organizational boundaries. Voluntary efforts of this sort can be difficult to sustain. Second, the success of many of the state's activities relied on developing a "shared vision" among many groups for criteria for good health in the state. That vision becomes the basis for assessing public health performance and outcomes.

---

[5]This section is based on a presentation by Kristine Gebbie.

Linking Academic Health Centers and Local Health Departments[6]

The School of Public Health at the University of Washington grew out of the medical school's department of preventive medicine. The school receives limited state support and relies heavily on federal research support and other grants and contracts to fund salaries and other activities. A 1990 grant from the Health Resources and Services Administration supported the creation of a Center for Public Health Practice. The Center's goals are to provide continuing education to public health practitioners, place students in practicum situations, and form linkages between the school and public health practice settings.

The Center has responded to training needs in local health departments with a two-week summer institute and, in collaboration with the state DOH, the local public health community, and several university programs, with a series of training modules that are offered via satellite in seven locations throughout the state. Training needs include: assessment techniques, data analysis, and community organizing.

In other collaborations, a tenured faculty member serves as health officer for a rural county in central Washington. This arrangement provides a training site for students and establishes a link for the faculty with local health officers. Ties with the state DOH have been strengthened by cross appointments. For example, the state health officer serves as assistant dean for public health practice. The links with public health practitioners are also adding new perspectives to the content of the academic program. Workshop discussion suggested that local and state health departments would benefit from easier access to the technical expertise of academic health centers, particularly in analytic areas such as biostatistics.

Private Sector Participation in Community Health Activities: The Role of Group Health Cooperative of Puget Sound[7]

Group Health Cooperative of Puget Sound (GHC), the nation's largest consumer-governed nonprofit health maintenance organi-

---

[6]This section is based on a presentation by James Gale.

[7]This section is based on a presentation by Bill Beery.

zation (HMO), was established in 1947 and has about 540,000 enrollees. GHC has an active program of performance monitoring that serves a variety of purposes, including HEDIS reporting to employers on health plan performance; accreditation requirements; data for an internal quality initiative; and feedback to individual clinicians. Performance measures are developed based on sources such as GHC's strategic plan and periodic vision statements. Eleven prevention and health promotion performance priorities have been specified.[8]

GHC has adopted a set of community service principles and a vision statement that calls for delivery of quality health care to the entire community, not just its enrolled population. Health promotion and disease prevention activities are currently focused on four areas: childhood immunization, the reduction of infant mortality, health care for homeless families, and the reduction and prevention of interpersonal violence. Several factors were considered in undertaking community programs. Improved community health is expected to lead to improved health for members. In some cases, members—or future members—may benefit as part of the target audience for specific programs. Some health problems (e.g., violence, alcohol abuse) require community-based programs because they are not easily addressed in a medical care framework. Community-based programs enhance GHC's competitive position for contracts with large employers and for services to Medicaid and Medicare populations. They also help fulfill community benefit obligations to maintain nonprofit status. Altruism is part of the motivation for these activities but will not outweigh long-term financial considerations.

Evaluating the impact of GHC's programs on community health and assessing costs and benefits for the organization will be challenging. GHC faces competition for resources within the organization, which creates pressures to focus exclusively on members' health care needs. No consensus exists on the extent of a health care organization's responsibilities in areas often considered "public health," and it may be difficult to sustain community efforts unless other health care organizations accept similar responsibilities, including public reporting on the extent to which

---

[8]The 11 prevention priorities are tobacco use, alcohol consumption and abuse, depression, cancer, high-fat diet, inactivity, diabetes, immunization and infectious disease, HIV/AIDS, heart disease, and injuries.

their efforts are meeting expectations. Communities may be able to promote an expectation for health plan participation.

Performance monitoring presents an opportunity to assess individual health care organizations and to encourage efforts such as health promotion rather than care for preventable illness. It may also be possible to monitor health plan partnerships with local health departments and other community groups. Some organizations (e.g., health plans, employers) may see their link to community service more readily than to public health.

The committee's vision statement was seen as an appropriate challenge for *all* health plans. Performance monitoring will, however, require developing explicit expectations in several areas: responsibilities of medical care organizations; public–private partnerships; contributions to community capacity-building; collaboration in community programs; how to monitor the extent to which partnerships exist; and the appropriate role of the consumer (individuals, groups, or the community).

The discussion highlighted concern that performance measures will focus attention on some tasks to the exclusion of others. Therefore, the selection of measures is a critical process that must be carefully and openly considered so that the implications of those selections are understood. Also noted was concern that measurement tasks are viewed very narrowly. Individual organizations may not be able to sustain more expansive approaches if competing groups do not make a similar effort.

Addressing Environmental Health Issues[9]

Although there are important links between environmental health issues and public health, some environmental health agencies have seen themselves as having separate responsibilities from what are perceived as personal health issues. The resulting organizational distance between the two fields has left many environmental health professionals out of the discussions about new approaches to public health practice and without an appreciation of their role in public health systems. Environmental health needs to develop new approaches to data collection and analysis that demonstrate the links between environmental health functions

[9]This section is based on a presentation by Carl Osaki.

and good health outcomes. In Seattle–King County, the focus has been on process measures (e.g., numbers of restaurant inspections conducted) without knowing the extent to which those activities contribute to disease prevention.

In Washington State, efforts are being made to bring environmental health clearly into the realm of public health. Environmental health directors in the state are working to develop clear and comparable definitions of terms and to address how to collect information that can be useful in efforts to improve community health status. An environmental health addendum has been developed for APEX*PH* materials for community assessments (Washington State Department of Health, 1993). A new model for the links between a community's health and environmental factors is emerging. This approach looks at health outcomes at the intersection of a population at risk, unsafe behavior, and an environmental hazard.[10] Each component of the model seems to have measurable elements that might guide preventive efforts to avert their intersection and an adverse health outcome.

The workshop participants saw how the model's concepts might apply beyond the traditional bounds of environmental health. Many thought, however, that the term "unsafe behavior" could be misunderstood as referring only to the behavior of the population at risk rather than to actions by a broad range of parties. Developing useful performance standards for environmental health will require further work to ensure that actions being measured have an impact on health. An important aim is to focus attention on issues beyond environmental hazards. It was emphasized that community-based assessments need approaches to performance monitoring that can link all of the determinants of a community's health, including the environmental and personal health care perspectives.

[10]Since the workshop, there has been further refinement of the model, influenced in part by comments offered at the workshop. It bases an assessment of health status on the interaction of environmental hazard(s), population(s) at risk, and public health protection factors. The model demonstrates the need to consider more factors than the regulation of hazards and to take a broad community perspective. The revised model has been endorsed by directors of environmental health in Washington State's local health departments and by the state Department of Health.

A Voluntary Approach to Public–Private Health Information Systems[11]

As part of its 1993 health care reform program, Washington State mandated creation of a statewide health data system to monitor and evaluate the effectiveness of reform efforts. Subsequently, the state has stepped back from the original mandates to adopt a more voluntary approach to health care reform. Health data system issues are now being addressed through a public–private partnership facilitated by the state. The change has overcome some of the resistance to a state-run system and may promote progress.

The state DOH has retained responsibility for considering data standards and quality improvement efforts. Several groups have been formed to address specific areas such as patient care, health status, and community assessment. Collaboration among the groups working on data on patient care, community assessment, health status, and enrollee measures has produced a proposal for a "clinical outcome measure amended HEDIS" strategy (COMAH). It combines clinical outcome measures with the more process-oriented HEDIS measures; only a few measures in this set will be community based. Data collection will be tested in a variety of settings including physicians' offices. These measures reflect the interests of the participating groups but not externally established or coordinated criteria for an appropriate or complete set of indicators. Other groups will be producing proposals that focus more on community health measures.

Communication between participants with a personal health care perspective and those with a public health perspective has made health care providers more interested in having access to population-based and clinical data. For community-oriented health plans such as GHC, Washington's collaborative approach to data systems development may offer a way to receive public recognition for some of their activities and to influence other health plans. Washington's experience with a voluntary public–private approach to developing data systems may be a useful reality check for the committee on the information health plans are willing to share.

---

[11]This section is based on a presentation by Elizabeth Ward.

Community Health Assessment in Seattle–King County[12]

The Seattle–King County health department's community health assessment program offers insights into the process of monitoring performance to improve the community's health. The program produces information on the community's major health problems and strengths, on perceptions about health-related concerns, and on health services. The results guide and motivate the development of policies and interventions, including action by community groups. The assessment program is a process, not just publishing a report. Data are reviewed with the community and with decision makers to understand whether the results seem reasonable, whether there are gaps between findings and perceptions, and whether there are concerns that have not been included. The review also identifies areas of special interest to the community and generates guidance on how to treat sensitive issues. In Seattle–King County, health department reports are released only after this kind of consultation.

Assessment Domains

The domains of the assessment process include health status, risk factors and other determinants of health, and health interventions. Standard measures are not available for social factors affecting health. Variables such as income, education, and race often serve as proxies. Other factors for which better measures are needed include stress, social support, and community values. In monitoring community health interventions, information is needed on the nature of the interventions, the targeted recipients (e.g., specific individuals, subpopulations, or the entire community), and providers (e.g., public health agencies, employers, schools). For many interventions, however, monitoring is hindered by limited evidence on their effectiveness.

Data Sources

In Seattle–King County, data for assessments come from sources such as vital statistics, hospital discharges, environmental inspections, and crime reports. No data are routinely available

---

[12]This section is based on a presentation by James Krieger.

on outpatient or emergency department care. Use of cancer registries is beginning. Some environmental data can be difficult to obtain in sufficient geographic detail for county analysis. Local surveys are used, but resources are not available to cover all areas of interest. Expanding the size of samples in state surveys, oversampling of some populations, or collecting additional information on residence could make state data more useful. Special studies, such as hospital record reviews, are used to obtain data on some health problems. Focus groups and selective interviews provide qualitative information to complement quantitative data. The value of combining data from multiple sources and making the best use of available data sources was emphasized.

Some recurring technical concerns related to the lack of clear standards for data and analysis were noted. Problem areas include classifying race and social status and inconsistent age-adjustment practices. Also mentioned were differences in diagnostic coding and in practices followed in statistical testing.

Populations of Interest

The health department has defined its population of interest on the basis of residence. Analyses of subgroups within the population are frequently valuable and require information on characteristics such as age, gender, race and ethnicity, educational attainment, and income. Experience has shown that "local" data on the county's 21 health planning areas generate greater interest and impact than countywide data. Determining the size of the denominator population, and relevant subpopulations, is an important and challenging task at the community level. Census data are supplemented with intercensal estimates from state and local agencies and from commercial vendors. Local health departments might benefit from access to additional expertise in making such estimates.

Selecting Indicators

Specific indicators used in the Seattle–King County assessment process reflect input from sources such as the statewide Community Data Task Force, various constituencies within the county, and the county health department. Factors considered in selecting indicators include the incidence or prevalence and the severity of a condition. The perceived importance in the community and likely community response are also considered. Other factors include the cost and availability of data and consistency with indicators used elsewhere (e.g., *Healthy People 2000* [USDHHS, 1991]).

Using Assessment Data

Information generated by the Seattle–King County health assessment program is being used for establishing priorities for health interventions and allocating state funds from the Public Health Improvement Plan. The assessments are also providing information needed to target interventions and are guiding program and policy development. County assessment data are used for comparisons with state and national data as well.

Some of the assessments that health agencies would like to make are complicated by resistance within the community due to the sensitive nature of some topics (e.g., data on sexual activity among teenagers). A suggestion at the workshop that health plans and other health care providers might be an alternative source of similar information brought the observation that sensitive information may be difficult to collect in that setting as well.

Promoting Community Participation

Seattle–King County has found that coalitions of community stakeholders (e.g., public health agencies, health plans, employers) need to be developed early in the assessment process. Such groups can provide valuable guidance on selecting indicators, interpreting assessment results, and understanding their policy implications. Public meetings that include community leaders can involve a broader segment of the community in health assessment and planning. Participation promotes community "ownership" of the process and the results.

Health departments are generally a resource for essential technical and organizational services for community health assessment. They can provide expertise and computing facilities needed to frame some indicators and to perform data management and analysis tasks. They can also help build community coalitions.

It was noted that health plans can be a source of information about their members and should be able to benefit from knowing more about the factors affecting health in the community. Their collaboration in community health assessment may encourage, and be encouraged by, the development of common goals for member and community health. Establishing common community practices in data standards and data interchange might promote health plan participation.

Observations to the Committee

Final remarks in this presentation highlighted several issues in monitoring community health. Monitoring needs to be a dynamic process and should promote local involvement. Indicators used for monitoring need to focus on risk factors with interventions known to be effective. Research is needed, however, to establish the effectiveness of a much broader range of interventions. Indicators should address not only health risk factors but also factors that promote good outcomes.

Some specific areas in which the committee might be helpful were noted: proposing indicators; encouraging the development of indicators for less developed domains such as environmental or social determinants of health; suggesting data standards for defining populations; and outlining processes for involving community stakeholders.

ACTIVITIES AT THE NATIONAL LEVEL

A variety of federal agencies and private sector organizations have programs that address monitoring and improving community health. The workshop gave the committee an opportunity to learn more about the work being done by some of these groups.

Federal Agencies

Office of the Assistant Secretary for Health[13,14]

The Office of the Assistant Secretary for Health in the U.S. Department of Health and Human Services (DHHS) has had broad responsibilities and interests in both health care and public health. Three activities have special relevance for the committee's work: (1) proposed performance partnership grants to states, (2) public health participation in the National Information Infrastruc-

[13]This section is based on a presentation by Roz Lasker.

[14]Following the workshop, a reorganization in the U.S. Department of Health and Human Services placed the activities described in this section under the direction of the Office of the Assistant Secretary for Planning and Evaluation.

ture (NII) initiative, and (3) development of comprehensive information on the nation's public health infrastructure.

Performance partnership grants Performance partnership grants (PPGs), are intended to combine the specificity and accountability of categorical programs with the flexibility of block grants. They are proposed for six areas: mental health, substance abuse, HIV/STD/TB, chronic diseases and prevention of disabilities, immunizations, and preventive health and health services. For each area, states would reach an agreement with DHHS on specific targets for improvement and the degree of improvement sought. Grants would provide states with funding for 3 to 5 years to achieve specific and measurable health status improvements.

A menu of health status objectives from which states can choose is to be developed in a collaborative effort organized by DHHS. Several factors will be considered in selecting PPG objectives: links to *Healthy People* 2000 (USDHHS, 1991); issues that are important and understandable to policymakers and the public; aspects of health status on which states can be expected to have an impact and for which change can be measured during the grant period; clearly specified measures; and timely availability of comparable data of good quality at a reasonable cost.

National Information Infrastructure Another important activity is bringing public health interests into the NII initiative, which is promoting the enhancement of the nation's computing and telecommunications infrastructure (see Lasker et al., 1995). Public health professionals are bringing to these discussions a familiarity with and interest in data issues that have not always been found in work with the health care community. Through its participation in the NII initiative, the public health community is gaining knowledge of and access to computing resources.

Information on the public health infrastructure The lack of, and need for, comprehensive information on the nation's public health infrastructure became clear during the development of health care reform proposals in 1993 and 1994. DHHS is funding a project to assemble a database on public health resources at the national, state, and local levels. This effort will include bringing together individuals and organizations already looking at these issues to develop a consensus on definitions and typologies for the elements of such a database.

Agency for Health Care Policy and Research[15]

The primary activities of the Agency for Health Care Policy and Research (AHCPR) relevant to performance monitoring include the development of clinical practice guidelines, technology assessment, support for outcomes research, and applied research on health care quality measurement and improvement.

One relevant project is collecting and classifying clinical performance measures being used by health care providers in the public and private sectors (Center for Health Policy Studies and Center for Quality of Care Research and Education, 1995). This "typology project" is producing a database with information on about 1,300 individual measures found in 40 measurement systems. The database will allow users to explore specific measures within the project's classification system and to identify measures linked to specific clinical conditions or patient populations. Anther project was aimed at producing information that can help consumers choose among health plans (Research Triangle Institute, 1995). It focused on developing questionnaires that could be used to collect information from and for health care consumers. Specific areas of attention include access to care, use of services, health outcomes, and satisfaction with care. The Consumer Assessment of Health Plans Study is following up the initial work.

Centers for Disease Control and Prevention: Activities in Managed Care[16]

Public health agencies have generally been responsible for broad community health needs but in many communities have also been providing personal health services. In the private sector, the growth of managed care organizations (MCOs) is shifting attention from individual patients to entire enrolled populations, including groups formerly served by public health agencies. The Centers for Disease Control and Prevention (CDC), guided by a Managed Care Working Group, is examining its role in this changing health care environment.

CDC is encouraging MCOs and other private sector health care providers, in collaboration with public health agencies, to

---

[15] This section is based on a presentation by Linda Demlo.

[16] This section is based on a presentation by Randolph Gordon.

give greater attention to prevention and community health. Concerns about the profitability of those activities may, however, encourage private sector health care organizations to focus their attention on their enrolled populations. There is need to create a new view of prevention as an investment in the quality of health services and not simply a means of avoiding treatment costs.

Among CDC's priorities is an effort to identify effective forms of community-based prevention and compile a guide to those interventions (similar to the report of the Clinical Preventive Services Task Force). CDC is also encouraging greater participation by state health agencies in the development and implementation of Medicaid Managed Care waiver programs. Another CDC priority is to enhance MCO contributions to public health activities and community health planning.

National Center for Health Statistics[17]

The National Center for Health Statistics (NCHS), a component of CDC, collects and reports national, state, and local health data. In addition to its role in assembling vital statistics data and conducting several long-standing surveys such as the National Health Interview Survey, NCHS has major responsibilities associated with *Healthy People 2000* (USDHHS, 1991). A particular focus is the set of 18 health status indicators selected in response to *Healthy People 2000* Objective 22.1, which calls for "a set of health status indicators appropriate for Federal, State, and local health agencies," and the summary indicator of years of healthy life (CDC, 1991; Erickson et al., 1995). A recent report prepared for NCHS compiled information on several sets of health care indicators, some of which are currently in use (see Lewin–VHI, 1995).

Among the points emphasized was making a careful assessment of data needed for performance monitoring. The cost of data collection could become a constraint as could the burden on those providing the data. Collecting some data less frequently or from a more limited population may be adequate. Also emphasized was the need to determine whether changes in health-related indicators signal real changes in health status.

---

[17]This section is based on a presentation by Ronald Wilson.

Private Sector Organizations

American Public Health Association[18]

Healthy Communities 2000: Model Standards (APHA et al., 1991) is a tool designed to help communities and local public health agencies monitor and improve health by translating the national health promotion and disease prevention objectives of *Healthy People 2000* into local objectives and developing community action plans to achieve those objectives. Use of *Model Standards* in conjunction with *APEXPH: Assessment Protocol for Excellence in Public Health* (NACHO, 1991) has been encouraged. In contrast to earlier versions, *Healthy Communities 2000* has built more directly on the national objectives of *Healthy People 2000* to provide an explicit link from the national level to state and local efforts. It also has expanded on some areas, such as environmental health, that received limited attention in *Healthy People 2000.*

Several suggestions about performance monitoring were offered to the committee. The recent collaboration among major businesses to negotiate with managed care organizations illustrates the diversity of perspectives on "community" health and the complexities in identifying relevant stakeholders for health improvement efforts (residents, enrollees, purchasers/employers, providers). Also stressed was seeing performance measures as part of a larger picture that includes other tools, such as practice guidelines and model standards, that can help guide community decision making.

National Association of County and City Health Officials[19]

The National Association of County and City Health Officials (NACCHO) is responsible for producing *APEXPH: Assessment Protocol for Excellence in Public Health* (NACHO, 1991). This workbook for local health officers has two parts. Part one is an organizational capacity assessment to identify strengths and weaknesses in a health department and develop a responsive action plan. The second part guides health departments in developing a community health planning committee that can identify health problems of concern to the community and mobilize the community to ad-

[18]This section is based on a presentation by Claude Hall.

[19]This section is based on a presentation by Nancy Rawding.

dress them. Also available is *APEXPH in Practice* (NACCHO, 1995a), which provides tools to facilitate use of APEXPH.

NACCHO recently published a profile of local health departments that presents, in the aggregate, information on their organization, resources, and activities (NACCHO, 1995b). NACCHO also plans to revise APEXPH, including enhancing the limited environmental health component.[20] NACCHO also is working through the Joint Council of Governmental Public Health Agencies on the role of state and local public health departments in issues of quality assurance and accountability as they affect population groups. Previously NACCHO collaborated with CDC to produce *Blueprint for a Healthy Community* (NACHO and CDC, 1994), which outlines 10 elements needed to protect and promote community health.

National Committee for Quality Assurance[21]

The National Committee for Quality Assurance (NCQA) focuses on quality in health care and on providing purchasers and consumers of health care services with information that helps them select among health plans offering those services. It uses accreditation to establish that health plans have structures and processes that should enable them to meet the needs of their enrolled populations.

NCQA has three aims for performance measurement. First, there should be national standardization of measures. Second, application of those measurement standards should be documented. Third, performance measurement should produce information that promotes quality improvement. NCQA is addressing these aims with HEDIS—the Health Plan Employer Data and Information Set—which provides a standard set of measures that helps purchasers compare health plans and helps health plans assess their own performance (NCQA, 1993).

NCQA is working with many health plans to help them improve their data collection and analysis capabilities for both external reporting and internal assessment. A pilot project involving 21 health plans with varying characteristics has demonstrated the feasibility of producing "report cards" but also has shown that the process is not easy. Work is also beginning on the HEDIS 3.0

---

[20]Since the workshop was held, a NACCHO committee has started this work.

[21]This section is based on a presentation by Cary Sennett.

update. Workshop participants expressed interest in the possibility that HEDIS could be expanded or adapted to meet community health information needs in addition to those of health plans and employers/purchasers. It was suggested that health plans could be gathering more information relevant to community health than they are currently asked to do, but NCQA questions the extent to which HEDIS and health plans should be expected to collect community health data.

Joint Commission on Accreditation of Healthcare Organizations[22]

The Joint Commission on Accreditation of Healthcare Organizations (JCAHO) assesses the qualifications and performance of hospitals and other types of health care facilities. Performance indicators are not considered sufficient by themselves since they can provide only an after-the-fact report.

The Joint Commission is developing preventive services standards, which extends the scope of the continuum of care beyond JCAHO's traditional focus on diagnosis and treatment. Primary, secondary, and tertiary prevention services are all within the scope of the new standards. These standards call for health networks to provide preventive services that are appropriate for their mission, that are considered efficacious, that are appropriate to the needs of the population they serve, and that are provided in an effective manner.

JCAHO also is addressing the development of indicators to monitor how well performance conforms with Joint Commission standards and to provide health care organizations with information needed for quality improvement efforts. The Indicator Measurement System (IM System), originally developed for hospitals, is being expanded to include other kinds of health care organizations and a broader range of indicators covering issues such as access to and satisfaction with care as well as clinical quality of care.

Rather than develop all additional indicators de novo, JCAHO will adopt some that are already available from other sources to address areas of care including substance abuse, mental health, cancer, diabetes, and pregnancy. Of about 800 indicators received from 24 organizations, about half are being evaluated for

---

[22]This section is based on a presentation by Margaret VanAmringe.

inclusion in the IM System for managed care networks. JCAHO also hopes to collaborate with other groups to assemble a collection of other indicator systems from which health care organizations can choose.

COMMITTEE COMMENTS ON PRESENTATIONS AND DISCUSSION

The workshop discussions made a valuable contribution to the committee's thinking about the general concept of health-related performance monitoring and about the specific tasks to be addressed in this study. They helped demonstrate the complexity of the issues and the need for further examination of many of the elements of the committee's vision for a performance monitoring system that can promote improvements in community health.

A phrase taken from the statement of the committee's aims, "examine public health performance monitoring from a systems perspective," contains several key terms requiring clarification. "Public" should be understood to mean the general population, the inclusive denominator for the measurement process. For some measures, the population of interest may vary but should be defined as comprehensively as possible. Addressing "health" raises concerns about boundaries on the continuum that ranges from obviously relevant morbidity and mortality to more complex issues of functional status and social constructs of well-being. A distinction must also be made between an individual's health and population-based health.

Trying to understand "performance" leads to questions about how to link it to either resource inputs or health outcomes. "Monitoring" emerges as an ongoing process of collecting, reviewing, and refining information. Finally, a "systems perspective" suggests looking for a way to see the constructive connections that could exist among activities and organizations.

Workshop discussions pointed to important issues that need further attention. The need to strengthen the evidence base for the health benefit—the efficacy—of many population-based health activities is of particular concern. It may not be possible, however, to identify "the" proper response to some health problems because circumstances and acceptable responses vary across communities. The concept of community will require further elaboration as well. Issues needing attention include determining who the community actors are or should be, understanding how they might be expected to change, and identifying strategies that can be used to promote change in a specific community.

The workshop also gave the committee an opportunity to learn about a substantial and diverse array of activities related to performance monitoring that are already in operation. A clear gap exists between the current outcomes and performance measurement work being done in many areas of medical care and that being done for various aspects of public health. Health-related data gathering and analysis activities in many communities are generally not integrated into a coherent system of sufficient quality and scope to support performance monitoring. The committee will have to consider not only the intellectual task of understanding the pieces that make up a performance monitoring system but also the practical realities of the organizational, social, and political context in which such a system will function. The committee will need to understand who the stakeholders are, what concerns they have, and how to promote their collaboration and commitment to making a system work. Within a community, the relationships may be complex: the organizational entity assuring that data are gathered may be different from the entity analyzing the data, which in turn may be different from the entity that has responsibility for developing or implementing changes.

In proposing how a performance monitoring system might work, the committee must take into account the political, economic, and organizational differences among states and communities. The committee's task is complicated further by the important changes occurring in the organization and delivery of public health and health care services. On some issues, such as improving linkages among health sectors and with areas outside the traditional scope of health (e.g., criminal justice, education, housing), the presentations suggested that opportunities exist but that progress has been limited so far.

Of concern to the committee is understanding how to achieve change in communities. What creates "readiness" or incentives to make the changes that address health problems in a collaborative way? What "levers" are available to promote constructive change at the federal, state, and local levels and in public and private sector organizations? The committee also faces the question of how a performance monitoring system fits into a process of community change. Data from a performance monitoring system may promote change, but change may be needed to create a setting in which a performance monitoring system can operate. Because performance monitoring systems will exist in an environment characterized by change, another question emerges for the committee to consider: What kind of system will be able to function successfully now and also be able to adapt to new circumstances?

The committee needs to consider what principles can serve as a guide toward its vision of a performance monitoring system and what some of the practical steps are that could be taken to move toward achieving that vision. The presentations making up the Washington State case study illustrated some of the possible accomplishments at the state and local levels and pointed out some of the obstacles that exist. The diversity of circumstances evident in the workshop presentations means that there will, of necessity, be different approaches to performance monitoring in different places.

As a result of the discussions during the workshop, the committee recognized the critical importance of presenting its ideas in a way that makes them understandable to the variety of audiences that need to participate in efforts to improve community health. A particular concern is ensuring that the phrase "public health" is understood in its broadest sense. As one step toward greater clarity, the committee changed the name of the study from "Public Health Performance Monitoring" to "Using Performance Monitoring to Improve Community Health."

REFERENCES

APHA (American Public Health Association), Association of Schools of Public Health, Association of State and Territorial Health Officials, National Association of County Health Officials, United States Conference of Local Health Officers, Department of Health and Human Services, Public Health Service, Centers for Disease Control. 1991. *Healthy Communities 2000: Model Standards.* 3rd ed. Washington, D.C.: APHA.

CDC (Centers for Disease Control and Prevention). 1991. Consensus Set of Health Status Indicators for the General Assessment of Community Health Status—United States. *Morbidity and Mortality Weekly Report* 40:449–451.

Center for the Advancement of Health and Western Consortium for Public Health. 1995. *Performance Indicators: An Overview of Private Sector, State, and Federal Efforts to Assess and Document the Characteristics, Performance, and Value of Health Care Delivery.* Washington, D.C.: Center for the Advancement of Health.

Center for Health Policy Studies and Center for Quality of Care Research and Education. 1995. *Understanding and Choosing Clinical Performance Measures for Quality Improvement: Development of a Typology.* AHCPR Pub. No. 95-N001. Columbia, Md.: Center for Health Policy Studies.

Erickson, P., Wilson, R., and Shannon, I. 1995. Years of Healthy Life. *Healthy People 2000: Statistical Notes,* No. 7. April. Hyattsville, Md.: National Center for Health Statistics.

Garfield, R.M., and Abramson, D.M., eds. 1994. *Washington Heights/Inwood: The Health of a Community.* New York: Health of the Public Program, Columbia University.

IOM (Institute of Medicine). 1988. *The Future of Public Health.* Washington, D.C.: National Academy Press.

Lasker, R.D., Humphreys, B.L., and Braithwaite, W.R. 1995. Making a Powerful Connection: The Health of the Public and the National Information Infrastructure. Public Health Data Policy Coordinating Committee. Mimeo. Washington, D.C.: U.S. Public Health Service.

Lewin–VHI, Inc. 1995. *Key Monitoring Indicators of the Nation's Health and Health Care and Their Support by NCHS Data Systems.* Fairfax, Va.: Lewin–VHI.

Miller, C.A., Moore, K.S., Richards, T.B., and McKaig, C. 1994a. A Screening Survey to Assess Local Public Health Performance. *Public Health Reports* 109:659–664.

Miller, C.A., Moore, K.S., Richards, T.B., and Monk, J.D. 1994b. A Proposed Method for Assessing the Performance of Local Public Health Functions and Practices. *American Journal of Public Health* 84:1743–1749.

NACCHO (National Association of County and City Health Officials). 1995a. *APEX-PH in Practice.* Washington, D.C.: NACCHO.

NACCHO. 1995b. *1992–1993 National Profile of Local Health Departments.* Washington, D.C.: NACCHO.

NACHO (National Association of County Health Officials). 1991. *APEXPH: Assessment Protocol for Excellence in Public Health.* Washington, D.C.: NACHO.

NACHO and CDC. 1994. *Blueprint for a Healthy Community: A Guide for Local Health Departments.* Washington, D.C.: NACHO.

NCQA (National Committee for Quality Assurance). 1993. *Health Plan Employer Data and Information Set and User's Manual, Version 2.0 (HEDIS 2.0).* Washington, D.C.: NCQA.

Research Triangle Institute. 1995. *Design of a Survey to Monitor Consumers' Access to Care, Use of Health Services, Health Outcomes, and Patient Satisfaction.* AHCPR Pub. No. 95-N003. Cary, N.C.: Research Triangle Institute.

Sofaer, S. 1995. *Performance Indicators: A Commentary from the Perspective of an Expanded View of Health.* Washington, D.C.: Center for the Advancement of Health.

Studnicki, J., Steverson, B., Blais, H.N., Goley, E., Richards, T.B., and Thornton, J.N. 1994. Analyzing Organizational Practices in Local Health Departments. *Public Health Reports* 109:485–490.

Turnock, B.J., Handler, A., Dyal, W.W., et al. 1994a. Implementing and Assessing Organizational Practices in Local Health Departments. *Public Health Reports* 109:478–484.

Turnock, B.J., Handler, A., Hall, W., Potsic, S., Nalluri, R., and Vaughn, E.H. 1994b. Local Health Department Effectiveness in Addressing the Core Functions of Public Health. *Public Health Reports* 109:653–658.

Turnock, B.J., Handler A., Hall W., Lenihan D.P., and Vaughn E. 1995. Capacity Building Influences on Illinois Local Health Departments. *Journal of Public Health Management and Practice* 1:50–58.

USDHHS (U.S. Department of Health and Human Services). 1991. *Healthy People 2000: National Health Promotion and Disease Prevention Objectives.* DHHS Pub. No. (PHS) 91-50212. Washington, D.C.: Office of the Assistant Secretary for Health.

Washington State Department of Health. 1993. *Environmental Health Summary and Background: APEX/PH Grant Environmental Health Addendum*. Olympia: Washington State Department of Health.

Washington State Department of Health. 1994. *Public Health Improvement Plan*. Olympia: Washington State Department of Health.

COMMITTEE VISION STATEMENT
August 1, 1995

The Institute of Medicine (IOM) Committee on Using Performance Monitoring to Improve Community Health intends to consider, from a systems perspective, the roles that the public health and personal health care systems and other stakeholders play in influencing community-wide health, how their performance of those roles can be monitored, and how a "public health performance monitoring" (PHPM) system can be used to foster collaboration among these sectors and promote improvements in community health. The committee's goal is to develop prototypical sets of indicators for specific public health concerns that communities can use to monitor the performance of public health agencies, personal health care organizations, and other entities with a stake in these matters. The committee will collect and analyze information on existing and planned systems related to public health performance monitoring, confer with experts in the field individually and through workshops, and prepare a written report that sets out principles of public health performance monitoring from a systems perspective, and illustrates these principles in a practical manner.

For PHPM to serve the core functions of public health—assessment, policy, and assurance—the committee foresees a need for an infrastructure for public health information. This information infrastructure would need to monitor diverse phenomena in the many sectors that contribute to the health of populations, including clinical care, environmental services, individual and public education, community social services, and public policy promoting behavioral change, among others. It also would need to employ measurement strategies far more sophisticated than those in current use; provide information on the health status of a community, including threats to its future health; inform decisions about how to improve the health of the public; and document change in community health and in performance of health-related functions. In such a PHPM system, individuals and programs concerned with the health of the public could coordinate data collection, trend and subgroup analyses, decision support, and program evaluation, successfully serving many organizational entities.

To guide its deliberations, the committee has framed an initial vision for PHPM. To affirm the potential future reality of this vision, the committee intends to take significant steps toward its initial specification. A central focus will be to

• Describe how to use a PHPM system to improve the public's health by identifying the range of actors that can affect community health, monitoring the extent to which their actions make a constructive contribution to the health of the community, and promoting policy development and collaboration between public and private sector entities that are responsible for components of the larger health enterprise of the nation.

To further develop its vision for PHPM, the committee aims to

• Specify an organizational and policy context for public health performance monitoring that unites the interests and authorities of the local, state, and national public and private sector entities that should be held accountable for the public's health;
• Advance a series of definitions to guide the development of a PHPM system;
• Document and critique the current state of the art in PHPM;
• Recommend innovations and priorities in the development of new measurement and data management systems to serve comprehensive PHPM;
• Provide detailed examples of several recommended performance indicator sets, illustrating the integration of data from multiple sources to assess various dimensions of the state of the public's health in relation to key health problems or risks. These dimensions would include (a) individual health status, (b) behavioral, biological, and environmental risk factors, and (c) the availability and use of individual- and population-focused interventions known to improve health;
• Recommend a set of performance indicators that would capture information on the most important health problems faced by the population so as to have a monitoring system that will continually assess the health status of the public;
• Specify recommended characteristics of the structure, resources, and reporting relationships among participants in the PHPM system; provide guidance on how public and private sector entities can work jointly to develop a PHPM system that is of use to the organizations as well as to the public's health; and
• Identify ways in which such a PHPM system can be continuously refined to accommodate emerging priorities in the nation's health.

Background

Performance measures have been used in assessing health status, personal health care services, as well as population-based public health activities with increasing sophistication for many years. Today, performance measures are gathered and used by a wide variety of sources: academic researchers, census takers, hospitals, public health and safety agencies, drug companies, insurance companies, employers and other health care purchasers, quality assurers, clinicians, and educators. Uses include resource allocation, monitoring of trends, cost containment, management, quality assurance, and accreditation.

In the personal health care area, for instance, *HEDIS: The Health Plan Employer Data and Information Set*, produced by the National Committee for Quality Assurance, is a defined set of performance measures used by employers and HMOs to compare health plans on the basis of quality, access and patient satisfaction, delivery of preventive services, membership and utilization, financing, and descriptive management information. The Joint Commission on Accreditation of Healthcare Organizations has used standards, the focus of which have in recent years been in keeping with a broader philosophy of performance monitoring.

Performance measurement has also been developed in public health. *Healthy People 2000: National Health Promotion and Disease Prevention Objectives*, produced by the Public Health Service with the collaboration of the Institute of Medicine, outlines 22 categories of measurable health objectives in health status, risk reduction, and services and protection, that is, both process and outcome measures. The objectives process has been implemented by a number of states and local health departments, in some cases using the tools provided by *Healthy Communities 2000* and earlier editions of the Model Standards, which is run with American Public Health Association (APHA) coordination. *Healthy Communities 2000* helps states and communities adapt *Healthy People 2000* objectives to their specific needs and frame the links between health outcomes and public health structure and process.

"America's Public Health Report Card," prepared by APHA, and *APEXPH: Assessment Protocol for Excellence in Public Health*, developed by the National Association of County Health Officials and others, illustrate other approaches. *APEXPH*, for example, offers local health officers a workbook for conducting an assessment of the strengths and weaknesses of their department. It also provides health departments with guidance on working with others in the community to assess and respond to community health needs. CDC's Public Health Practice Program Office (PHPPO) is leading efforts to respond to objective 8.14 in *Healthy People 2000*, which calls for measuring the extent of effective public health practice at the local level. This work derives not only from *Healthy People 2000* and *Healthy Communities 2000*, but also from definitions of public health core functions in the IOM report *The Future of Public Health* and CDC's earlier work on "public health practices."

Taken together, these activities provide a good foundation for monitoring key health outcomes and public health practices. What is needed, and will be the centerpiece of the IOM study, is a way to use the available systems and others to assess how well the providers of population-based core public health services, in conjunction with providers of personal health services, perform and interact in protecting and improving the health of communities.

PHPM Examples

If public health performance monitoring is to develop into an important tool used by many and varied entities, an ongoing conceptual development process is critical. Each user will face its own decisions, look at a health question from its own vantagepoint, and scrutinize particular opportunities to influence the health of the public it serves. Not only will different users have different priorities, they will have different budgets, time frames, and values, all influencing the balance of measures to be chosen. Ongoing changes in emerging technologies in clinical medicine, improving informatics, new biophysical technology, and evolutions in marketing, governance, and benefits coverage, along with redefined values, will compel the PHPM system to anticipate and help shape, as well as respond to, changes in health and health care in the United States. For these reasons, the committee will not offer a full prescriptive set of PHPM indicators, but will develop a framework for such a system and practical examples of its application in about ten critical areas.

In its report, the committee will illustrate the process it recommends for the development of a PHPM system, using examples suitable for diverse potential users and situations. Those seeking to use performance monitoring could include local, state, or federal government public health agencies; employers; private health industries; community organizations; budget analysts; accrediting organizations; health-related workforce planners and educators; and research agenda setters. Specific community health concerns to be addressed might be selected from broad categories such as environmental toxins, infectious disease, injury control, quality of life in chronic disease, mental illness, and vulnerable populations (such as children, the elderly, and those with financial or geographic access difficulties).

Selection of these specific examples will depend on various considerations including the extent to which meaningful health improvements can be promoted by appropriate and measurable actions taken by identifiable parties within a community. The appropriate actions and actors to monitor are likely to vary across communities because of factors such as differences in the organization of the public and private health sectors and in the political, economic, and cultural contexts.

For each specific health concern chosen for detailed consideration, the committee will suggest a set of indicators that, taken together, can be used to monitor health status in relation to actions that should have an influence on it. Indicators should be selected so as to promote constructive actions that are expected to have a positive influence on community health. For example, monitoring smoking rates among health plan members might encourage a plan to avoid enrolling smokers rather than to offer smoking cessation programs. The committee also will identify some of the information sources for particular indicators and will address methods for presenting and analyzing that information. An example might be a set of indicators on tobacco and health that can be used to monitor health effects associated with tobacco use and factors that can influence the use of tobacco. The indicators could include elements such as:

- traditional vital statistics (e.g., lung cancer and heart disease mortality and morbidity rates),
- results from behavioral risk and attitude surveys,
- use rates for tobacco and other substances (e.g., excise taxes collected on tobacco products, sales figures, survey data),
- quit rates,
- smoking cessation program availability (location, price, enrollment),
- business policy actions (e.g., advertising budgets and strategies),
- local government actions (e.g., regulation of tobacco use in public places),

• youth access to tobacco products,

• economic costs of tobacco use (e.g., morbidity, mortality, work loss), and

• the implementation of public and private tobacco control programs.

Implementation

To achieve its goals, the committee will prepare a book-length report that would introduce a vision of a PHPM system that can monitor and improve the production of health in communities; clarify the vision and its value to stakeholders, including the public; and document the current reality of scientific cultures, political environments, and gaps in knowledge in our current understanding of health and its determinants. The report will recommend guiding principles and who can do what to move us toward the vision.

The report will include examples that demonstrate how a PHPM system can be used by a community to characterize and monitor the actions that the agencies, organizations, individuals, and other entities in a community could be expected to take to contribute to health improvement, and to apply the information generated to encourage entities to take those actions that promote improvements in the community's health. These examples will demonstrate tools that communities can use to address other health concerns.

Sections in the report (as it is currently planned) will address:

• The committee's vision, and PHPM definitions and concepts.

• The current reality of the political and cultural environment in which PHPM must take place, including the need for better links between medical care and public health; differences of language, culture, conflicting goals and interests; many stakeholders with different needs/perceptions; diversity and complexity; and problems with accountability.

• Health and its biologic and social determinants, including basic questions such as the definition of health and ways to measure it in the determinants of health; the interconnectedness of health, public, and social systems.

• Health systems, including capacities of well-functioning health systems such as problem identification and monitoring; relations among public health systems, care providers, and so on;

capacities for measuring health system effectiveness; well-functioning processes of change and improvement and feedback.

- Detailed examples, as suggested above, of indicator sets that can be used for public health performance monitoring directed toward specific health concerns.
- Detailed examples of public health performance monitoring as it currently exists or can exist in particular states or localities; each would focus on the system as a whole, how problems are identified, and how specific problems are managed.
- Recommendations regarding guiding principles and operationalizing the vision.

WORKSHOP AGENDA

May 24–25, 1995
Cecil and Ida Green Building
2001 Wisconsin Avenue, N.W.
Washington, D.C.

Wednesday, May 24, 1995

9:00 a.m. **Welcome**
Michael Stoto
Director, IOM Division of Health Promotion and Disease Prevention

9:10 a.m. **SESSION I: Workshop Introduction and Goals**
Thomas Inui
Professor and Chair, Department of Ambulatory Care and Prevention, Harvard Medical School
Co-Chair, IOM Committee on Public Health Performance Monitoring
Susan Thaul
Study Director, IOM Committee on Public Health Performance Monitoring

9:40 a.m. **SESSION II: Connecting with the Community**
Facilitator: Thomas Inui

Richard Garfield
Professor, Columbia University School of Nursing
Shoshanna Sofaer
Associate Professor, George Washington University
Member, IOM Committee on Public Health Performance Monitoring

11:00 a.m. **SESSION III: Public Health Practice and Process Measurement in the Community**
Bernard Turnock
Clinical Professor of Community Health Sciences, University of Illinois at Chicago

12:00 p.m. Lunch

1:00 p.m.	**SESSION IV: Public Health Performance Monitoring: A Case Study from the State of Washington** Introduction and Facilitator: Bobbie Berkowitz *Deputy Secretary, Washington Department of Health* *Co-Chair, IOM Committee on Public Health Performance Monitoring*
1:15 p.m.	**Overview** Kristine Gebbie *Faculty, Columbia University School of Nursing* *Former Commissioner of Health, Washington* *Member, IOM Board on Health Promotion and Disease Prevention*
1:30 p.m.	**Academic Health and Local Health Departments** James Gale *Professor, University of Washington School of Public Health, Health Officer, Kittitas County, Washington* *Member, IOM Committee on Public Health Performance Monitoring*
1:50 p.m.	**Public–Private Cooperation for Health Improvement Activities** Bill Beery *Director, Center for Health Promotion, Group Health Cooperative of Puget Sound*
2:20 p.m.	**Environmental Risk Assessment and Data at Local Health Departments** Carl Osaki *Director, Environmental Health, Seattle–King County Department of Health*
2:40 p.m.	**Data Systems/Quality** Elizabeth Ward *Assistant Secretary, Epidemiology and Health Statistics, Washington Department of Health*
3:25 p.m.	**Community Health Assessment and Information Use by Local Health Departments** James Krieger *Chief of Epidemiology, Planning, and Evaluation, Seattle–King County Department of Health*
4:25 p.m.	**Discussion**
5:00 p.m.	**Summary Comments** Alan Cross *Director, Center for Health Promotion and Disease Prevention, University of North Carolina* *Vice Chair, IOM Committee on Public Health Performance Monitoring*
6:00 p.m.	Adjourn

Thursday, May 25, 1995

9:00 a.m. **SESSION V: Revisit Yesterday's Discussion and Broaden Scope**
Facilitator: Thomas Inui

10:00 a.m. **SESSION VI: National Activities: Other Involvement with Performance Monitoring and Reaction to Committee Draft Vision**
Facilitator: Alan Cross

Linda Demlo
Acting Director, Center for Quality Measurement and Improvement, Agency for Health Care Policy and Research
Randy Gordon
Associate Director for Managed Care, Centers for Disease Control and Prevention
Claude Hall
Director, Model Standards Project, American Public Health Association
Roz Lasker
Deputy Assistant Secretary for Health Policy Development, Office of the Assistant Secretary for Health
Nancy Rawding
Executive Director, National Association of County and City Health Officials
Cary Sennett
Vice President, National Committee for Quality Assurance
Margaret VanAmringe
Washington Office Director, Joint Commission on Accreditation of Healthcare Organizations
Ronald Wilson
Special Assistant, Office of Analysis, Epidemiology, and Health Promotion, National Center for Health Statistics

12:00 p.m. **Committee Challenge, Wrap Up and Thank You**
Facilitator: Bobbie Berkowitz

12:30 p.m. Adjourn

WORKSHOP SPEAKERS AND GUESTS

Speakers

BILL BEERY, Director, Center for Health Promotion, Group Health Cooperative of Puget Sound, Seattle, Washington

LINDA DEMLO, Acting Director, Center for Quality Measurement and Improvement, Agency for Health Care Policy and Research, Rockville, Maryland

RICHARD GARFIELD, Professor, Columbia University School of Nursing, New York, New York

RANDOLPH GORDON, Associate Director for Managed Care, Public Health Practice Program Office, Centers for Disease Control and Prevention, Atlanta, Georgia

CLAUDE HALL, JR., Director, Model Standards Project, American Public Health Association, Washington, D.C.

JAMES KRIEGER, Chief of Epidemiology, Planning, and Evaluation, Seattle–King County Department of Health, Seattle, Washington

ROZ LASKER, Deputy Assistant Secretary for Health Policy Development, Office of the Assistant Secretary of Health, Department of Health and Human Services, Washington, D.C.

CARL OSAKI, Director, Environmental Health, Seattle–King County Department of Health, Seattle, Washington

NANCY RAWDING, Executive Director, National Association of County and City Health Officials, Washington, D.C.

CARY SENNETT, Vice President for Planning and Development, National Committee for Quality Assurance, Washington, D.C.

BERNARD TURNOCK, Clinical Professor of Community Health Sciences, University of Illinois at Chicago

MARGARET VANAMRINGE, Director of the Washington Office, Joint Commission on Accreditation of Healthcare Organizations, Washington, D.C.

ELIZABETH WARD, Assistant Secretary, Epidemiology and Health Statistics, Washington State Department of Health, Olympia, Washington

RONALD WILSON, Special Assistant, Office of Analysis, Epidemiology and Health Promotion, National Center for Health Statistics, Hyattsville, Maryland

Invited Guests

CYNTHIA ABEL, Program Officer, Division of Health Promotion and Disease Prevention, Institute of Medicine, Washington, D.C.

MIKE BARRY, Project Manager, Public Health Foundation, Washington, D.C.

CHERYL BEVERSDORF, Executive Vice President, Association of State and Territorial Health Officials, Washington, D.C.

JUDITH MILLER JONES, Director, National Health Policy Forum, Washington, D.C.

NANCY KAUFMAN, Vice President, The Robert Wood Johnson Foundation, Princeton, New Jersey

JORDAN RICHLAND, Executive Director, Partnership for Prevention, Washington, D.C.

JOSEPH THOMPSON, Luther Terry Fellow, Office of Disease Prevention and Health Promotion, U.S. Public Health Service, Washington, D.C.

ALISON WOJICIAK, Manager of Practice Programs, Association of Schools of Public Health, Washington, D.C.

D

Using Performance Monitoring to Improve Community Health: Conceptual Framework and Community Experience

Workshop Summary[1]

INTRODUCTION

In recent years, performance monitoring has gained increasing attention as a tool for evaluating the delivery of personal health care services and for examining population-based activities addressing the health of the public. This attention to performance monitoring is related to several factors, including concerns about ensuring the efficient and effective use of health care dollars in providing high-quality care and achieving the best possible health outcomes. Also contributing are a wider recognition that the health of the population depends on many factors beyond medical care and heightened concern about accountability for use of resources and whether desired results have been achieved.

An interest in understanding how monitoring the activities performed by health care and public health agencies and organizations might contribute to improving the health of entire communities is the basis of a study by the Institute of Medicine (IOM) Committee on Using Performance Monitoring to Improve Commu-

[1]This appendix is a workshop summary that has been published separately as *Using Performance Monitoring to Improve Community Health: Conceptual Framework and Community Experience* (Institute of Medicine [1996], E.M. Weissman, ed.; Washington, D.C.: National Academy Press).

nity Health. The study is being funded by the U.S. Department of Health and Human Services and The Robert Wood Johnson Foundation.

The Committee's Charge

The committee was asked to examine how performance monitoring can be used to promote improvements in community health. In particular, the committee was asked to consider the roles that public health and personal health care systems and other stakeholders play in influencing community-wide health, how their performance in connection with health improvement goals can be monitored, and how a performance monitoring system can be used to foster collaboration among these sectors and promote improvements in community health.

The committee brought together expertise in state and local health departments, epidemiology, public health indicators, health data, environmental health, adult and pediatric clinical medicine, managed care, community health and consumer interests, quality assessment, health services research, and employer concerns. The group met six times between February 1995 and April 1996. Workshops held in conjunction with two of these meetings gave the committee an opportunity to learn more about conceptual and applied work relevant to performance monitoring and to hear about a variety of community experiences.

The Workshop

The committee's second workshop, held on December 11, 1995, is summarized here. The purpose of this workshop was to discuss both conceptual models underlying performance monitoring and its use in specific communities. Workshop presentations on conceptual models addressed the determinants of health, social change, and accountability. Presentations and a panel discussion gave five professionals working in communities an opportunity to bring to the committee comments and observations based on practical experience in health improvement programs and performance monitoring.

This summary of the workshop presentations and discussions is based on notes from the presentations, a transcript of the taped proceedings, and comments from the speakers. It does not present opinions, conclusions, or recommendations of the committee. Conclusions and recommendations, which will reflect consideration of the workshop discussions, will be presented in the committee's final report.

BACKGROUND[2]

As used by the committee, the term performance monitoring refers to a continuing community-based process of selecting indicators that can be used to measure the process and outcomes of an intervention strategy for health improvement, collecting and analyzing data on those indicators, and making the results available, to the community as a whole and specifically to those segments of the community engaged in health improvement activities, to inform assessments of the effectiveness of an intervention and the contributions of accountable entities. Performance monitoring should promote health improvement in a context of shared responsibility and accountability for achieving desired outcomes. Many parties within a community share responsibility for health (e.g., consumers, health care providers, businesses, government agencies, public service groups); those with responsibility for accomplishing specific tasks are accountable to the community for their performance.[3]

Several assumptions underlie the committee's approach to performance monitoring. First, it is increasingly necessary to use resources efficiently, that is, to accomplish tasks with a minimum of waste. Performance monitoring is expected to facilitate efficient approaches to improving the health of communities at a population level. Second, a performance monitoring system should have

[2]This section is based on comments by Thomas Inui.

[3]The committee's approach to performance monitoring relies on the public health "core functions" of assessment and assurance (IOM, 1988) and the health care activities related to quality assessment, assurance, and improvement (see IOM, 1990). From a public health perspective, assessment is the regular collection, analysis, and dissemination of information on the health of the community. Assurance refers to a governmental responsibility to ensure that services necessary to achieve agreed upon goals are provided. Quality assessment refers to measurement of processes and outcomes of health care and their comparison against a standard. Quality assurance employs such measurement within the context of a broader set of activities that includes steps to identify and correct problems. Quality improvement uses continuous measurement and analysis of processes and outcomes not only to address problems but also to maintain and enhance good performance. The health improvement activities envisioned by the committee combine a responsibility to the community for achieving health goals with techniques like those used in quality improvement.

a broad enough perspective to monitor diverse factors that influence a community's health, including ones that may not appear obviously health related. Third, a wide range of actors share a stake in community health; thus, social action and changes that involve many sectors of the community are necessary. Finally, special attention to vulnerable populations is important, because equity is valued in community health.

The application of performance monitoring presents problems at the current level of knowledge and infrastructure. Although tools for indicator development exist, the conditions for creating operational monitoring systems at the community level may not. Furthermore, measurement strategies for an array of health issues are not universally available, and measures that are available may not always be applicable at the community level. In addition, most information systems are not yet able to support the identification and analysis of health problems and to track interventions.

A central task for the committee is the development of indicators suitable for community-based performance monitoring.[4] Ideally, performance indicators measure states or critical processes that are potentially alterable and thought to have a demonstrable relationship to health outcomes. Those indicators may be measures of capacity, resources, processes, or actual health outcomes. Committee discussions suggest that indicator selection should be based on a community process that includes identification of stakeholders, adoption of a shared conceptual framework to analyze the community's health, selection of indicators appropriate to fundamental concerns, operational development of indicators, and field testing of indicators. Indicators should be descriptive; reliable, valid, and sensitive to changes in the community's health; important to stakeholders; sensitive to declines in the health of vulnerable subpopulations; and useful in monitoring health initiatives.

DETERMINANTS OF HEALTH[5]

Health encompasses physical and psychosocial well-being, not simply the absence of disease. Because many factors influence health and well-being, understanding the nature and scope of

[4]The indicators proposed by the committee will appear in the final report for this study.

[5]This section is based on a presentation by Jonathan Fielding.

these determining factors is an essential element in developing health improvement strategies and in determining what indicators may be appropriate elements of a performance monitoring effort. The workshop's opening presentation used the framework of the Health Field Model for examining the determinants of health.

Health Field Model

A model of the determinants of health proposed by Evans and Stoddart—the health field model—provides a broad conceptual framework for considering the factors that influence health in a community (Evans and Stoddart, 1990). Unlike a biomedical model that views health as the absence of disease, the field model includes functional capacity and well-being as health outcomes of interest (see Figure D-1). The model also emphasizes general factors that affect many diseases or the health of large segments of the population, rather than specific factors that account for small changes in health at the individual level. It takes a multidisciplinary approach, uniting biomedical sciences, public health, psychology, statistics and epidemiology, economics, sociology, education, and other disciplines. Social, environmental, economic, and genetic factors are seen as contributing to differences in health status and, therefore, as presenting opportunities to intervene.

Although this type of model is not an entirely new paradigm, its implications for designing health improvement programs deserve attention. For example, the way in which (health) behavior is understood fundamentally changes. Rather than a voluntary act amenable to direct intervention, behavior can be seen as an *intermediate* factor that is itself shaped by multiple forces, particularly the social and physical environments and genetic endowment. At the same time, behavior remains a relevant target for intervention. The model also differentiates among disease, health and function, and well-being. They are affected by separate but overlapping factors, and therefore, indicators selected to monitor health improvement programs may need to differ depending on which outcome is of primary interest. The model also reinforces the interrelatedness of many factors. Outcomes are the product of complex interactions of factors rather than of individual factors operating in isolation. It was suggested that the interactions among factors may prove to be more important than the actions of any single factor.

Each of the factors included in the model is considered briefly in turn.

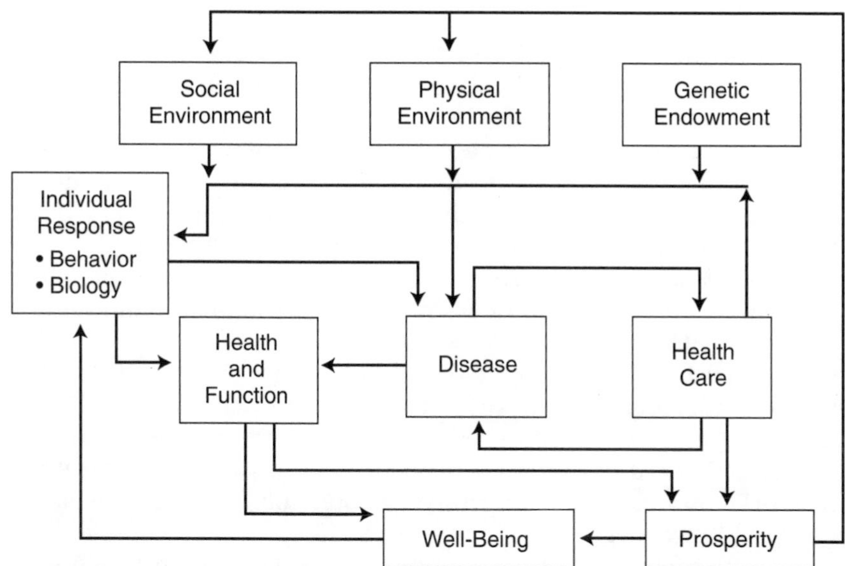

FIGURE D-1 A model of the determinants of health. Source: Reprinted from R.G. Evans and G.L. Stoddart, 1990, Producing Health, Consuming Health Care, *Social Science and Medicine* 31:1359, with permission from Elsevier Science Ltd, Kidlington, UK.

Social Environment

Among the elements of the social environment that have been linked to health are family structure, the educational system, social networks, social class, work setting, and level of prosperity.

Family structure, for example, is known to affect children's physical and mental health. On average, children in single-parent families do not do as well on measures of development, performance, and mental health as children in two-parent families. Children's relationships with their parents, social support, nurturance, and sense of self-efficacy have been shown to be related to their mental and physical health and even to their future economic productivity (Schor and Menaghan, 1995).

Education has an effect on health status separate from its influence on income. Years of formal education are strongly related to age-adjusted mortality in countries as disparate as Hungary, Norway, and England and Wales (Valkonen, 1989). Although most research is based on years of formal schooling, evidence suggests a broader relationship that includes the preschool period. An assessment at age 19 of participants in the Perry Preschool Study, which randomized children into a Head Start-like program, showed that participation in the preschool program was correlated with better school performance, attending college, and avoiding involvement with the criminal justice system (Weikart, 1989). Critical periods for education, particularly at young ages, may prove to be important in determining health. In addition, studies show that maternal educational attainment is a key determinant of child welfare and survival (Zill and Brim, 1983).

"Social networks" is a term that refers to an individual's integration into a self-defined community and the degree of connectedness to other individuals and to institutions. There is a strong inverse correlation between the number and frequency of close contacts and mortality from all causes, with odds ratios of 2:1 or higher and a clear "dose–response" relationship (Berkman and Syme, 1979). Although it is possible to see the impact of social networks on health, the pathways responsible for those effects are not yet known.

Social class is another well-described determinant of health, independent of income. Major studies have been done in Britain, where social class is defined more explicitly than in the United States. In the Whitehall study of British civil servants, Marmot et al. (1987) demonstrated a clear relationship between social class (based on job classification) and mortality. The relationship persists throughout the social hierarchy and is unchanged after adjusting for income and smoking. The effect of social class may raise uncomfortable issues in the United States but is important to consider in dealing with issues of health and equity.

The health effects of work-related factors are seen in studies of job decision latitude, autonomy, and cardiovascular mortality (Karasek and Theorell, 1990). Involuntary unemployment negatively affects both mental and physical health. Economic prosperity is also correlated with better health. Throughout history, the poor have, on average, died at younger ages than the rich. The relationship between prosperity and health holds across the economic spectrum. For every decile, quintile, or quartile of income, from lowest to highest, there is a decline in overall age-adjusted mortality. In international comparisons by the Organization for Economic Cooperation and Development, the difference in income between the highest and lowest deciles of income shows a stronger relationship with overall mortality rates than does median income (Wilkinson, 1992, 1994).

Genetic Endowment

Genetic factors are recognized as having a significant influence on health, and it will be important to gain a better understanding of these influences. For the most part, genetic factors are currently understood as contributing to a greater or lesser *risk* for health outcomes, rather than determining them with certainty. Briefly highlighted in the presentation was the link seen between genetics and behavior. Studies of twins separated at birth demonstrate a high concordance rate in alcoholism, schizophrenia, and affective disorders (Baird, 1994). Even so-called voluntary behaviors such as smoking and eating habits may be subject to genetic predispositions (e.g., Carmelli et al., 1992; de Castro, 1993; Falciglia and Norton, 1994). Health behaviors are complex, and the influences that determine them are likely to be extremely complex.

Genetic factors also interact with social and environmental factors to influence health and disease. It will be important to understand these interactions to learn why certain individuals with similar environmental exposures develop diseases whereas others do not (e.g., why most smokers do not develop lung cancer).

Physical Environment

The physical environment affects health and disease in diverse ways. Examples include exposures to toxic substances that produce lung disease or cancers; safety at home and work, which influences injury rates; poor housing conditions and overcrowding, which can increase the likelihood of violence, transmission of infectious diseases, and mental health problems; and urban–rural differences in cancer rates.

Behavior

In the field model framework, behavior is a response to the other determinants and can be seen as an "intermediate" determinant of health. It is shaped by many forces, particularly the social and physical environments and genetic endowment, as previously described. Behaviors related to health care, such as adherence to treatment regimens, are influenced by these forces as are behaviors that directly influence health, such as smoking.

Health Care

Health care has a limited but not negligible role as a determinant of health. Approximately 5 years of the 30-year increase in life expectancy achieved this century can be attributed to improved health services (Bunker et al., 1994). Of these 5 years, it has been estimated that curative services contribute about 3.5 and clinical preventive services about 1.5 years. The greatest share of this gain from health care can be attributed to diagnosis and treatment of coronary heart disease, which contributes 1 to 2 of these additional years of life.

Linking the Determinants

According to the presenter, the Evans and Stoddart field model helps in conceptualizing factors affecting health. Substantial evidence is available to support the relationship that many of these factors have with health. Currently incomplete, however, are descriptions of mechanisms underlying the linkages among the various determinants and full characterizations of the interactions among factors. Some evidence is available to demonstrate that these interactions exist. For example, high socioeconomic status is a buffer against the negative impact of perinatal stress on developmental outcomes in children at age 20 months (Werner, 1989). Similarly, high socioeconomic status reduces the negative impact of high umbilical lead levels on mental development (Bellinger et al., 1993). What is not yet available is an understanding of why the interactions occur.

INTERVENTIONS TO IMPROVE HEALTH

Many factors can influence the impact of interventions to improve health. It is possible to target various determinants of health to produce change at an individual level, a community level, or both. All aspects of each broad determinant of health are not equally amenable to intervention, however. For example, the social environment of isolated senior citizens can be improved by increasing contact with others, but their genetic endowment is not changeable.

Time frames for change following interventions can vary widely, from days to decades. Some successful interventions will produce observable results within a year or two, but others may be followed by long latency periods before significant changes can be observed in health status. The impact of an intervention may also be influenced by when it reaches an individual because there appear to be "critical periods" in human development. Certain interventions in childhood, for example, may have long-delayed yet long-lasting results. In addition, the population effects of interventions are important to consider. Small changes at the individual level may have important ramifications when applied to a whole community (Rose, 1992).

Community Interventions

The literature on community interventions is diffuse and difficult to summarize. A few observations based on that literature were shared with the committee. For example, the Healthy Cities/Healthy Communities activities demonstrate that a high level of interest in community interventions exists, but these activities have not yet generated a body of evidence that will allow them to be replicated in other settings. Study designs rarely meet high scientific standards. Although literature on advocacy and the process of community change abounds, validation through outcomes research is often lacking. Information linking process with outcome is inadequate, as are details describing implementation of interventions.

It was suggested that evidence that interventions have had a positive impact on the population is more likely to emerge in narrowly defined areas such as increasing immunization rates or decreasing workplace smoking. Similarly, one-time accomplishments are easier to document than what is needed to sustain activities. Literature examining the difference between attaining goals and maintaining them is lacking, and this issue requires more attention.

Targets for Intervention

The traditional targets for intervention have been specific diseases or behaviors. The field model of the determinants of health suggests consideration of a wider array of targets. For example, if adolescents' sense of well-being can be improved by reducing their feelings of alienation and hopelessness, can unintended pregnancies, alcohol and other drug use, crime, and the school dropout rate all be reduced? A multidimensional approach would be required, focusing on education, social and community involvement, family preservation, and improved social networks for teens and their parents. Community-level interventions might include after-school programs, athletics (e.g., midnight basketball), and church-based programs.

The multidimensional approach may be unfamiliar to health professionals because it is new and relies on partnerships with people from fields beyond those traditionally encompassed by a medical model. It is, however, consistent with the field model and may provide expanded opportunities for performance monitoring and improving the community's health. The variety of ways in which community can be defined, such as geography, politics, or social networks, was also noted (Patrick and Wickizer, 1995). The committee was encouraged to consider all kinds of communities in seeking solutions to health needs.

Implications for Performance Monitoring

Performance monitoring should make use of measures of inputs, process, and outcomes so that their interrelationships can be studied.[6] It was suggested that key determinants of health should be monitored, regardless of whether they are amenable to change at the local level, so that communities can understand the range of important factors.

The value of both individual- and community-level data was emphasized. Subjective individual-level data may contribute important information about community needs. For example, information on social support, perceived barriers to service utilization, and attitudes toward the community and its resources is all relevant to health and to performance monitoring and can be obtained from community surveys.

The quality of cooperation among organizations is an often-neglected consideration for which community-level measures might be developed. The success of multiple organizations serving

---

[6]In the context of the committee's work, *outcome* measures describe a state of health or well-being (e.g., immunization rates) that is the product of factors that can be characterized on the basis of the field model. To monitor outcomes that change slowly, *intermediate outcome* measures may be used (e.g., monitoring changes in prevalence of smoking rather than changes in incidence of lung cancer). *Process* measures describe activities that are being performed in connection with efforts to achieve a desired outcome. *Input* measures (also referred to as measures of structure or capacity) describe the characteristics of resources (e.g., funds, personnel, equipment, time, policies) available or in use (e.g., number of doses of vaccine available).

a particular community may depend on how well their services are coordinated. For example, senior citizens may be served by separate programs providing meals, transportation, outreach, and mental health services. Each program may be meeting its own goals, but if they are not working together, their overall impact may be diminished.

It was suggested to the committee that an initial step in performance monitoring is to determine which organizations and institutions in a community can affect health and disease. Those institutions can then be described with respect to goals and objectives, resources, and activities. What problems are being addressed? How effectively? What other activities might be added? Are these institutions educating the community about the problems and their responses?

Although organizations themselves can benefit from internal monitoring systems to determine their efficiency in resource utilization and whether desired outcomes are being achieved, they often lack the tools to adequately monitor their activities. If available, however, such tools may contribute to performance monitoring activities in the community. Important measures include units of services delivered, costs of services, proportion of need met, percentage of resources used to meet objectives, and impact. Community members can provide feedback, measuring how well individuals external to an organization rate the organization's efforts. In addition, an organization should consider how well its programs and services compare with "best practices." It was noted that efforts to identify best practice in developing and using community report cards are under way.

Performance monitoring provides an opportunity for a community to define and articulate expectations for organizations' contributions to the population's health. Although organizations might disagree with the appropriateness of the expectations, a useful dialogue may ensue. It was suggested that communities may want to focus special attention on expectations regarding managed care organizations (MCOs) and business. MCOs have improved provider education efforts and information tools such as clinical records, but "community" is often defined as their enrollees. Historically, MCOs have not considered the entire community or public health as their area of concern. A community expectation that part of their corporate and social responsibility is the health of the entire local population could encourage their broader involvement in public health activities.

Businesses, including MCOs, that have strong historical ties with a city or region may have greater interest in local health issues. However, as corporations expand to multiple regions, they may be less involved in the local communities where they have a presence. It was suggested that larger corporations operating in many locations should be encouraged to be involved in those communities. At the same time, smaller businesses with strong local bases should be educated and encouraged to become involved in community health efforts.

The presentation concluded with mention of another framework for assessing the community and health that translates the determinants of the field model into community terms (see Figure D-2). Community social and physical environments are affected by cultural, political, policy, and economic systems and in turn, influence community response, activation, and social support, and ultimately community outcomes including social behaviors, community health, and quality of life (Patrick and Wickizer, 1995). Therefore, performance monitoring might also benefit from attention to the underlying cultural, political, and economic forces represented in this framework.

COMMUNITY EXPERIENCE WITH PERFORMANCE MONITORING

The committee heard presentations from five panelists describing health improvement programs in their communities. A moderator-led discussion followed the presentations.

McHenry County Project for Local Assessment of Need[7]

The McHenry County Project for Local Assessment of Need (McPLAN) is a framework for improving the community's health. McHenry County is the fastest growing county in Illinois and consists of 29 individual municipal areas. Although the county enjoys good health overall, certain subpopulations have less favorable health indicators.

The panelist noted that the State of Illinois was a pioneer in local community health assessment and planning through its network of local health departments. In 1993 and 1994, the Illinois Department of Public Health (IDHP), using a process patterned after the Assessment Protocol for Excellence in Public Health

[7]This section is based on a presentation by J. Maichle Bacon.

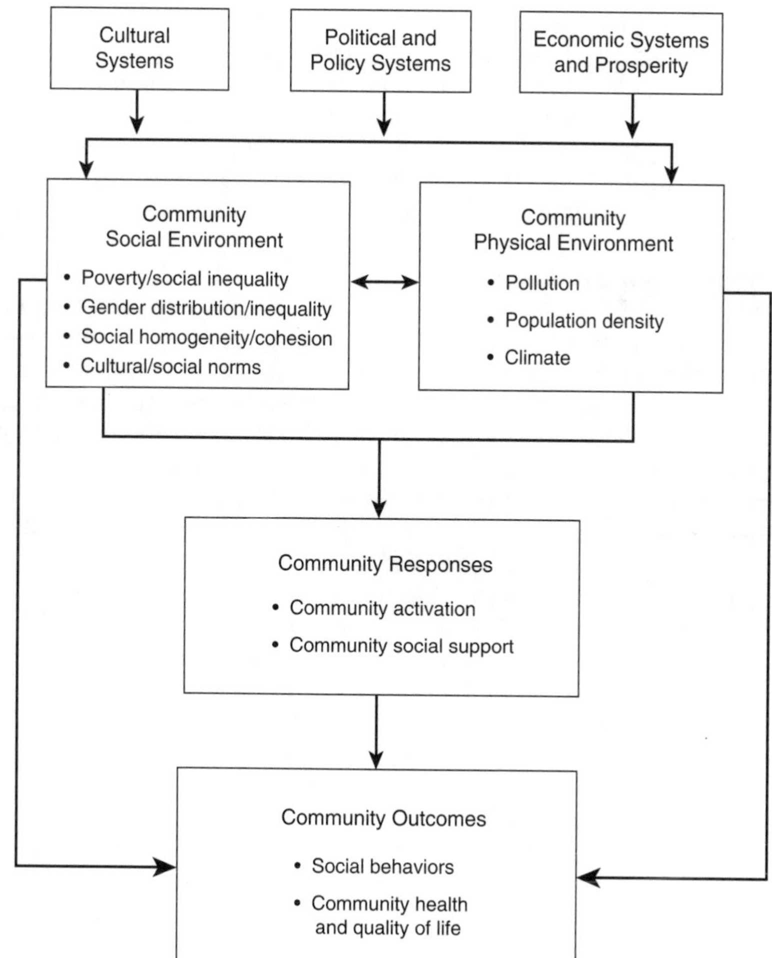

FIGURE D-2 An organizing framework for studying community and health (illustrative factors for community social environment and community physical environment). Source: From D.L. Patrick and T.M. Wickizer, "Community and Health," p. 67, in *Society and Health*, B.C. Amick et al., eds. Copyright 1995 by B.C. Amick et al. Used by permission of Oxford University Press, Inc.

(APEX*PH*) (NACHO, 1991), coordinated a statewide project to assess the needs of local populations. McPLAN is part of this initiative. The process involved local health agencies and other health-related community organizations that promote health or work in related areas that contribute to health (e.g., education, jobs, housing). Institutionalization of the assessment process now requires that local health departments respond to local health priorities and maintain services in four basic areas (communicable disease, private sewage, private water, and food protection) rather than offer a standard set of 10 programs specified by the state. IDPH provides training and has developed a data system to better enable local health departments to conduct an effective assessment process.

In developing and implementing McPLAN, the McHenry County Department of Health has applied its experience over the past nine years in performance-based budgeting and community health needs assessment. These processes have been empowering for staff as well as community stakeholders. In the budgeting process, problem statements are developed based on local needs assessment, and indicators are selected to serve as markers for appropriate public health interventions. Staffing and other resources needed to address these problems plus an annual review of the health department's mission and goals become the basis for developing a program budget. Each quarter, a review of indicator status and resource utilization allows further refinement of staffing and resource needs. Under McPLAN, both staff and community representatives are active participants in the process through advisory committees and the Community Health Committee. The health priorities selected for the county through the first application of the McPLAN process were environmental health, unintentional injuries, and cardiovascular disease.

The performance-based budgeting process has been used to incorporate health assessment findings into local public health programming and other stakeholder organization initiatives. The use of such a process over the past nine years in McHenry County has (1) aided in the training, focus, confidence, and perspective of staff; (2) led to a clearer understanding of the roles of the Board of Health, County Board, and related community organizations; (3) allowed movement toward allocation of a more appropriate level of resources to address identified issues (grants, appropriate fees, etc.); (4) led to greater involvement and understanding of other community providers; and (5) resulted in community-wide efforts to address childhood immunizations, improve access to health care for the medically indigent, develop joint grant applications, and begin discussion about a community-wide human services needs assessment in McHenry County.

City of Escondido Health Care and Community Services Project[8]

The goal of the Health Care and Community Services Project is to reduce the harmful effects of alcohol and other drug use in the community of Escondido, California (population, 120,000; county population, 2.6 million). The project coordinates a cross section of community services, including law enforcement, hospital emergency rooms, and community agencies. Integration of data systems, administrative coordination, financing, and training are other integral elements of the project's success. The municipal government functions as a facilitator for the community collaboration but does not provide services directly. Its interest is to reduce the cost of alcohol and drug use to the city and to improve the city's health.

Unlike most alcohol or drug control programs, which target individuals who are already dependent on alcohol or drugs, the Escondido project seeks to identify users who are at high risk of *becoming* dependent in the future. The objective is to influence drinking behavior before it reaches a critically destructive level, not to identify those already in need of specialized services (although such referrals are made when necessary). This approach is consistent with population data showing that the majority of alcohol and drug incidents involve users, not addicts. The program involves routine screening for alcohol or drug use in high-volume, high-risk situations. It includes a three- to five-minute screening interview and brief intervention. It is administered to all adults in hospital emergency rooms, health centers, and law enforcement settings. A new component of the program is the "Sobering Service," which provides services to individuals who would otherwise be sent to the police or to the emergency room for alcohol- or drug-related care.

Three important lessons were emphasized to the committee. First, the ability to cross sectors and create an integrated program made it possible to capture savings in one sector and make these resources available to the program. For example, the city is saving the money normally spent on booking people for alcohol-related offenses and investing it in the project. The project may become self-sustaining, because local private funds may soon be raised from managed care firms and combined with ongoing public fund-

[8]This section is based on a presentation by Dennis Kelso.

ing for uninsured participants. (Initial funding for the project came from local city general funds, county government funds, and a matching grant from The Robert Wood Johnson Foundation.)

Second, the importance of data was emphasized. The availability of data helped to identify the stakeholders and to create a collaborative value system, based on community participation. Third, development of a data system will be important in monitoring and maintaining the integration of screening and brief intervention services within multiple collaborating agencies.

North Shore Community Health Network Area[9]

The Massachusetts state health department has designated 27 Community Health Network Areas (CHNAs) across the state with the goal of improving health at the community level. In each CHNA, representatives from provider groups, boards of health, community health centers, and neighborhoods work together to review community health needs, set priorities for health interventions, and help implement those interventions. The state is making available to the CHNAs data on community characteristics and health status that can be used in assessing health needs and setting priorities.

Experiences of the North Shore Community Health Network Area (NSCHNA), which encompasses eight towns north of Boston, were reviewed with the committee. The NSCHNA was one of three pilot efforts for the CHNA initiative, which began in 1992. It serves as an advocate for public health ideals, strengthens the public health team, focuses on the consumer, increases affiliations by integrating services with larger health systems, and de-emphasizes specific illnesses. It was noted that through the NSCHNA it has been possible to pool resources, which has stretched funds and may make more money available for efforts in areas such as prevention.

A variety of traditional health status indicators are monitored by the NSCHNA. These include economic and demographic statistics, cause-specific mortality, incidence of infectious diseases, maternal and child health indices, substance abuse rates, and hospital discharge data. High rates of lung cancer deaths and asthma hospitalization pointed to tobacco use as an area of particular concern. Thus, tobacco control emerged as the NSCHNA's

[9]This section is based on a presentation by Tony Traino.

initial priority. Activities that have achieved some success include promoting the removal of cigarette vending machines from areas accessible to children and adolescents and promoting expansion of smoke-free space in establishments such as malls and restaurants. Other CHNAs in the state have chosen to focus on issues such as immunization and a reduction in sexually transmitted diseases among 15- to 19-year olds.

Arizona Partnership for Infant Immunization[10]

The goal of the Arizona Partnership for Infant Immunization is to improve the preschool immunization rate in Arizona by influencing provider behavior. In 1991, initial efforts were made to address immunization of preschool children. Available data showed that providers' perceptions that they were immunizing all their patients were inaccurate. Despite a historic lack of collaboration between the physician and HMO communities, representatives from each sector were convened as stakeholders. Other identified stakeholders were advocacy groups, businesses, and foundations. Participation by pediatricians was high. Because influencing 2,000 providers directly would be very difficult attention was focused on the state's 25 health plans, hoping to influence providers via the payers.

To take further action, a formal partnership, the Arizona Partnership for Infant Immunization (TAPII), was formed. Collecting data on immunization rates was recognized as essential to the project, but reaching agreement on measurement methodology was difficult. Finally, CASA (Clinic Assessment Software Application), a tool of the Centers for Disease Control and Prevention (CDC, 1992), was chosen. Once a methodology was chosen, data collection and interventions were relatively easy to plan. Health plans are now using HEDIS (NCQA, 1993) and CASA methodologies to measure and collect data.

In 1993, only 46 percent of 2-year-olds were fully immunized. In 1994, the rates increased by 10 percent. These rates were determined from medical records but may have understated immunization levels if vaccine doses given by other providers were not recorded. In 1995, immunization rates measured by the National Immunization Survey were 77 percent.[11] Provider education is a

---

[10]This section is based on a presentation by Laurie Carmody.

[11]These results are based on parents' records, which typically show rates 15–20 percent higher than doctors' records.

key component of the program. Once an immunization rate of 80–90 percent is reached, TAPII activities may be expanded to include parent education.

The panelist emphasized the importance of clearly defining a problem that motivated stakeholders to work together. Partners in the coalition have not yet agreed to work together on other problems but have been able to collaborate effectively on this clearly defined task.

Calhoun County Health Improvement Program[12]

The Calhoun County Health Improvement Program (CCHIP) is a community-based program that began in 1993. Its mission is to improve community health in Calhoun County, Michigan. The county has a population of 136,000, with a minority population of 17,000. The county's health status indicators fall below statewide averages. CCHIP was developed with funding from the W.K. Kellogg Foundation. A participatory approach that includes providers, consumers, and payers is taken. It views "health care" more broadly than merely the provision of "medical care." Personal responsibility and primary prevention are central to its vision. Its organizational structure is conceived as a circle with improved health at the intersection of four quadrants: neighborhood groups, membership organizations, a governing board, and implementation teams.

Health assessment is conducted through collaboration between the Community Assessment Implementation Team (a CCHIP-based team) and the Calhoun County Health Department. Together, they have developed a health outcomes report and have shared responsibility for community response to the report.

The program has developed long-range goals based on a five-year plan with six focus areas: (1) community decision making, (2) community-wide health care coverage, (3) a comprehensive delivery system, (4) an integrated administrative structure, (5) a community-based health care information system, and (6) community assessment. The goals include decreasing the risks to health, increasing access to cost-effective health care through the establishment of a purchasing cooperative, improving decision making through a community health information network, and changing

[12]This section is based on a presentation by Bonnie Rencher.

local and state policy to reflect community values and community decision-making processes.

DISCUSSION

In response to questions from the committee, workshop panelists discussed their experiences with performance monitoring. They specifically addressed identifying stakeholders, selecting health priorities and indicators, using indicators for accountability, gaining community support for performance monitoring, and implementing a performance monitoring system.

Identification of Stakeholders

As described by the panelists, identification of stakeholders proceeds in one of two ways, depending on whether the stakeholders are involved in defining or responding to the problem. When stakeholders are involved in problem identification, it is best to cast a wide net, leading particular groups to self-identify as stakeholders and become active collaborators. The stakeholder group may evolve as the process moves from problem identification to intervention to evaluation. It was noted that in the public sector different agencies or different personnel within agencies may become involved depending on the stage of the program.

When a problem is already defined and an intervention is suggested by existing data (as in TAPII), the participation of key stakeholders able to produce the desired results can be actively sought. In Arizona, the process was facilitated by participation of the governor, who convened a meeting of identified stakeholders. Groups with divergent interests may be able to cooperate in implementing solutions to defined problems when data and interventions are available to focus their joint efforts.

Participation by "consumers," that is, members of the general public, was mentioned as an important stakeholder issue. Ideally, participants should reflect the various population groups in the community, based on factors such as age, race or ethnicity, and neighborhood. All members of coalitions are consumers in a sense, but most participants are invested in particular interests. Engaging those participants who are not affiliated with particular stakeholder groups can be difficult. Barriers include the difficulty in identifying interested individuals and the commitment in time and energy that is required. Other barriers to participation can include meetings scheduled for normal working hours or added costs such as transportation and child care. TAPII found that because consumers participated for only a short period of time focus groups and community surveys were helpful for bringing their perspectives into the process.

Selecting Health Issues and Performance Indicators

Epidemiologic data are often used to guide the selection of performance indicators, but community interest may argue for focusing attention on specific issues or indicators, even in the absence of supporting epidemiologic data. It was noted that in some cases, a "triggering event" may focus attention on a particular health issue. The trigger might be a severe adverse event such as a measles epidemic or a more positive stimulus such as the availability of funds and other resources earmarked for specific topics.

Social determinants of health (e.g., income, family structure) and epidemiology are sometimes viewed as separate issues because epidemiology traditionally is associated with the biomedical model. However, the scope of epidemiology has expanded to include measurement of social factors, and epidemiologic data can drive the development of interventions in the social realm. Some workshop participants believe that the distinction between the two is artificial.

A discussion of the utility of epidemiologic health status data based on small sample sizes generated dissenting views. Some participants commented that sampling error is too large to make detailed follow-up measurements a worthwhile use of resources. Changes on the order of a few percent per year are extremely difficult to measure at the community level. Even if changes are measurable, communities may lack the resources to collect such data accurately. Other participants suggested that although measurement error can be a problem, it is essential to quantify problems and the effects of interventions. Otherwise, efforts to solve problems could be completely misguided. They suggested that combining quantitative and qualitative information can provide a more meaningful picture of a community's health.

Should Performance Indicators Be Standardized?

Workshop participants noted that there is tension between the need for standardized performance indicators and the need for community flexibility in defining indicators. Standardized indicators are advantageous for making comparisons within and between communities, for simplifying the synthesis of data from different sources, and for developing data systems. However, in designing and monitoring interventions in individual communities, the development of more specific indices may be helpful and standardization may be less important.

It was also suggested that the dichotomy between standardization and individualization is artificial. Most programs would benefit from a combination of the two. A basic set of indicators could be developed, with modifications based on specific community needs. Alternatively, a broad spectrum of questions could be developed from which communities could choose appropriate subsets. The selection of indicators may be especially difficult in a diverse community. Participants pointed out that performance indicators could be coordinated with currently existing health indicators in the private and public sectors such as HEDIS 2.0 (NCQA, 1993), APEX*PH* (NACHO, 1991), *Model Standards* (APHA et al., 1991), and *Healthy People 2000* (USDHHS, 1991).

Development of performance indicators requires stakeholder involvement. Some participants emphasized the importance of including private-sector stakeholders early in the planning stages in order to frame questions in a manner compatible with existing data bases. Distinguishing performance indicators from overall program evaluation was raised as an important distinction. The speaker suggested that performance monitoring should focus on the component parts of an intervention whereas program evaluation should examine the overall outcome.

Role of Performance Indicators in Stakeholder Accountability

Workshop participants agreed that defining accountability—which "actors" are responsible for what functions—is extremely important. Accountability for both process and outcome goals needs to be determined. The programs described at the workshop vary in how they hold groups accountable. For example, TAPII has led to ties between capitation and immunization rates, which fosters competition among health plans. Competition as a mechanism to gain accountability may be especially useful in the private sector. The Escondido program addresses accountability through formal written agreements detailing participation in the project, contract arrangements with providers, target rates for screening and performance, and management information systems for the integrated services. In other programs represented at the workshop, accountability is less explicitly defined. According to one panelist, it is hoped that "providers (will) come forward and increase their provision of services or education as it relates to the objectives."

Community Responses to Performance Indicators

The workshop participants reported that positive outcomes engender positive community response and that achievement of short-term objectives serves to cement community cooperation. They also commented on the importance of communicating realistic expectations to prevent discouragement with slower progress toward long-term objectives. Balancing short-term and long-term objectives helps maintain motivation.

Strong leadership is necessary to prevent coalitions from splintering into groups with self-serving agendas. On the other hand, outside leadership cannot substitute for communities' developing their own momentum to maintain programs. It was suggested that community groups need to be involved from the start in order for a community to be empowered and to continue projects regardless of changes in political personnel.

Tension between health problems articulated by the community and health problems identified by data analysis can potentially undermine community support for performance monitoring and health improvement activities. Participants suggested that the specific approach to selecting health issues should involve a larger community collaborative. However, the conceptual bases for selecting health issues should be founded on research that suggests that effective interventions will be possible.

Implementation: What Does It Take?

Issues common to the five programs discussed with the committee are availability of resources, leadership, training, and the development of organizational knowledge. The balance between data-driven and community-driven processes varies among the five programs, as does the degree of community involvement in defining problems and interventions. All use performance indicators in some form.

SOCIAL CHANGE AND ACCOUNTABILITY[13]

Recognizing that health improvement activities and performance monitoring imply the need for change in communities, the committee sought to explore some of the theories of social change and how they might relate specifically to health and health care. It was noted that change is ubiquitous today in health care systems, health care policy, and social policy and is occurring in multiple dimensions. Emphasis is shifting from individual health to population-based health; from tertiary to primary care; from preventive care to health promotion. Tension between controlling costs and improving health complicates change in all dimensions.

Change is not linear. It occurs in a specific context and is subject to complicated interactions. Change is a process of transition; therefore, it is fruitful to study both the change process and its outcome. To determine whether an outcome is causally related to a particular intervention, it is necessary to study the process of change linking the intervention and the outcome. The suggestion was made that natural experiments provide unique opportunities to study change and deserve more scrutiny than they currently receive.

The committee was reminded that people frequently resist change and that change can both arise from and contribute to conflict and tension. Although admittedly uncomfortable, conflict and tension may be necessary prerequisites for constructive change.

Models of Change

Three theoretical contructs that can be used in formulating models of change were noted. Structural functionalism is a positivist approach and is consistent with an epidemiologic orientation. Conflict theory views change as subjective and value laden. Its naturalistic approach parallels community development and participatory action orientations. Symbolic interactionism involves developing consensus to produce change (Thompson and Kinne, 1990).

---

[13]This section is based on a presentation by Ann Casebeer.

Individual Change

Change at the individual level is described by several models. The "stages of change" model was developed to describe smoking cessation (Prochaska and DiClemente, 1986). Readiness for change progresses through stages of precontemplation, contemplation, action, and maintenance. For maximum impact, health interventions are chosen with attention to the individual's stage of readiness.

The Health Belief Model views behavioral change as the result of "triggers" (Rosenstock et al., 1988). Beliefs about susceptibility, severity, benefits of treatment, and barriers to treatment contribute to individuals' willingness to change their behavior. The committee was told that this concept, along with other models of behavioral change, may also be important in studying the change process at an organizational level.

Organizational Change

An organizational model of change described by Lewin (1976) is based on a three-stage process that includes "unfreezing" the old behavior, cognitive recognition of the need for a new behavior, and "refreezing" the new behavior. This description is accurate for many organizational change processes. In health care, however, change is currently so rapid that behavior is in a seemingly constant state of unfreezing and refreezing.

Other models also describe organizational change as a staged process (Beckhard and Harris, 1987; Bridges, 1980). Thompson and Kinne (1990) offer a community development model of change that considers change on a continuum from individual to community. The PRECEDE–PROCEED model developed by Green and Kreuter (1991) is also frequently used in health promotion. It approaches change through factors that are grouped as predisposing, enabling, or reinforcing.

Change in Health Care: Case Study of Alberta, Canada

Both initiating performance monitoring and responding to the problems identified by performance monitoring systems require changes in the community and on the part of various stakeholders. Alberta, Canada, provides an example of the change process in health care.

Several tensions are influencing health care: individual versus population health; treatment of illness versus health promotion; meeting health needs versus managing health care costs; traditional versus new organizational models; current social conditions versus societal goals; and maintaining the status quo versus shifting paradigms (Casebeer and Hannah, 1995). Regionalization of the health care system in the province of Alberta constitutes a significant change in the arrangements for managing and providing health services. The change is largely an attempt to control increased health care spending, which grew from 20 to 32 percent of the provincial government's budget between 1980–1981 and 1993–1994, and to alter the orientation of health care provision (managing the system regionally and shifting to a population-based, community-based, health-promoting focus for care).

A study of change in health care and health policy identifies processes of change used by managers, as well as expected and actual health outcomes (Casebeer, 1996). Managers have suggested that successful change depends on the development of structures, processes, and outcomes that encourage the system to change in positive and sustainable ways.

With regard to structures, these managers are attempting to work with

- new and broader governance roles;
- leaner, flatter, more horizontal management of the system;
- new working arrangements for health care providers and managers; and
- new participatory roles for communities.

In relation to process issues, managers emphasized several critical aspects of change:

- the importance of sustaining political will;
- the pace of change;
- the capacity for shifting resources;
- the need for a renewed commitment to positive change;
- improved communication capabilities;
- better information;
- effective planning; and
- time for learning and adjusting.

Managers articulated a range of hopes and concerns in relation to short-term and long-term outcomes. For example, they expect that new management structures and savings would be short-term outcomes, new ways of developing services for better information would be medium-term outcomes, and improved services and health status would be long-term outcomes.

Gaining a better understanding of health care change such as that taking place in Alberta will require additional longitudinal and comparative experience as well as targeted research.

COMMENTARY[14]

The workshop discussions served as the basis for a commentary on community-based performance monitoring and issues to which the committee should give further attention. It was noted that the day's discussions focused broadly on community health improvement and community activation, rather than focusing more narrowly on performance indicators. This perspective is consistent with many community-based efforts to reduce health risks and prevent disease, such as the National Heart Lung and Blood Institute's cardiovascular risk reduction programs or the Kaiser Family Foundation's community health promotion grants program. Coalition building was central to these programs. They emphasized ensuring community involvement and participation of key stakeholders; needs assessment; project implementation based on the needs assessment; and program monitoring and evaluation.

It was suggested that although this approach, which is based on collaboration and community empowerment, is consistent with public health values, the evidence to date suggests that the model, as implemented in the past, may not work. Coalitions include varied interest groups and may be swayed by political concerns. The process may not select the most effective interventions at a population level. Efforts are being made, however, to bridge the gap that seems to exist between the community activation approach and the science of health improvement (Wandersman et al., 1995).

In contrast, the HEDIS approach relies on central planning and oversight. Although its top-down approach may conflict with the values and instincts of public health practitioners, it appears to be effective in promoting change. Its effectiveness was attributed to its visibility, its evidence-based approach, and its use of measures that lend themselves to managerial action.

The speaker proposed a new paradigm for community health

[14]This section is based on comments by Edward Wagner.

improvement based on a synthesis of community partnerships with an evidence-based approach. First, cooperation with the private sector, particularly medical care, would be a key element. Second, the private sector requires a business reason such as competition to participate. Third, performance indicators should be used to focus attention on those health issues and interventions supported by scientific evidence, as well as to generate and sustain accountability. Finally, the partnership should generate specific implementation strategies. In sum, performance indicators should support a community participation model by helping community partnerships set priorities and design interventions based on evidence.

Also critical to consider is the issue of accountability. In the speaker's view, accountability should be clearly assigned within the community. It must also rest on all who have responsibility to act. For there to be true accountability, performance must be monitored.

The workshop discussions suggested that performance indicators are used for multiple purposes: to identify problems and generate hypotheses, as political tools for mobilization in the community, to suggest ideas for improvement, and in fact, to monitor the performance of specific sectors of the community. Among the characteristics of useful performance indicators is a focus on populations and rates, rather than on absolute numbers of contacts involved in the interventions. In other words, the denominator is as important as the numerator.

Indicators were described as most useful when they focus on areas where improvement is possible. Global health status indicators often have little practical use for guiding health improvement strategies. More useful are indicators that incorporate a "theory of improvement"—that is, they suggest a clear means of moving from measurement to action. Indicators that have been shown to change in intervention studies should be preferred over those that may be more conceptually elegant but may not be able to capture the impact of an intervention. "Responsive" indicators of this sort allow real change to be distinguished from random variation.

The value of standard epidemiologic health needs assessments was questioned. Often, needs assessments merely document problems that are already well known. On the other hand, needs assessments focused on factors in the community that influence program implementation—politics, resources, barriers, key players—may be very useful. The speaker also emphasized that although coalitions are an essential component of community-based health improvement projects, they can consume substantial resources. Participants may, for example, spend an average of 3–4 hours a month conducting coalition-related work. It has also proved difficult to document a relationship between the characteristics of coalition operations and health outcomes achieved. The contributions that coalitions make to health improvement activities need to be better understood.

The committee was urged to articulate a model (or models) of health improvement that specifies use of performance indicators and holds social and nonclinical improvement strategies to the same evidence base as clinical strategies. Such a model should

- help communities clarify accountability and consider ways in which to include the private and public sectors as accountable entities;
- identify performance indicators in the model of health improvement; indicators should not be expected to generate models of community improvement;
- illustrate its concepts with the selection of a limited number of "performance areas" that are characterized by (a) evidence that services affect health status, (b) a clear theory of improvement, and (c) some reasonable ideas about how to reach the entire population; and
- identify key input processes and intermediate outcomes within each performance area.

CONCLUDING OBSERVATIONS[15]

The workshop concluded with a review of lessons for the committee, beginning with comments on the field model. The field model appears especially useful from a public health perspective. The model facilitates focusing on population effects, and its broad inclusion of disease, well-being, health, and function provides a basis for expanding monitoring systems to include these areas.

The field model also provides a useful basis for addressing the committee's concern for equity in health and how to promote equity in health through a performance monitoring system. The model makes it possible to study equity as it relates to social class, family structure, education, and social networks. The model's treatment of genetics in interrelationship with other de-

[15]This section is based on comments by Bobbie Berkowitz.

terminants and its view of behavior as an intermediate determinant are also helpful. Considering behavior as a product of various factors encourages users of the model to avoid blaming victims. Still needed, however, is better information regarding which determinants are actually amenable to intervention and whether community processes really lead to measurable community outcomes. Ways to measure cooperation are also lacking.

The panel's presentations and discussion illustrated differences among programs in the degree to which goals, performance measurement, and stakeholder roles have been articulated. The discussion also pointed out that community process can be catalyzed by a triggering event. This might be the availability of funding or public outcry when a situation is unacceptable. Different communities will require different approaches to the selection and use of performance indicators. It will be a challenge for the committee to propose a system that satisfies both "cookbook" and "menu" approaches.

Stakeholder identification appears to occur in two parallel tracks based on different responsibilities in some programs. One set of stakeholders is more involved in developing the information infrastructure, while the other set of stakeholders is involved in decision making or policy development. Potential trouble exists if the two groups do not communicate adequately. It was suggested that well-constructed coalitions of stakeholders can "keep the process honest." Ensuring meaningful consumer participation is another challenge shared by the programs, and is a topic that requires more attention. Panelists were sensitive to the need to listen both to stakeholders who are active participants and to those who are not before reaching conclusions about intervention strategies or performance indicators.

Concern about the potential for harmful use of data provided by performance monitoring was raised. There is a possibility that data could be misused in resource allocation if overly simplistic formulas are applied, and the committee must remain aware of these risks. Communities with multiple needs and few resources might lose funding for doing poorly, or communities that are achieving positive results might be at risk of losing funding if needs are assumed to be met. A community that is addressing a difficult problem may be doing a good job if it can *maintain* a given level of performance. For some health issues, prevalence of HIV/AIDS infection, for example, finding only a small increase might represent progress over higher increases in the past. It is also important to monitor "what is going right" rather than just looking for poor outcomes.

Final comments addressed social change issues. The models described to the committee contribute to the notion that the process of change is as important as the outcome. They also emphasize that the role of each stakeholder in the process is important for the committee to consider.

REFERENCES

APHA (American Public Health Association), Association of Schools of Public Health, Association of State and Territorial Health Officials, National Association of County Health Officials, United States Conference of Local Health Officers, Department of Health and Human Services, Public Health Service, Centers for Disease Control. 1991. *Healthy Communities 2000: Model Standards.* 3rd ed. Washington, D.C.: APHA.

Baird, P.A. 1994. The Role of Genetics in Population Health. In *Why Are Some People Healthy and Others Not? The Determinants of Health of Populations.* R.G. Evans, M.L. Barer, and T.R. Marmor, eds. New York: Aldine de Gruyter.

Beckhard, R., and Harris, R.T. 1987. *Organizational Transitions: Managing Complex Change.* 2nd ed. Don Mills, Ontario: Addison Wesley.

Bellinger, D., Leviton, A., Waternaux, C., Needleman, H., and Rabinowitz, M. 1993. Low-Level Lead Exposure, Social Class and Infant Development. *Neurotoxicology and Teratology* 10:497–504.

Berkman, L.F., and Syme, S.L. 1979. Social Networks, Host Resistance, and Mortality: A Nine Year Follow-up Study of Alameda County Residents. *American Journal of Epidemiology* 109:186–204.

Bridges, W. 1980. *Transitions: Making Sense of Life's Changes.* Reading, Mass.: Addison Wesley.

Bunker, J.P., Frazier, H.S., and Mosteller, F. 1994. Improving Health: Measuring Effects of Medical Care. *Milbank Quarterly* 72(2):225–255.

Carmelli, D., Swan, G.E., Robinette, D., and Fabsitz, R. 1992. Genetic Influence on Smoking: A Study of Male Twins. *New England Journal of Medicine* 327:829–833.

Casebeer, A.L. 1996. The Process of Change Related to Health Policy Shift. Unpublished Ph.D. dissertation. Department of Community Health Services, University of Calgary.

Casebeer, A.L., and Hannah, K.J. 1995. Evaluating the Process of Change Related to Health Policy Shift. Presented at *Evaluation 1995—Evaluation for a New Century: A Global Perspective*, Vancouver, British Columbia. November 1–5.

CDC (Centers for Disease Control and Prevention). 1992. *Guidelines for Assessing Vaccination Levels of the 2-Year-Old Population in a Clinic Setting.* Atlanta: U.S. Department of Health and Human Services, Public Health Service.

de Castro, J.M. 1993. Genetic Influences on Daily Intake and Meal Patterns of Humans. *Physiology and Behavior* 53:777–782.

Evans, R.G., and Stoddart, G.L. 1990. Producing Health, Consuming Health Care. *Social Science and Medicine* 31:1347–1363.

Falciglia, G.A., and Norton, P.A. 1994. Evidence for a Genetic Influence on Preference for Some Foods. *Journal of the American Dietetic Association* 94(2):154–158.

Green, L.W., and Kreuter, M.W. 1991. *Health Promotion Planning: An Educational and Environmental Approach.* 2nd ed. Mountain View, Calif.: Mayfield.

IOM (Institute of Medicine). 1988. *The Future of Public Health.* Washington, D.C.: National Academy Press.

IOM. 1990. *Medicare: A Strategy for Quality Assurance.* Vol I. K.N. Lohr, ed. Washington, D.C.: National Academy Press.

Karasek, R.A., and Theorell, T. 1990. *Healthy Work: Stress, Productivity and the Reconstruction of Working Life.* New York: Basic Books.

Lewin, K. 1976. *Field Theory as Human Science.* Compiled by J. de River. New York: Gardner Press.

Marmot, M.G., Kogevinas, M., and Elston, M.A. 1987. Social/Economic Status and Disease. *Annual Review of Public Health* 8:111–135.

NACHO (National Association of County Health Officials). 1991. *APEXPH: Assessment Protocol for Excellence in Public Health.* Washington, D.C.: NACHO.

NCQA (National Committee for Quality Assurance). 1993. *Health Plan Employer Data and Information Set and User's Manual, Version 2.0 (HEDIS 2.0).* Washington, D.C.: NCQA.

Patrick, D.L., and Wickizer, T.M. 1995. Community and Health. In *Society and Health.* B.C. Amick., S. Levine, A.R. Tarlov, and D.C. Walsh, eds. New York: Oxford University Press.

Prochaska, J.O., and DiClemente, C.C. 1986. Toward a Comprehensive Model of Change. In *Dealing with Addictive Behaviors.* W. Meller, and N. Healhen, eds. New York: Plenum.

Rose, G. 1992. *The Strategy of Preventive Medicine.* New York: Oxford University Press.

Rosenstock, I.M., Strecher, V.J., and Becker, M.H. 1988. Social Learning Theory and the Health Belief Model. *Health Education Quarterly* 15(2):175–183.

Schor, E.L., and Menaghan, E. 1995. Family Pathways to Child Health. In *Society and Health.* B.C. Amick, S. Levine, A.L. Tarlov, and D.C. Walsh, eds. New York: Oxford University Press.

Thompson, B., and Kinne, S. 1990. Social Change Theory: Applications to Community Health. In *Health Promotion at the Community Level.* N. Bracht, ed. Newbury Park, Calif.: Sage Publishing.

USDHHS (U.S. Department of Health and Human Services). 1991. *Healthy People 2000: National Health Promotion and Disease Prevention Objectives.* DHHS Pub. No. (PHS) 91-50212. Washington, D.C.: Office of the Assistant Secretary for Health.

Valkonen, T. 1989. Adult Mortality and Level of Education: A Comparison of Six Countries. In *Health Inequalities in European Countries.* J. Fox, ed. Aldershot, England: Gower.

Wandersman, A., Morrissey E., Crusto, C., et al. 1995. Bridging the Gap Between the State of the Science and the State of the Practice in Prevention: Program Improvement Through Program Evaluation. Presented at *Community-Based Health Promotion: State of the Art and Recommendations for the Future,* Seattle, Wash. October.

Weikart, D.P. 1989. Early Childhood Education and Primary Prevention. *Prevention in Human Services* 6(2):285–306.

Werner, E.E. 1989. Children of the Garden Island. *Scientific American* 260(April): 106–111.

Wilkinson, R.G. 1992. Income Distribution and Life Expectancy. *British Medical Journal* 304(6820):165–168.

Wilkinson, R.G. 1994. The Epidemiological Transition: From Material Scarcity to Social Disadvantage? *Daedalus* 123(4):61–77.

Zill, N. II, and Brim, O.G., Jr. 1983. Development of Childhood Social Indicators. In *Children, Families, and Government: Perspectives on American Social Policy*. E.F. Zigler, S.L. Kagan, and E. Klugman, eds. New York: Cambridge University Press.

WORKSHOP AGENDA

December 11, 1995
Foundry Building—Room 2004
1055 Thomas Jefferson Street, N.W., Washington, D.C.

8:30 a.m. **Welcome and Overview of the Committee's Approach to Performance Monitoring**
Thomas Inui, *Harvard Medical School*

9:00 a.m. **Presentation and Discussion on Determinants of Health**
Jonathan Fielding, *University of California at Los Angeles*

10:00 a.m. **Community Experience with Performance Monitoring**
Moderator: Alan Cross, *University of North Carolina*

Brief Program Descriptions
J. Maichle Bacon, *McPlan, the McHenry County (Illinois) Project for Local Assessment of Need*
Dennis Kelso, *Health Care and Community Services Project (Escondido, California)*
Tony Traino, *North Shore Community Health Network (Massachusetts)*
Laurie Carmody, *Arizona Partnership for Infant Immunization*
Bonnie Rencher, *Calhoun County (Michigan) Health Improvement Program*

11:00 a.m. **Panel Discussion:**
Committee Questions on Performance Monitoring Experience and Perspectives

12:30 p.m. Lunch

1:30 p.m. **Continue Panel Discussion**

3:15 p.m. Break

3:30 p.m. **Presentation and Discussion on Issues of Social Change and Accountability**
Ann Casebeer, *University of Calgary*

4:15 p.m. **Commentary and Response**
Edward Wagner, *Group Health Cooperative of Puget Sound and University of Washington*

4:45 p.m. **Concluding Discussion and Comments**
Bobbie Berkowitz, *Washington State Department of Health*

5:15 p.m. Adjourn

WORKSHOP SPEAKERS AND GUESTS

Speakers

J. MAICHLE BACON, Public Health Administrator, McHenry County Department of Health, Woodstock, Illinois
LAURIE L. CARMODY, Public Health Consultant, Group Health Association of America, Washington, D.C.
ANN CASEBEER, Doctoral Candidate, University of Calgary, Department of Community Health Sciences, Calgary, Alberta
JONATHAN E. FIELDING, Professor of Health Services and Pediatrics, University of California at Los Angeles, Los Angeles, California
DENNIS J. KELSO, Director, Health Care and Community Services Project, Escondido, California
BONNIE RENCHER, Community Outreach Coordinator, Calhoun County Health Improvement Program, Battle Creek, Michigan
TONY TRAINO, Associate Director, Home Care Operations, Visiting Nurse Association of Greater Salem, Salem, Massachusetts
EDWARD H. WAGNER, Director, Center for Health Studies and W.A. (Sandy) MacColl Institute for Healthcare Innovation, Group Health Cooperative of Puget Sound, Seattle, Washington

Invited Guests

DENNIS P. ANDRULIS, National Public Health and Hospital Institute, Washington, D.C.
MICHAEL BARRY, Public Health Foundation, Washington, D.C.
GEORGES C. BENJAMIN, Public Health Services, Department of Health and Mental Hygiene, Baltimore, Maryland
CHERYL BEVERSDORF, Association of State and Territorial Health Officials, Washington, D.C.
JACKIE BRYAN, Association of State and Territorial Health Officials, Washington, D.C.
LINDA K. DEMLO, Agency for Health Care Policy and Research, Rockville, Maryland
PATRICIA A. EBENER, Behavioral Scientist, RAND, Santa Monica, California
MARGO EDMUNDS, Institute of Medicine, Washington, D.C.
SARA GARSON, Center for the Advancement of Health, Washington, D.C.
CAREN GINSBERG, National Public Health and Hospital Institute, Washington, D.C.
SUSANNA GINSBURG, Lewin-VHI, Inc., Fairfax, Virginia
HOLLY GRASON, Child and Adolescent Health Policy Center, Johns Hopkins School of Hygiene and Public Health, Baltimore, Maryland

CLAUDE H. HALL, JR., Public Health Innovations Project, American Public Health Association, Washington, D.C.
RICHARD HEGNER, National Health Policy Forum, Washington, D.C.
PHYLLIS E. KAYE, American Health Planning Association, Washington, D.C.
ROZ LASKER, The New York Academy of Medicine, New York, New York
J. MICHAEL MCGINNIS, National Research Council, Washington, D.C.
CATHY MERCIL, National Committee for Quality Assurance, Washington, D.C.
MICHAEL MILLMAN, Health Resources and Services Administration, Rockville, Maryland
NANCY RAWDING, National Association of County and City Health Officials, Washington, D.C.
JORDAN RICHLAND, Partnership for Prevention, Washington, D.C.
JAMES SCANLON, U.S. Department of Health and Human Services, Washington, D.C.
JOSEPH THOMPSON, U.S. Department of Health and Human Services, Washington, D.C.
KAREN TROCCOLI, National Association of County and City Health Officials, Washington, D.C.
JAMES WEED, National Center for Health Statistics, Hyattsville, Maryland
RONALD WILSON, National Center for Health Statistics, Hyattsville, Maryland

E

Committee Biographies

BOBBIE BERKOWITZ, Ph.D., R.N. (*Co-Chair*), joined the faculty at the University of Washington School of Public Health and Community Medicine in July 1996 as Deputy Director of The Robert Wood Johnson Foundation "Turning Point" National Program Office. She came to the University of Washington from the Washington State Department of Health where she served as Deputy Secretary from May 1993 until July 1996. Prior to that, she served as Chief of Nursing Services for the Seattle–King County Department of Public Health. She currently holds appointments as Senior Lecturer with the Department of Health Services at the University of Washington School of Public Health and Community Medicine and as Assistant Professor with St. Martin's College Department of Nursing. She is also an Assistant Clinical Professor at the Seattle University School of Nursing. Dr. Berkowitz served on the Washington State Board of Health from 1988 until 1993. She was appointed by the Governor to the Washington Health Care Commission from 1990 through 1992 where she served as chair of the Health Services Committee. Dr. Berkowitz is a member of the Board of Directors for the Hanford Environmental Health Foundation and serves on the Editorial Advisory Board of the journal *Public Health Nursing*. She is a fellow in the American Academy of Nursing. Dr. Berkowitz holds a Ph.D. in Nursing Science from Case Western Reserve University, and a Master of

Nursing and Bachelor of Science in Nursing from the University of Washington.

THOMAS S. INUI, M.D., Sc.M. (*Co-Chair*), received his undergraduate degree in philosophy from Haverford College, his M.D. from the Johns Hopkins School of Medicine, and his Sc.M. in public health from the Johns Hopkins School of Hygiene and Public Health. In 1992, Dr. Inui was appointed head of a new Harvard Medical School/Harvard Pilgrim Health Care Department of Ambulatory Care and Prevention, which oversees community-based ambulatory care education for all Harvard medical students and provides oversight for a required course in prevention. Dr. Inui is also Director of the Health of the Public Program, which was established in 1986 by the Pew Charitable Trusts and the Rockefeller Foundation to introduce population-based perspectives into academic medical centers. He holds academic appointments as Professor of Ambulatory Care and Prevention at Harvard Medical School and Professor, Department of Health and Social Behavior, Harvard School of Public Health. Dr. Inui's special emphases in teaching and research have included physician–patient communication, health promotion and disease prevention, the social context of medicine, and medical humanities. He became a member of the Institute of Medicine in 1990 and is a past president and council member of the Society of General Internal Medicine.

ALAN W. CROSS, M.D. (*Vice Chair*), is a professor in the Departments of Social Medicine and Pediatrics in the School of Medicine at the University of North Carolina at Chapel Hill and serves as Director of the university's Center for Health Promotion and Disease Prevention. Since joining the faculty in 1978, virtually all of Dr. Cross' work has been interdisciplinary and oriented toward communities. His research interests include assessing the effectiveness of community-based strategies for reducing infant mortality, testing methods for improving adolescent health through school and community interventions, improving the delivery of preventive health services to low-income populations, and exploring the dimensions of medical ethics in the doctor–patient relationship. Both in his teaching and as director of the Center for Health Promotion and Disease Prevention, Dr. Cross is dedicated to facilitating interdisciplinary, collaborative approaches to health problems, including research involving communities across North Carolina.

LARRY W. CHAMBERS, Ph.D., is a professor in the Department of Clinical Epidemiology and Biostatistics and was appointed to the faculty at McMaster University in 1978. Since 1978, he has held a number of positions within the faculty and its partner community agencies, including the Hamilton–Wentworth Regional Public Health Department, a teaching health unit affiliated with McMaster University and the University of Guelph. At present, he is Epidemiology Consultant and Coordinator of the Teaching Health Unit Program in the department. His research, education, consultation, and administrative responsibilities focus on epidemiology and program evaluation issues related to aging, community health, and local-level health policy development. Dr. Chambers' recent research has included studies on maintaining independence for seniors with dementia and their care givers, transfer of research to decision makers, and community health indicator development. Dr. Chambers is a Fellow of the American College of Epidemiology.

ELLIOTT S. FISHER, M.D., M.P.H., is Associate Professor of Medicine and Community and Family Medicine at Dartmouth Medical School, where he codirects the health policy program in the Center for the Evaluative Clinical Sciences. He is a staff internist at the Department of Veterans Affairs Medical Center in White River Junction, Vermont, and codirector of the VA Outcomes Group, a research and training program for physicians. His research and writing focus on use of large databases for health care research, population-based assessment of health system performance, and development of methods to support improved resource allocation in health care. He has served on the Institute of Medicine's committee responsible for the report *Health Data and the Information Age* and on national advisory committees for both the Department of Veterans Affairs and the Health Care Financing Administration.

JAMES L. GALE, M.D., M.S., is Professor, Department of Epidemiology, and Adjunct Professor, Department of Health Services, at the University of Washington School of Public Health and Community Medicine. He is also Director of the Northwest Center for Public Health Practice at the University of Washington. He has been a faculty member since 1969. In addition, he is the health officer for the Kittitas County (Washington) Health Department. Among his research interests are infectious disease epidemiology, vaccines and their adverse effects, and the uses of surveillance information by state and local health departments. He has served on various National Institutes of Health review committees. He is a member of the Washington State Association of Local Public Health Officials and of national organizations including the American Public Health Association, American Epidemiological Society, and Infectious Disease Society of America. He is a past president of the Society for Epidemiological Research. He received his B.A. from Harvard University, his M.D. from Columbia University, and a Master of Science in Preventive Medicine (Epidemiology) from the University of Washington.

KRISTINE GEBBIE, Dr.P.H, R.N., is the Elizabeth Standish Gill Assistant Professor of Nursing at Columbia University School of Nursing. Her teaching and research focus is health policy and health services, with particular attention to population-based public health services. Dr. Gebbie previously served as the first National AIDS Policy Coordinator, as Secretary of the Department of Health for the State of Washington, and as Oregon Health Division Administrator. In addition to her academic responsibilities, Dr. Gebbie currently serves as Senior Advisor on Public Health Initiatives in the Office of Disease Prevention and Health Promotion, Office of Public Health and Science, U.S. Department of Health and Human Services. She became a member of the Institute of Medicine in 1992. Dr. Gebbie's career has included practice and academic posts in nursing as well as public health and public policy.

FERNANDO A. GUERRA, M.D., M.P.H., is Director of Health for the San Antonio Metropolitan Health District and has been a practicing pediatrician in San Antonio for many years. He has a longstanding commitment to pediatric care, public health, and health policy. He is a fellow of the American Academy of Pediatrics (AAP) and has served on many national committees for the AAP, including its Committee on Community Health Service. He is a member of the Board of Trustees of the Urban Institute; the Board on Children, Youth, and Families of the National Research Council and Institute of Medicine; the Advisory Committee on Immunization Practices of the Centers for Disease Control and Prevention; and The Robert Wood Johnson Foundation's All Kids Count Advisory Committee. Dr. Guerra currently serves on the Secretary of Health and Human Service's Advisory Committee on Infant Mortality and previously served on the Pew Health Professions Commission. He has published numerous articles on community health and pediatric medicine. He received his bachelor's degree from the University of Texas–Austin, his medical degree from the University of Texas at Galveston, and a Master of Public Health from the Harvard School of Public Health.

GARLAND LAND, M.P.H., is the director of the Center for Health Information Management and Epidemiology in the Missouri Department of Health. In that capacity, he supervises the Center for Health Statistics, the Office of Information Systems, and the Office of Epidemiology. He has worked for the Missouri Department of Health for 25 years. Mr. Land has served on many national public health committees and has authored many articles in public health journals. He has an M.P.H. in biostatistics from the University of Michigan.

SHEILA T. LEATHERMAN, M.S.W., is Executive Vice President of United HealthCare Corporation (UHC). She is also founder and President of the Center for Health Care Policy and Evaluation, United HealthCare Corporation. Ms. Leatherman's expertise is in health care quality measurement and the design and application of methods for performance evaluation of managed care delivery systems. Prior to joining UHC, she was chief executive officer of a large group-network model health maintenance organization; vice president of Medical Affairs for PARTNERS National Health Plans; and had held positions in the Minnesota State Health Department and the Veterans Administration. Ms. Leatherman was appointed Senior Fellow at the Institute of Health Services Research of the School of Public Health at the University of Minnesota in 1994. She is currently a member of the Board of Directors of the Minnesota State Data Institute and a member of the National Committee on Vital and Health Statistics. In addition, she has served as chair of the Rand Corporation National HMO Consortium on Quality and as a director on the board of the National Committee for Quality Assurance.

JOHN R. LUMPKIN, M.D., M.P.H., was appointed Director of the Illinois Department of Public Health in January 1991, after appointment as acting director in September 1990. Previously he served as associate director of the department's Office of Health Care Regulation. Before joining the state health department, Dr. Lumpkin practiced emergency medicine at several Chicago hospitals. From 1987 to 1990, he served as the U.S. Public Health Service project officer for emergency medical services and injury prevention aid to the Arab Republic of Egypt. His areas of expertise include injury prevention and public health information systems. Dr. Lumpkin was the 1996 president of the Association of State and Territorial Health Officials (ASTHO). He is a member of the Health Resources and Services Administration's HIV/AIDS Advisory Committee and the Centers for Disease Control and Prevention's Advisory Committee on Childhood Lead Poisoning Prevention. Dr. Lumpkin received his medical degree from Northwestern University Medical School and a master's degree in public health from the University of Illinois School of Public Health. He currently holds academic appointments at both schools.

WILLIAM J. MAYER, M.D., M.P.H., is President and General Manager of the functional foods division of the Kellogg Company in Battle Creek, Michigan. Previously he was Vice President for medical affairs. Prior to joining the Kellogg Company, he was a medical consultant for the Wyatt Company in Washington, D.C. Dr. Mayer received his bachelor's degree from Amherst College and his M.D. from the State University of New York at Buffalo School of Medicine. Following an internship in internal medicine, he earned his M.P.H. from the Johns Hopkins University School of Hygiene and Public Health. Dr. Mayer is board certified in preventive medicine. He served as a medical staff fellow and program director at the National Cancer Institute and is currently a faculty member of the National Cancer Institute's Cancer Prevention Fellowship Program. He is also a lecturer at the Johns Hopkins University School of Hygiene and Public Health.

ANA MARIA OSORIO, M.D., M.P.H., is Chief of the Occupational Health Branch in the California Department of Health Services and Assistant Clinical Professor in the Division of Occupational and Environmental Medicine at the University of California at San Francisco. Her prior experience includes service as an epidemic intelligence officer for the Centers for Disease Control and Prevention and an occupational medicine residency at the University of Southern California. She received her M.D. and M.P.H. (emphasis on epidemiology) from the University of California at Los Angeles. Dr. Osorio's research has included reproductive health, lead-associated disease, construction industry hazards, international labor issues, repetitive trauma disorders, child labor, agricultural hazards, and epidemiologic methods. She serves as a member of the Board of Scientific Counselors for the Agency for Toxic Substances and Disease Registry, the Advisory Committee for Construction Health and Safety for the Occupational Safety and Health

Administration, and the Interagency Coordination Committee for U.S.–Mexico Border Environmental Health for the Public Health Service and the Environmental Protection Agency. Dr. Osorio is a member and official consultant for environmental and occupational health issues of the Council of State and Territorial Epidemiologists.

SHOSHANNA SOFAER, Dr.P.H., is Associate Professor, Department of Health Care Sciences, and Director of the Center for Health Outcomes Improvement Research at the George Washington University (GWU) Medical Center. Dr. Sofaer received her doctorate at the University of California–Berkeley, and served on the faculty of the UCLA School of Public Health for six years prior to joining GWU in 1991. Dr. Sofaer's research interests include health care decision making, with special emphasis on the development of effective materials and strategies for providing information on health care coverage options to consumers. A related set of activities addresses the development of performance indicators to support more informed decision making about health plans by consumers, purchasers, and providers. She is particularly concerned about developing indicators that reflect an expanded view of health that takes into account not only traditional biomedical concerns but also public health, psychosocial, and behavioral issues. Dr. Sofaer's other research interests include the use of community coalitions to pursue community health improvement objectives such as tobacco control and cancer control. She has also examined the impact of interorganizational interactions on the quality and continuity of care for older persons and others with chronic conditions.

DEBORAH KLEIN WALKER, Ed.D., is Assistant Commissioner for the Bureau of Family and Community Health in the Massachusetts Department of Public Health. She is responsible for maternal and child health, health promotion and disease prevention, primary care, and community health programs. Dr. Walker is currently president-elect of the Association of Maternal and Child Health Programs, chair of the Maternal and Child Health Section of the American Public Health Association, and a member of the Secretary of Health and Human Service's Advisory Committee on Infant Mortality. Before assuming her current position, she was Associate Professor in the Departments of Behavioral Sciences and of Maternal and Child Health at the Harvard School of Public Health and a faculty member at the Harvard Graduate

School of Education. Dr. Walker received her B.A. from Mount Holyoke College and an Ed.D. in human development from the Harvard Graduate School of Education. She has authored policy and research articles on a wide range of issues in child development, education and measurement, and public health practice.

RICHARD A. WRIGHT, M.D., M.P.H., is Director of Community Health Services for Denver Health Medical Center and in this capacity serves as the manager of professional service for Denver's community health centers. Dr. Wright is a professor in the Departments of Medicine and Preventive Medicine and Biometrics, University of Colorado Health Sciences Center. He has 21 years experience in managing community-oriented primary care service delivery, teaching, and research programs. He is board certified in general internal medicine, infectious disease, and medical management. He received advanced training in epidemiology from the Centers for Disease Control and Prevention and received his master's degree in public health administration in 1995 from Loma Linda School of Public Health. Dr. Wright's areas of expertise include health services administration, applied epidemiology and needs assessment, and health policy and planning related to primary and preventive care services. He serves on local and national boards and on committees related to health care reform and community health services. He lectures and teaches on community-oriented primary care, epidemiology, and health policy.

Acronyms

AAPCC	adjusted average per capita cost (Medicare)
ACS	ambulatory care sensitive
AFDC	Aid to Families with Dependent Children
AHA	American Hospital Association
AHCPR	Agency for Health Care Policy and Research
AIDS	acquired immune deficiency syndrome
ALA	American Lung Association
AMA	American Medical Association
AMBHA	American Managed Behavioral Healthcare Association
AMI	acute myocardial infarction
AOA	American Osteopathic Association
APEX*PH*	Assessment Protocol for Excellence in Public Health
APHA	American Public Health Association
ASTHO	Association of State and Territorial Health Officials
BRFSS	Behavioral Risk Factor Surveillance System
CABG	coronary artery bypass graft
CASA	Clinic Assessment Software Application
CCHIP	Calhoun County Health Improvement Program
CCN	Community Care Network
CDC	Centers for Disease Control and Prevention

CHA	Catholic Health Association
CHART	Community Health Assessment and Resource Team
CHIP	community health improvement process
CHNA	Community Health Network Area
CHP	comprehensive health planning
CME	continuing medical education
COMAH	Clinical Outcome Measure Adjusted HEDIS
COMMIT	Community Intervention Trial (for Smoking Cessation)
COPC	community-oriented primary care
COPD	chronic obstructive pulmonary disease
CQI	continuous quality improvement
DNA	deoxyribonucleic acid
DTP	diphtheria–tetanus–pertussis
DSM-IV	*Diagnostic and Statistical Manual of Mental Disorders*, Fourth Edition
EAP	employee assistance program
EPA	Environmental Protection Agency
ERISA	Employee Retirement Income Security Act
ETS	environmental tobacco smoke
HDO	health data organization
HEDIS	Health Plan Employer Data and Information Set
Hib	*Haemophilus influenzae* type b
HIV	human immunodeficiency virus
HMO	health maintenance organization
HPV	human papilloma virus
HUD	U.S. Department of Housing and Urban Development
ICD-9	International Classification of Diseases, 9th Revision
ICU	intensive care unit
IM System	Indicator Measurement System
INPHO	Information Network for Public Health Officials
IOM	Institute of Medicine
IPLAN	Illinois Project for Local Assessment of Need
IRS	Internal Revenue Service

JCAHO	Joint Commission on Accreditation of Healthcare Organizations
LHD	local health department
MassCHIP	Massachusetts Community Health Information Profile
MCO	managed care organization
McPLAN	McHenry County Project for Local Assessment of Need
MMR	measles–mumps–rubella
NACCHO	National Association of County and City Health Officials
NCHS	National Center for Health Statistics
NCQA	National Committee for Quality Assurance
NHANES	National Health and Nutrition Examination Survey
NHLBI	National Heart, Lung, and Blood Institute
NII	National Information Infrastructure
OSHA	Occupational Safety and Health Administration
PATCH	Planned Approach to Community Health
PHPPO	Public Health Practice Program Office
PKU	phenylketonuria
PPG	Performance Partnership Grant
PTA	parent–teacher association
SAMMEC	smoking-attributable morbidity, mortality, and economic costs
SIDS	sudden infant death syndrome
SMHA	state mental health agency
STD	sexually transmitted disease
TANF	Temporary Assistance to Needy Families
TAPII	the Arizona Partnership for Infant Immunization
WHO	World Health Organization
WIC	Special Supplemental Food Program for Women, Infants, and Children
YRBSS	Youth Risk Behavior Surveillance System

Index